Cannabis

by Kim Ronkin Casey with Joe Kraynak

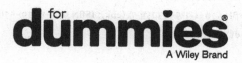

for
dummies®
A Wiley Brand

Contents at a Glance

Table of Contents

Introduction

Welcome to *Cannabis For Dummies*, your definitive guide to all things cannabis. Cannabis has a long history. Human use dates back to the third millennium BCE according to the earliest written records. In the U.S., its popularity rose among subcultures and countercultures in the 1950s and 60s. However, cannabis didn't break through the subculture barriers to enter the mainstream until relatively recently. Now, with several countries and many states in the U.S. legalizing it for medical or adult recreational use (or both), cannabis has exploded onto the national and international stage. Interest and excitement are growing fast, whether you're a consumer, entrepreneur, investor, or someone who's just curious about it.

Depending on your experience with cannabis, you may know a lot, a little, or virtually nothing about it or about certain facets of it. For example, you may know all about buying it and consuming it but very little about growing, harvesting, and curing it. You may know something about concentrates and extracts but nothing about the business side of cannabis. Likewise, you may have used cannabis recreationally but have little or no idea of its potential health benefits.

Regardless of your interest in cannabis and your motivation for finding out more about it, you've come to the right place.

About This Book

In *Cannabis For Dummies* we cover the science behind the effects cannabis has on people; the rules and regulations governing its purchase, possession, and use; how to buy and consume it; how to grow it and make your own concentrates and marijuana infused products (MIPs); how to reap its potential health benefits for you and your pets; the basics of starting and running a cannabis business; how to invest in it; and how to find work in the industry.

To make the content more accessible, we divided it into six parts:

>> Part 1, "Getting Started with Cannabis" brings you up to speed on the basics. We take you on a tour of the entire book, covering each key topic in a nutshell. Then, we give you a primer on cannabis rules and regulations to keep you out of legal trouble and explain the politics and culture surrounding cannabis,

>> Part 2, "Buying, Storing, and Using Cannabis," guides you through the process of choosing and visiting a cannabis dispensary, provides instructions on various methods for consuming cannabis, and provides insight on how to use cannabis safely and responsibly.

>> Part 3, "Reaping the Potential Benefits of Medical Marijuana," explains the potential health benefits of cannabis and provides guidance on how to use cannabis for potential symptom relief connected to a wide range of medical conditions. You also find out about the potential benefits of cannabis products for pets along with guidance for how to use these products more safely.

>> Part 4, "Grasping the Basics of Cannabis Cultivation, Post-Harvest, and Production," is for the do-it-yourselfers among the audience. Here, we lead you through the process of growing cannabis indoors or outdoors; how to harvest, dry, and cure it properly; and how to make your own cannabis concentrates and marijuana infused products (MIPs).

>> Part 5, "Getting Down to Business," offers insight into starting your own cannabis business, finding work in the industry, and investing in cannabis — the various ways to earn a buck from a potentially lucrative industry.

>> Part 6, "The Part of Tens," features ten tips for growing more and better weed, ten tips for enhancing your cannabis experience, and ten tips for ensuring that you get what you paid for when buying cannabis.

As an added bonus, the appendix provides a number of recipes for cooking up your very own cannabis edibles, including Infused Lavender Lemonade, Michelle's Medicated Blueberry Pie, No-Guilt Nosh, and Chocolate Chip Oatmeal Cookies.

In short, this book serves as your A–Z guide to all things cannabis.

Foolish Assumptions

All assumptions are foolish, and we're reluctant to make them, but to keep this book focused on the right audience and ensure that it fulfills our purpose in writing it, we had to make the following foolish assumptions about you:

>> You're old enough to buy, possess, and consume cannabis wherever you happen to live. If you're not of legal age, don't read this book.

>> You're committed to complying with the cannabis rules and regulations in whatever jurisdictions you live. We don't condone breaking any laws, which is why we have an entire chapter on rules and regulations and plenty of warnings sprinkled throughout the book.

>> If you consume cannabis, we assume that you're committed to doing so safely and responsibly, which includes not driving high, preventing children and pets from accessing your cannabis, and consuming in moderation.

>> You're eager to find out more about cannabis. While you may know a great deal already, our hope is that you will learn something new, especially if you're returning to cannabis after a long absence.

Other than those four foolish assumptions, we can honestly say that we can't assume much more about you. The vast number of people who have experience with cannabis or are curious about it represent a diverse demographic. You may be 21 or 90 years old or somewhere in between, a white collar or blue collar worker, a housewife or house husband, a doctor, a lawyer, rich or poor. Regardless of the demographic, we applaud you for being open-minded and willing to explore what we feel is a fascinating world.

Icons Used in This Book

Throughout this book, icons in the margins highlight certain types of valuable information that call out for your attention. Here are the icons you'll encounter and a brief description of each.

REMEMBER

We want you to remember everything you read in this book, but if you can't quite do that, then remember the important points flagged with this icon.

TIP

Tips provide insider insight. When you're looking for a better, faster way to do something, check out these tips.

WARNING

"Whoa!" Before you take another step, read this warning. We provide this cautionary content to help you avoid the common pitfalls that are otherwise likely to trip you up.

Beyond the Book

In addition to the abundance of information and guidance related to cannabis that we provide in this book, you get access to even more help and information online at Dummies.com. Check out this book's online Cheat Sheet for handy info regarding different strains of cannabis, cannabinoids, and terpenes; tips for growing more and better cannabis plants, and pros and cons of starting your own cannabis business. Just go to www.dummies.com and search for "Cannabis For Dummies Cheat Sheet."

Where to Go from Here

You're certainly welcome to read this book from cover to cover, but we wrote it in a way that facilitates skipping around. For a quick tutorial on cannabis that touches on all the key topics, turn to Chapter 1. For a brief tour of cannabis anatomy and its unique chemical properties, check out Chapter 2. Chapter 3 is a must-read; we included it to help you avoid getting into legal trouble.

If you're looking to buy cannabis and consume it medically, recreationally, or both, turn to the chapters in Part 2. We want to be sure you're buying the products that are most likely to deliver the experience you desire without getting ripped off, and we want you to know about the various ways of consuming cannabis, so you can make well-informed choices.

Those who are looking to reap the medical benefits of marijuana or use it for their pets should turn to the chapters in Part 3. If you want to grow your own cannabis and use it to make concentrates and other products, turn to Part 4. And if you want to find gainful employment or explore other ways to make money in the cannabis industry, turn to the chapters in Part 5.

Consider Part 6 and the appendix bonus items — tips and recipes for getting the most out of your cannabis experience!

1

Getting Started with Cannabis

IN THIS PART . . .

Wrap your brain around the multifaceted topic of cannabis — from consumption and cultivation to law and culture.

Explore the cannabis plant, its chemical composition, and the many extracts and concentrates derived from it.

Find out where cannabis is legal for medical and adult recreational use and figure out where to go to find out more about specific rules and regulations.

Get up to speed on cannabis politics and culture to increase your awareness of the ever-evolving landscape regarding accessibility and acceptance.

» Checking out the unique chemical properties of cannabis

» Differentiating among a variety of cannabis strains

» Starting on the road to becoming a savvy shopper and consumer

» Understanding the path from farm to final product

Chapter **1**

Taking the Nickel Tour

C annabis is a multifaceted topic, which is one of the reasons it's so fascinating. You can approach it from many different angles, discussing consumption (both medical and adult use), law (as it applies to individuals and businesses), the science behind it (in terms of both biology and chemistry), how to buy it without getting ripped off, the various ways to consume it, how it's made, and even different ways to make money in and from the industry.

In this chapter, we touch on each of these topics and more to provide you with a broad introduction to the fascinating world of cannabis and refer you to other parts and chapters in the book where you can find more in-depth discussions. Think of this chapter as cannabis orientation day and your roadmap to discovering more about cannabis all rolled into one.

Exploring the Basics of Marijuana Consumption

People have been ingesting marijuana in various forms (mostly by smoking it) for more than 5,000 years. The plant has unique chemical properties that make it attractive for use in certain religious and cultural ceremonies, adult recreational activities, and medicinal regimens (to potentially alleviate symptoms of a wide range of medical conditions).

In this section, we explore some of the potential benefits of cannabis for medical and adult recreational use along with some of the potential drawbacks, so you can begin to develop well-informed opinions and decisions regarding its use.

Considering medical use

Some of the chemical components of cannabis have unique properties that mimic certain chemical messengers found naturally in the body that help to regulate certain bodily functions, such as appetite, digestion, and immune function. (See the later section "Knowing What Makes Cannabis So Special" for details.) As a result, two countries and the majority of states in the U.S. have legalized medical marijuana use for certain medical conditions. Qualifying medical conditions vary from one jurisdiction to another but may include the following:

>> Acute or chronic pain

>> Anxiety and/or stress

>> Arthritis

>> Asthma

>> Epilepsy

>> Gastrointestinal disorders

>> Glaucoma

>> Inflammation

>> Loss of appetite or wasting syndrome

>> Movement disorders (dystonia, Huntington's disease, Parkinson's disease, Tourette's syndrome, and spinocerebellar ataxias)

>> Multiple sclerosis (MS)

>> Nausea and vomiting (particularly when associated with chemotherapy)

>> Opioid withdrawal

>> Palliative care

>> Post-traumatic stress disorder (PTSD)

>> Sleep disorders

REMEMBER

Unfortunately, by classifying marijuana as a Schedule I drug, the U.S. federal government has declared that it has "no currently accepted medical use and a high potential for abuse." As a result, and because of the lack of research supporting cannabis' potential health benefits, we need to be careful about how we approach this topic. We can't say it cures any disease or illness, that it helps to cure a disease or illness, or even that it provides symptomatic relief. All we can say is that it has the potential to alleviate symptoms of certain medical conditions, which means maybe it works and maybe it doesn't.

A LACK OF RESEARCH

One of the big factors preventing doctors and veterinarians in many states from recommending medical marijuana to patients is the lack of research proving or disproving its effectiveness and risks. The lack of research can be traced to several causes, including

- **Regulatory hassles:** Researchers must navigate through complex regulatory barriers put in place by the Food and Drug Administration (FDA), the Drug Enforcement Administration (DEA), the National Institute on Drug Abuse (NIDA), and state regulatory agencies.

- **Restricted supply of cannabis for research:** NIDA is the only source of cannabis available for research scientists, and until recently, the University of Mississippi had the sole contract to grow it, and the strains it grows have a potency that's too low for high-quality studies and much lower than current products available in the legal market.

- **Funding limitations:** Federal funding for cannabis research is primarily allocated to study its possible adverse effects and much less so to study its potential therapeutic effects.

- **Challenges with dosing and placebos:** Study participants may not accept any consumption method other than smoking or vaping, which makes dose control in studies especially difficult. Also difficult is finding a suitable placebo for the control group.

- **Research controls:** Tremendous variations in cannabinoid content and potency in different strains as well as consumption methods are difficult to control for researchers using current cannabis consumers as subjects.

Although some challenges are outside the scope of government control, the big reasons for lack of research in this area can be traced back to the fact that cannabis is federally illegal in the U.S. This results in a Catch-22, in which the government denies the potential health benefits of cannabis while preventing the studies necessary to provide any evidence.

The one big exception is at least three clinical studies have shown that low-dose cannabidiol (CBD) is useful in reducing seizures in people who suffer from two rare forms of epilepsy — Lennox-Gastaut syndrome and Dravet syndrome. Proof for alleviating symptoms related to a host of other medical conditions is restricted to either anecdotal evidence or evidence from limited clinical trials.

See the chapters in Part 3 for details about using medical marijuana for yourself and possibly even your pets.

Looking into adult recreational use

THC (short for *tetrahydrocannabinol*) has strong psychoactive properties, meaning it can alter brain function to create changes in perception, mood, consciousness, cognition (thinking and memory), and behavior. Other substances that are psychoactive include caffeine, nicotine, alcohol, ephedrine, cocaine, and a number of pharmaceutical drugs used for treating psychiatric conditions. At low doses, THC tends to create a sense of well-being or euphoria and relaxation, which is largely responsible for making cannabis such an attractive adult recreational drug. At higher doses, it can create anxiety, impaired thinking, and loss of coordination.

When looking at cannabis as an adult recreational drug, it's best compared to alcohol, which also produces intoxicating effects and tends to lower anxiety in the short term. Some argue that cannabis is actually safer than alcohol because cannabis isn't associated with physical addiction and because it may not be as harmful to the body as alcohol. However, cannabis is associated with psychological addiction, and long term use or overconsumption may be associated with long-term adverse side effects, so it is not totally safe. In addition, because it's intoxicating, a consumer should never drive or operate machinery when using cannabis.

WARNING

Use cannabis only legally and responsibly. Follow the same precautions as you would (should) when consuming alcohol recreationally — use it in moderation, and don't drive under the influence.

Acknowledging the potential drawbacks

Cannabis isn't a totally safe miracle drug as some present it to be. Nor is it a highly addictive and dangerous drug as others think. It's not nearly as addictive or potentially dangerous as opioids, for example. Cannabis offers many potential benefits when consumed responsibly. However, it also has some potential drawbacks, including the following:

>> Heavy underage use is associated with impaired thinking, memory, and learning functions. One study from New Zealand conducted in part by Duke

University researchers showed an average loss of 8 IQ points among those who smoked marijuana heavily in their teenage years. (Those who started consuming cannabis as adults didn't show notable declines.)

>> Increased heart rate, which may increase the chances of heart attack in susceptible populations.

>> Lung irritation, coughing, and potential breathing problems if the cannabis is smoked, including problems associated with secondhand smoke.

>> Increased risk of serious accidents, including car accidents caused by those who consume illegally and irresponsibly.

>> Worsening of symptoms in people with schizophrenia, such as paranoia, hallucinations, and disorganized thinking.

>> Problems with childhood development during and after pregnancy in the form of lower birth weight and increased risk of both brain and behavioral problems, including attention deficits.

Check out Chapter 9 for additional details on the possible adverse side effects of cannabis.

Knowing What Makes Cannabis So Special

Mammals, including humans, are equipped with a chemical messenger system called the *endocannabinoid system (ECS)*, which plays a role in regulating appetite, pain, inflammation, immune function, digestion, reproduction, memory, motor learning, stress, and so on. The ECS contains cannabinoid receptors distributed throughout the central and peripheral nervous systems along with *endocannabinoids*, which serve as chemical messengers to enable communication across the system.

The ECS plays a key role in helping the body maintain *homeostasis* — healthy equilibrium. When an imbalance occurs, the body engages the ECS to help correct it. Certain endocannabinoids are dispatched, and they lock into designated cannabinoid receptors, fitting into the receptors like keys in a lock. The receptors then engage the nervous system to take action to correct the imbalance. The two main cannabinoid receptors are CB1 and CB2:

>> **CB1** receptors are located primarily in the brain and central nervous system and, to a lesser extent, in other tissues. They play a role in regulating appetite and pain and in memory and emotional processing.

>> **CB2** receptors are located primarily in the peripheral organs, especially cells associated with the immune system. When activated, they work to reduce inflammation. Because many chronic conditions, including pain, are associated with inflammation, many of the potential health benefits of cannabis are thought to be linked to the CB2 receptor.

Cannabis contains *phytocannabinoids* — a type of exogenous (as opposed to endogenous) cannabinoid — along with *terpenes* — aromatic chemical compounds commonly found in plants and essential oils made from plants. Here's a list of the chemical compounds in cannabis most strongly associated with its effects:

>> **Tetrahydrocannabinol (THC)** is the psychoactive chemical compound in cannabis that creates the high. It affects thinking, memory, pleasure, physical movement, concentration, coordination, and sensory and time perception.

>> **Cannabidiol (CBD)** is mostly associated with cannabis' potential health benefits. CBD is often used by patients seeking relief from pain, inflammation, anxiety, and seizures. It's not psychoactive, so it won't make you feel intoxicated. In fact, it may help to counteract the psychoactive properties of THC. CBD can also be extracted from hemp, and in this form, it's federally legal; hence, hemp-derived CBD products are generally more available across the U.S.

>> **9-tetrahydrocannabinol acid (THCa)** is the precursor to THC that doesn't have psychoactive properties, so it won't make you high. When cannabis is heated to above 220 degrees Fahrenheit, THCa is converted into THC through a process called *decarboxylation*. THCa may help to stimulate appetite, reduce nausea and vomiting, prevent or reduce inflammation, inhibit prostate growth, and slow the progression of certain neurodegenerative diseases, such as Parkinson's disease.

>> **Tetrahydrocannabivarin (THCv)** is similar to THC and does have some psychoactive properties in high doses, but it has some unique effects that differ from those of THC. It is an appetite suppressant, stimulates bone growth, and may help with diabetes, Alzheimer's, and panic attacks in PTSD. It needs to be heated higher than THC to about 428°F when vaporizing.

>> **Cannabigerol (CBG)** is a non-psychoactive cannabinoid. It has analgesic, muscle relaxant, anti-erythemic (reduces redness is skin), antifungal, anti-depressant, anti-proliferative, anti-psoriatic, and anti-bacterial properties. As an antibacterial, it can be a powerful weapon against the methicillin-resistant Staphylococcus aureus (MRSA) virus.

>> **Cannabinol (CBN)** is a mildly psychoactive cannabinoid that comes from the degradation of THC after an extended period of time due to exposure to oxygen and heat. CBN has analgesic, antibacterial, anti-inflammatory, anti-insomnia, antiemetic, appetite stimulant, and bone stimulant properties.

It's also effective in treating burns. CBN is only 10 percent as psychoactive as THC, but it can produce a very mild high.

>> **Terpenes** are aromatic chemical compounds in plants that give them their unique aroma and flavor. They may also work synergistically with cannabinoids and other terpenes to enhance the overall effect of the cannabis — a phenomenon commonly referred to as the "entourage effect."

REMEMBER

All cannabis products you purchase at a dispensary are labeled with concentrations or amounts of the various active ingredients, which usually includes amounts and/or percentages of THC and CBD. The label may also include a terpene profile or other ingredients. See Chapter 2 for more about cannabinoid and terpene chemistry.

Recognizing the Diversity of Cannabis Strains

Not all cannabis plants are the same. They vary in structure, cannabinoid and terpene content, and the conditions they require for optimal growth. However, the diversity of strains can all be traced back to one or more of the following strains:

>> **Indica:** Indicas are short, bushy plants that reach a maximum height of 10 feet and have rounder leaves (than sativas). They flower relatively quickly and are sensitive to changes in light. Indicas have a higher concentration of CBD-to-THC than sativas, so they produce a more relaxed effect and are more likely to make you drowsy. The high CBD content also makes indicas more attractive for their potential medicinal properties.

>> **Sativa:** Sativas are taller and less bushy than indicas and can reach a maximum height of about 19 feet. Their leaves are more slender. Sativas tend to have a higher concentration of THC-to-CBD, which tends to create a more active, energetic, and creative high.

>> **Ruderalis:** Ruderalis plants are very short and bushy, reaching a maximum height of about two feet. They have a shorter growing season and are auto-flowering instead of photoperiod plants. While *photoperiod* plants require about 12 hours of total darkness over several weeks to form buds, *auto-flowering* plants flower after a certain amount of time regardless of the amount of light to which they're exposed. Ruderalis plants aren't nearly as psychoactive as indicas and sativas, so you'll rarely see them on product labels, but you will see them on labels when you're shopping for seeds to plant. A ruderalis is commonly cross-bred with an indica and a sativa (or an existing hybrid) to make the latter plants auto-flowering.

REMEMBER

Sativas and indicas are cross-bred to create many of the popular hybrids, such as Blue Dream, Pineapple Express, and Lemon Kush. See Chapter 2 for more about the different strains.

Buying Cannabis

Buying cannabis has never been easier or less risky, at least in places where it's legal. You enter a cannabis dispensary, show your ID to prove you're of age and show your medical marijuana card (when applicable), and consult with a sales associate (sometimes referred to as a *budtender*) to find the products that meet your needs and desires. The only big difference from other retail purchases is that when you're buying cannabis, you usually have to pay cash. Of course, the process is somewhat more involved, which is why we devoted an entire chapter to choosing and visiting a cannabis dispensary (Chapter 5).

In this section, we bring you up to speed on how to buy cannabis in order to reinforce the rationale behind buying legally and steer you clear of common scams.

Knowing where and where not to get it

One of the biggest benefits of marijuana legalization is the accompanying regulation that's put in place to protect consumers. When you buy from a legal, reputable dispensary or other retailer, you're benefiting from those protections. Some of the value delivered by the dispensary or retailer is quality assurance. All products are tested and clearly labeled to show the ingredients and potencies along with the levels of any contaminants. You can purchase products with the assurance that you're getting what you paid for.

If you choose to buy from a friend or from a black market seller, which we highly discourage, you increase your exposure to risks, including the following:

>> **Getting robbed or ripped off:** A thief may either steal your money outright or sell you a poor quality product that's not worth the money.

>> **Buying and consuming a potentially dangerous product:** You may be sold something other than cannabis, something laced with a dangerous substance, or something that inadvertently contains high levels of pesticides, mold, fungi, solvents, or other harmful contaminants.

>> **Not knowing the potency of the product:** Because black market sellers don't lab test their products and label them, you may have little to no idea how potent it is, what the CBD-to-THC ratio is, or what dose to take.

>> **Supporting crime:** By buying on the black market, you're supporting crime, which increases safety risks not only for you but also for others in your community.

Because the seller plays such a key role in quality assurance, your choice of where to buy may be even more important than your choice of what to buy. Buy from a medical marijuana or adult recreational dispensary and not from a black market seller.

WARNING

Placing an order online or over the phone for pickup or delivery is fine, but only if you're ordering from a licensed and reputable retailer with whom you've already established a relationship. Otherwise, you're exposing yourself to a significant risk of getting ripped off or passing your credit card information to someone who'll use it for his personal spending spree.

Understanding what you're buying

Although the sales associate at your chosen cannabis dispensary can be your greatest ally in understanding what you're buying, you still need to be able to read and understand product labels and, if you're buying bud/flower, be able to judge its quality by looking at it and smelling it.

The information printed on product labels for flower, edibles, vape oils, tinctures, and other cannabis products is very useful for understanding what you're buying and for comparison shopping. Product labels are usually required to contain the following details:

>> **Universal THC logo:** If the product contains more than 0.03% THC, it needs to display the universal THC logo.

>> **Cannabinoid content:** For bud/flower, the label may indicate the percentages or ratios of CBD, THC, THCa, and other cannabinoids. In processed products, such as edibles and tinctures, cannabinoid content may be presented in milligrams (mg) for the entire package and broken down by serving.

>> **Strain(s):** The strain(s) of the bud/flower or the plants used to create the product.

>> **Organic:** If the product is organic, the label usually has some indication of that fact.

>> **Terpene content:** Percentages or milligrams of the various terpenes.

>> **Test results:** Some indication that the product doesn't contain harmful levels of pesticides, molds, fungi, solvents, or other contaminants.

>> **Expiration, sell-by, or best-used-by date:** The date on which the freshness of the product can't be guaranteed.

Additionally, you can usually tell the quality of flower by looking at it and smelling it. It should be colorful, mostly green, and have a pleasantly pungent odor. If it looks brown and dry, smells moldy or like wet hay, or it has little to no aroma, don't buy it. For additional guidance on buying quality cannabis, check out Chapters 8 and 19.

REMEMBER

Hemp-derived CBD products are widely available, but they contain no more than 0.03 percent of THC. If you buy a hemp-derived CBD product expecting some sort of high, you're going to be very disappointed. However, these products should have similar medicinal properties to the CBD in cannabis.

Avoiding rip-offs

Cannabis rip-offs generally fall into two categories:

>> **Investment schemes:** The promise of big returns in a short period of time by investing in cannabis businesses makes eager investors susceptible to investment scams.

>> **Illegal sales:** These are most commonly online sales from sellers who promise to ship product across state lines (a federal offense) and who never have the intention of doing so. Illegal sales also include black-market sales, which increase exposure to several risks, as explained in the earlier section "Knowing where and where not to get it."

REMEMBER

To avoid stock market scams, perform your due diligence in researching any cannabis company or fund carefully before investing in it. If you don't understand the industry, the company's management, and its financials, don't invest in it. To avoid illegal sales scams, simply shop for your cannabis at a legal, reputable dispensary or other licensed retail outlet.

Exploring Different Consumption Methods

Traditionally, consumers smoked cannabis in a pipe, a bong, or rolled as a joint. Edibles, primarily brownies or cookies, provided another common method. However, the legalization of cannabis, along with new technologies such as vaping devices, have given rise to a plethora of new consumption methods. In this section, we briefly describe your options. (See Chapter 6 for details along with instructions.)

Smoking or vaping

The two most common methods of consuming cannabis are smoking and vaping. With smoking, you burn (combust) the cannabis and inhale the smoke. With vaping, a device heats the plant matter or (usually) a concentrate such as oil to a point at which it vaporizes, and you inhale the vapor. The benefits of both methods are fast onset and intensity of the effect. Some consumers claim that smoke is more aromatic and flavorful and delivers longer-lasting effects, but vaping offers a few advantages:

>> **More efficient:** Vaping releases a higher percentage of THC from the plant than does combustion.

>> **More discreet:** People can't tell whether you're vaping cannabis or nicotine oil, and you don't have the lingering odors that result from smoking cannabis.

>> **Easier to do:** All you do is press a button and inhale. However, you do need to charge the battery, and if you're vaping plant matter (as opposed to oil), you need to load the chamber and clean it after each use.

>> **Probably healthier:** Vapor doesn't contain the tar and other carcinogens produced by burning plant matter. We're not saying vapor is healthy, only that it's probably not as unhealthy as smoke.

Edibles

Edibles include chocolates, gummies, baked goods, and beverages infused with cannabis. They provide the most discreet means for consuming cannabis, and they enable you to enjoy two or more of your favorite indulgences at the same time.

WARNING

Don't consume too much too quickly. You may not begin to feel the effects for up to two hours, so start low and go slow until you get a feel for how a certain dose affects you.

REMEMBER

Eating raw cannabis plant matter won't produce the desired effects. Decarboxylation (usually through heating the cannabis) is required to convert the THCa into the THC that makes you high.

Tinctures

A *tincture* is a concentrated herbal extract. You commonly consume tinctures by placing a few drops under your tongue, holding them there a few seconds, and then swallowing. You can also add tinctures to your favorite foods, beverages, or lotions (for topical application). Cannabis tinctures take effect fairly quickly; the speed of onset is second only to smoking or vaping.

TIP

Tinctures are great for avoiding overconsumption with edibles. Because tinctures take effect much more quickly than edibles, you can use a tincture to figure out how many milligrams (mg) of THC you need to take to feel the desired effects. Then you'll know the maximum amount of THC to consume when you're using edibles.

Topical or transdermal applications

Topicals are cannabis-infused lotions, creams, oils, and balms that are applied to the skin to relieve pain and inflammation. They don't reach the bloodstream, so they don't deliver the intoxicating effects of other consumption methods. However, transdermal patches applied to the skin, do deliver cannabinoids to the bloodstream. While topicals are generally used to relieve localized pain and inflammation, transdermal patches are the better choice for more systemic relief.

Getting Up to Speed on Cannabis Laws

As of the writing of this book, cannabis is federally illegal in the U.S., but legal throughout Canada and Uruguay and in certain states in the U.S. In states where cannabis is legal, it may be legal for medical use only or for both medical and adult recreational use. To find out where cannabis is legal in the U.S. and where it's not, check out the map at thecannabisindustry.org/ncia-news-resources/state-by-state-policies.

Cannabis laws vary by state and even within the states where it's legal, because various jurisdictions within the state can set their own laws and even prohibit dispensaries from operating in their jurisdiction. While laws vary, the laws that apply to consumers are typically broken down into the following categories:

>> **Purchase:** Laws that pertain to purchasing cannabis specify a minimum age, identification and age verification, purchase limits, and purchase locations in addition to certain rules governing the sales transaction; for example, in some jurisdictions, customers are prohibited from pooling their money to buy products.

>> **Possession:** Like purchase laws, possession laws specify a minimum age, identification and age verification, and possession limits. For example, in Colorado, if you're 21 years or older, can you legally possess one ounce (about 28 grams) of THC in flower form.

>> **Consumption:** Driving under the influence of cannabis is illegal everywhere, and public consumption is generally illegal. You're not allowed to simply light

up when you're walking down the street. Some areas have legal bring-your-own-cannabis clubs or lounges and other establishments, such as cannabis-friendly motels. One key to steering clear of trouble is to be discreet — edibles and vape pens may be your best options when consuming away from the privacy or your own home.

Don't consume on federal property, such as a national park.

WARNING

>> **Transportation:** Cannabis laws contain rules similar to open container laws for alcohol. You're not allowed to have cannabis in the passenger area of a vehicle if it is in an open container (manufacturer's seal is broken) or if there's evidence of consumption. Also, you're prohibited from transporting or shipping product over state lines, even across state lines that separate two legal states, because it constitutes drug trafficking, which is a federal offense.

>> **Cultivation:** These laws typically stipulate that you must be a certain age to grow marijuana, that you're allowed to grow only a certain number of plants, that only a certain number of those plants can be in the flower stage, and that plants must be in an enclosed, private, and locked space on private property you own.

Many more rules and regulations govern commercial operations, including growers, manufacturers, sellers, and delivery services. See Chapter 3 for more detailed coverage of cannabis laws and advice for staying out of legal trouble.

Being a Safe and Responsible User

Being a safe, responsible cannabis consumer is important for two reasons: First, it ensures your health and safety and that of others. Second, irresponsible and inconsiderate use runs the risk of spoiling legalization for everyone. To be a safe and responsible cannabis consumer, follow these guidelines:

>> **Protect minors and pets.** Keep your cannabis out of the reach of children and teenagers, along with your pets.

>> **Don't drive high.** Stay at home or designate a driver.

>> **Be discreet and considerate.** Smoking or vaping in the company of others may or may not be appropriate or welcome. Consider the setting, the people, and the situation.

>> **Don't overconsume.** Excessive long-term consumption isn't healthy and may negatively affect various aspects of your life.

>> **Don't mix cannabis and alcohol.** These two substances can intensify the intoxicating effects of one another in unexpected ways.

>> **Be careful with edibles.** Until you know the dose required to produce the desired effects, start with a low dose and wait at least two hours before taking any more.

See Chapter 7 for additional guidance on how to consume safely and responsibly.

Grasping the Basics of Cannabis Production

Take a stroll through a cannabis dispensary and you'll be amazed at the diversity of products — bud/flower, pre-filled vape pens, concentrates, tinctures, lotions, sprays, gummies, chocolates, and more. If you're wondering how all this stuff gets made or you want to grow your own bud or make your own cannabis infused products, you've come to the right place. Here, we cover the bare-boned basics. Turn to Part 4 for detailed coverage.

Growing cannabis

In most areas where cannabis is legal, it's legal to grow, too, assuming you follow the rules and regulations and your grow operation doesn't offend the neighbors. Cannabis is as easy to grow as a tomato plant. Assuming you give it all the nutrients it needs — rich soil, clean water, and plenty of sunshine and fresh air — you can expect to have a bountiful crop ready to harvest in six to ten weeks (typically eight weeks).

We devoted an entire (long) chapter (Chapter 11) to growing cannabis, which covers indoor and outdoor grows, lighting, ventilation, fertilizers, and much more, but here are the key takeaways:

>> Start with good quality soil that absorbs moisture but drains well, too.

>> Provide enough water but not too much.

>> If you're growing in containers, make sure the container is large enough to accommodate the roots of the plant you're growing. Some cannabis strains are much larger than others, and a pot that's too small will stunt the plant's growth or even kill it.

>> Start with feminized seeds, which are much more likely to grow into female plants, which eventually develop the buds you want to harvest. Seeds sold at dispensaries are feminized.

>> A single male plant can pollinate all the female plants in your grow room and ruin your entire crop, so identify each plant's sex as early as possible and isolate the males. (See Chapter 2 for guidance on telling the difference between male and female plants.)

>> Plants can be photoperiod or auto-flowering. Photoperiod plants are sensitive to changes in light and require at least 12 hours of darkness daily to enter the flowering stage. Auto-flowering plants develop flowers on schedule even if they get less than 12 hours of darkness. With photoperiod plants, you need to be much more diligent about ensuring that they're getting at least 12 hours of darkness starting about halfway through the grow cycle. Seed package labeling indicates whether the seeds are for auto-flowering plants.

>> During the vegetative stage of the growth cycle (the first four to eight weeks) feed the plants a fertilizer that's higher in nitrogen. When the plant is nearly half its adult size, switch to a fertilizer that's lower in nitrogen and higher in potassium and phosphorous. (If you're starting with soil that has fertilizer mixed in, don't fertilize for the first four or five weeks.)

>> When your plant starts getting bushy, start pruning it to remove growth near the center stalk and lower branches that aren't receiving much growth. The goals are to redirect the plant's energy to the buds/flowers and open the plant up to light and fresh air.

Harvesting and curing cannabis

When the pistils (hair-like structures) on about half the buds on your plant turn orange or red, the plant is ready to harvest. You can cut down the entire plant or cut off all the branches that contain buds. Remove the fan leaves, and hang the branches (with flowers attached) upside down in a dark room with a temperature of 60–70 degrees Fahrenheit, relative humidity between 45 and 55 percent, and a small fan to gently circulate the air. Be sure to leave space between the branches to prevent mold and mildew.

This initial drying period usually takes a week or two. When the flowers are a little crunchy on the outside but feel a little spongy (not squishy wet) and the smaller branches snap when bent rather than folding over, the flowers are ready to be cured.

To cure the flowers, remove them from the branches and trim any leaves that stick out of the flowers. Place the trimmed flowers in glass jars (loosely packed), seal the jars, and place them in a cool, dry place. During the first week, open the jars once a day for a few minutes to air out the flowers. Over the next four to seven weeks, open the jars for a few minutes once per week.

When your cannabis is fully cured, it's suitable for smoking or creating concentrates and other products.

REMEMBER

Drying and curing isn't necessary if you're making certain concentrates. As explained in Chapter 13, you can use a couple of different extraction methods to collect the trichomes from the flower and use it to create hash and other concentrates. (Trichomes are sticky crystal structures on the outside of the flowers that contain the highest concentrations of cannabinoids and terpenes.)

Creating cannabis, extracts, concentrates and infused products

From cannabis flower, you get extracts, concentrates, and infused products:

» **Extracts** are oils of various consistency that contain high concentrations of cannabinoids and terpenes. They're used to vape, dab, and create other marijuana infused products (MIPs). Extracts are typically made in special facilities using pressure, heat, and potentially dangerous solvents and processes.

» **Concentrates** are made through various mechanical processes with or without the use of heat or cold to collect the trichomes from the flower. The goal is to remove as much of the inert plant matter as possible, leaving behind the cannabinoids and terpenes. Common concentrates are hashish (hash) and rosin.

» **Marijuana infused products (MIPs)** include edibles, tinctures, topicals, and other products that contain flower or an extract or concentrate. Making an infused product is usually a process of adding flower or an extract or concentrate to an existing recipe.

REMEMBER

Decarboxylation is required to convert the non-psychoactive THCa to the psychoactive THC, so if you're making your own infused products, you need to make sure this process takes place. If you're creating a baked good, such as brownies, decarboxylation occurs during the baking process. However, if the product doesn't require heat, you need to bake the cannabis first. See Chapter 13 for details.

Making Money in the Cannabis Industry

According to a 2018 article in *Forbes* magazine, spending on legal cannabis worldwide is expected to reach $57 billion by 2027. You can claim your piece of this potentially lucrative cannabis pie in various ways — by getting a job in the industry, starting your own cannabis business or an ancillary business, or investing in the industry. In this section, we introduce these options, but first, we look at some of the challenges that may make you think twice about seeking your fortune in cannabis.

Recognizing the challenges

Although $57 billion is certainly a lot of money, it's not necessarily easy money, especially in the U.S. where cannabis is still federally illegal. However, even in areas where it's legal, governments tax it heavily and have rules and regulations in place that make compliance difficult and costly. In addition, because cannabis is a drug, and because it's primarily a cash business (in the U.S.), it's very attractive to criminals. Everyone wants a piece of their cannabis pie, and some people aren't afraid to simply take it.

Due to these challenges, you need to be ready to manage your expectations by reminding yourself of the following:

>> Due to the high costs of starting and running a cannabis business, profit margins can be slim. A dispensary license application alone can cost more than $60,000, and U.S. federal tax laws prohibit cannabis businesses from deducting a host of business expenses.

>> Because profit margins are low, don't expect wages to be any higher in the cannabis industry than they are in other industries. They're likely to be a little lower in most cases.

>> Cannabis stocks can go from boom to bust in a hurry, and cannabis investment scams are rampant. Currently, cannabis investing is highly speculative. You can certainly earn a handsome return, but just as easily and quickly lose your shirt.

Getting a job in the industry

The easiest way to begin your foray into the cannabis industry is to get a job in the industry. Given the growth of the industry, a variety of positions need to be filled, including the following:

>> Accountant

>> Buyer

>> Communications director

>> Compliance manager

>> Courier/delivery driver

>> Cultivation technician

>> Cure associate

>> Dispensary manager

>> Dispensary receptionist or cashier

>> Edibles chef

>> Extractor

>> Facilities manager

>> Grower or grow master (head grower)

>> Human resources (HR) managers

- >> Joint roller
- >> Laboratory worker
- >> Marketing managers or team members
- >> Nutrient chemist
- >> Packager
- >> Public affairs administrator
- >> Quality assurance manager

- >> Sales associate (budtender)
- >> Sales representative
- >> Security personnel
- >> Technology director
- >> Trainers
- >> Trimmer

TIP

Before you start looking for a job in the industry, consider getting a state badge. A cannabis company may deem you a more attractive candidate if you already have your documentation. If a company hires someone and that person's application for a badge is denied, they need to start their candidate search all over again.

Openings are posted on traditional job sites, such as indeed.com. Some job sites, such as www.vangsters.com, are dedicated to the cannabis industry. Also consider visiting the websites of cannabis companies you're interested in to see whether any job openings are posted on those sites.

Starting your own cannabis business

If you're considering starting your own cannabis business, you have numerous opportunities to consider in the various industry segments:

- >> **Grow:** Grow operations cultivate, harvest, and cure cannabis to supply it to dispensaries/retail locations and to MIPs.

- >> **MIP:** MIPs obtain cannabis from grow operations and use it to create concentrates, extracts, edibles, and other marijuana infused products supplied to dispensaries/ retail locations. MIPs may be broken down further into extraction operations and industrial kitchen operations, both of which can be a distinct business.

- >> **Dispensary/retail:** Dispensaries (and perhaps other retailers) obtain products from growers and/or MIPs and sell them to consumers.

Vertically-integrated cannabis businesses are those that contain all three operations — grow, MIP, and dispensary/retail.

REMEMBER

Many failed cannabis businesses have been started by very smart people who are passionate about the plant but lacking in the knowledge and skills to start and run a business and unprepared for the costs and regulatory pressures. Don't start a business until you have all the pieces in place to give yourself a reasonable chance of success. This industry can be brutal.

Exploring ancillary business

Ancillary businesses are those that operate on the periphery of the cannabis industry and supply it with goods and services. These businesses can profit from cannabis without the risks and hassles, because they can also serve businesses and individuals outside the cannabis industry. Ancillary businesses include the following:

>> Fertilizer manufacturers

>> Nurseries

>> Manufacturers and sellers of grow lights

>> Heating, ventilation, and air conditioning (HVAC) companies

>> Breweries that sell their CO_2 to grow facilities

>> Packaging and labeling services

>> Security services and manufactures and sellers of security equipment

>> Technology, and software companies

>> Marketing, public relations, and advertising firms

>> Real estate companies and investors

>> Law firms and consulting agencies

REMEMBER

Success in any business requires both competence in the industry and business management skills. However, ancillary businesses don't have the high costs (including high taxes) and regulatory requirements that make success in the cannabis industry so challenging.

Investing in the industry

Cannabis businesses are expensive to start and maintain, and because it's federally illegal in the U.S., entrepreneurs have difficulty finding bank loans to finance their startups. They often need to use either their own money or money from private lenders or investors. If you have money available to invest and you can afford to let that money ride, you may be able to earn a sizeable long-term return. However, you may also lose your entire initial investment.

The key to success is performing your due diligence. Before investing, research the industry as a whole so you have a general understanding of it and can recognize the major players. Also research individual companies thoroughly. Invest in only those companies with solid leadership and financials.

WARNING

Cannabis investment scams are rampant. Don't rely solely on articles, blog posts, incoming email messages, or press releases for guidance on finding cannabis companies in which to invest. These sources may be promoting scams or highlighting the good news and downplaying any negatives for ulterior motives.

See Chapter 16 for more about investing in the cannabis industry.

Chapter 2

Brushing Up on Cannabis Anatomy and Chemistry

Whether you're consuming, growing, harvesting, or selling cannabis, you should be familiar with the plant from which products are derived, the active ingredients the plant contains (and their effects), and the various extracts and concentrates produced from plants. This familiarity with the plant and its chemicals may be essential when growing and harvesting cannabis, or it may simply make you a more educated consumer and enhance your experience.

In this chapter, we bring you up to speed on cannabis anatomy and chemistry, describe the two major strains of cannabis (indica and sativa), and introduce you to the numerous extracts and concentrates derived from the plant.

Getting to Know the Plant from Top to Bottom

At its most basic level, cannabis is a plant or, as some like to call it, a "weed." Like most plants, it's made up of roots, a stem (stalk), branches, leaves, and buds/flowers. The leaves extend out from areas called *nodes* along the stem.

In this section, we break down the plant into its component parts and describe each part in greater detail, but first we distinguish between the two primary strains of cannabis plants.

Examining the structure of the two primary strains

Marijuana plants come in two primary strains along with a host of hybrid strains produced through cross-breeding. Traditionally, consumers have chosen end products based on the common effects inherent in the different strains — sativa for a more energetic high and indica (often referred to as "inda couch") for its relaxation and sedative properties. The evolved genetics of the two strains have produced these differing properties. While consumable buds from each strain are similar in appearance, the plants have unique properties that distinguish the two strains:

>> **Indica** plants have a shorter and wider plant profile with a bushy appearance. The leaves are also shorter and wider. Indica plants have a shorter flowering cycle and are more suitable for colder climates with shorter growing seasons.

>> **Sativa** plants appear taller and slimmer overall with thinner leaves. Sativa plants have a longer flowering cycle and are better suited for warm climates with longer growing seasons.

Checking out the buds and flowers

Male and female plants differ in respect to their buds/flowers. As a female plant matures, a large *cola* (a cluster of buds) forms at the *apex* (top) of the plant and thus is commonly referred to as the *apical bud*. Smaller colas may form on lower branches that extend out from the stem. The *pistil* contains the reproductive parts of the flower. Hair-like strands of the pistil, called *stigmas*, collect pollen from male plants.

A *bract* (a collection of tiny leaves) encases the female's reproductive parts, including the *calyx* (the translucent layer that that covers the ovule at each flower's base). Bracts are covered with resin glands, called *trichomes* (pronounced "trick-combs" or "try-combs"), which produce the highest concentration of *cannabinoids* — the active ingredients of the plant. As cannabis buds mature, they're commonly covered in this crystal resin. (See the later section "Combing through the trichomes" for details.)

In male plants, the flowers produce pollen for fertilizing the female plants.

REMEMBER

Because the cola contains the highest concentration of cannabinoids, growers generally want to grow female plants, especially in a commercial enterprise, which is why they typically start plants from cuttings or clones instead of seeds. However, when a female plant is highly stressed, it may turn *hermaphrodite* (serving the role as both female and male plant) to pollinate itself.

When grown for marijuana product, the plant is harvested at the bud stage and not allowed to fully flower. Within the industry, the budding flower may be referred to as either "flower" or "bud," though technically it's a flower.

The bud is the harvested product that creates almost all the marijuana products on the market. In some states it is the only part of the plant that can be legally sold. It is also the part of the plant that has the majority of THC and other cannabinoids, including *cannabidiol* (CBD) and *cannabinol* (CBN).

Taking a peek at the seeds

Female plants that are allowed to flower and are pollinated by male plants produce seeds, which can be used to grow new plants. Seeds contain almost no THC and aren't generally used in marijuana products. In fact, most states with medical marijuana laws don't consider seeds to be a usable part of the plant. However, in most states, seeds, as well as plants, are strictly regulated. Seeds typically play a role in the following applications:

>> Home growers may start their plants from seeds.

>> Growers may cross-breed plants to create seeds for growing hybrid plants.

>> Growers may also use seeds to refresh older mothers/clone stock. (Generally, strains that are closest to the seed generation are healthier than ones that have been cloned over multiple generations.)

REMEMBER

Commercial growers as well as most home grows strive to avoid seeding because it's undesirable in the final flower product. To avoid seeding, most operations allow only female plants in the grow room; a single male plant in a growing room can cause the entire room to seed! They grow new plants from clippings or clones, a practice that delivers the following benefits:

>> Controls the sex of the plant. While seeds have about a 50/50 chance of growing a male or female plant, a clipping or clone has a 100 percent chance of being the same sex as the parent. (Note, however, that some seed banks offer feminized seeds, which can have about a 90 percent chance of growing into more desirable female plants.)

>> Ensures that new plants are genetically pure, which is important for the consistency of the end product and the desired effects it creates.

>> Ensures that only the healthiest and most effective plants continue to be grown.

>> Shortens the time to produce a flowering bud and, hence, a harvestable bud.

Combing through the trichomes

As cannabis plants mature, the leaves and buds become covered by what appear to be tiny crystals but are actually large collections of trichomes — fine, hair-like, glandular outgrowths on a plant's surface (see Figure 2-1). They may appear shiny or frosty, look like orange hairs, or cover the buds like a layer of frost.

Trichomes are a common part of plant anatomy. They may be a single cell or two to three cells viewable only through the use of a microscope or multi-cell structures that are visible to the naked eye. Located on all parts of the plant, from stems to leaves to buds, trichomes protect plants from animals (especially insects) and from environmental effects, such as wind and heat. They can be prickly, sticky, stinky, and bitter, making the plant unpalatable. On some carnivorous plants, trichomes play a role in catching prey.

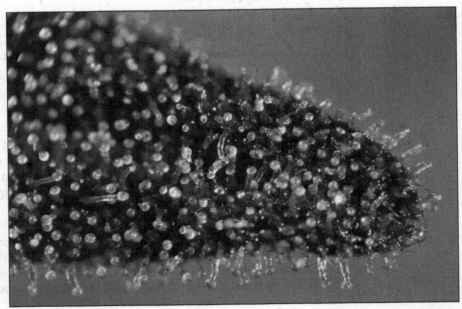

FIGURE 2-1: Trichomes protect the plant and are the largest source of cannabinoids.

gleti/Shutterstock.com

A great deal of the cannabinoids THC and CBD are found in the trichomes. They also contain the terpenes that carry the aroma of the cannabis plant and indicate expected effects beyond the definition of strain. Large numbers of trichomes indicate high levels of cannabinoids, which equates to potency:

REMEMBER

Trichome volume = Potency of all cannabinoids

Trichomes exist in many shapes and sizes, but these three appear most often on cannabis plants:

>> **Bulbous trichomes** form on the entire surface of the plant. They typically have a stalk consisting of 1–4 cells and a mushroom-shaped top consisting of another 1–4 cells. They're so small, only 10–15 micrometers (mcm) wide, that you need a microscope to see them. (The width of a human hair is 40–50 mcm.)

>> **Capitate sessile trichomes** are slightly larger than the bulbous trichomes and significantly more abundant.

>> **Capitate-stalked trichomes** are between 50–100 mcm wide, making them large enough to be seen by the naked eye. Their structure consists of a stalk topped off by a large, waxy glandular head, which serves as the epicenter for cannabinoid and terpenoid synthesis.

REMEMBER

Over time, trichomes change in appearance from clear to cloudy and may change color. These changes in appearance help growers identify optimal harvest times to ensure maximum potency — when the volume of cannabinoids is highest and just before the chemicals begin to break down.

Considering the lesser parts of the plant

Although the bud/flower is the primary source of active ingredients used to make medical marijuana and adult recreational cannabis products, the plant contains a few other parts worthy of mention:

>> **Stems and branches:** Stems and branches are important for supporting the plant, but they contain very little THC and other cannabinoids. They are generally considered unusable parts of the plant.

>> **Stalk:** Like the stems and branches, the stalk contains very little THC and other cannabinoids and is generally considered an unusable part of the plant for cannabinoid products. However, the fibers in the stalk, called hemp, are often used to make paper, rope, fabric, and oil.

>> **Leaves:** Marijuana plants have two types of leaves — vegetative leaves that power plant growth and have a very low concentration of cannabinoids, and

sugar leaves that grow within the bud and have high THC content. Sometimes growers remove large leaves to allocate more of the plant's energy to bud growth, a process commonly referred to as *de-fanning*.

>> **Roots:** Obviously, the roots are essential for plant growth, but they contain little THC and are generally not considered a usable part of the plant for cannabinoid production.

Taking a Crash Course in Cannabinoid Chemistry

Cannabis affects each person differently depending on the chemical composition of the product and how the chemicals (cannabinoids and terpenes) interact with the individual's biology and physiology. With a better understanding of the biological and physiological factors and the chemical composition of cannabis, you can more closely align product choices to your desired experience.

TIP

This section covers the basics of cannabinoid chemistry and the human endocannabinoid system, but the best resource for guiding product selection is a well-trained budtender at your dispensary of choice. A *budtender* is a person who serves customers at a cannabis dispensary. A qualified budtender can recommend products that most closely align with your needs and the experience you desire. (See Chapter 5 for more about choosing and visiting a cannabis dispensary.)

Assessing factors impacting individual effects

Even when two people consume the same cannabis product at the same time in the same place, they can have vastly different experiences due to factors such as the following:

>> **Altitude:** Consuming weed at high altitudes may not increase the high, but it will make you feel higher, and not necessarily in a good way. Until you're acclimatized to the higher altitude, consider reducing the amount you usually take by half as a starting point. (See Chapter 7 for more about dosing.)

>> **Age:** Your biology and physiology change with age. As a result, the same cannabis may affect you differently at different stages of your life. While using a product may have calmed you when you were younger, it may make you feel anxious later in life or vice versa. The same is true about quantity — you

may have different effects from the same amount, though the commercial product of today is vastly more potent than in decades past.

>> **Recent food eaten (stomach contents):** Various foods contain ingredients that interact with cannabinoids or terpenes to change the experience. Fat-soluble meals have been shown to increase the onset time and heighten the effects of cannabis. Sweet potatoes, nuts, and broccoli can also enhance or prolong the experience. Mangoes, which contain myrcene terpenes (also present in cannabis), may intensify the effects. The smell of black pepper may help to lessen the intensity or duration of the effects.

>> **Environment:** Whether you use cannabis at home alone, at a party with friends, on a serene beach near the ocean, out in the woods, or in the hustle and bustle of a large city, the experience can differ considerably.

>> **Emotional status:** How you feel emotionally can significantly impact how you feel when you consume cannabis. While cannabis may calm you when you're feeling stressed, for example, it may also exacerbate your anxiety. What you expect from the experience may also impact how you feel.

>> **Frequency of consumption:** People who consume cannabis frequently build up a tolerance for it, so the experience may not be quite as intense as it is for a new or infrequent user.

REMEMBER

The variations that occur in these situations are mainly in the intensity of the experience and the time required to feel the effects rather than changes in the experience itself, such as a relaxing experience becoming an overly energetic one.

Exploring the endocannabinoid system

Nature has provided humans with a specific internal system for processing cannabis called the *endocannabinoid system (ECS)* — a chemical messaging network that helps to regulate certain bodily functions, including fertility and pregnancy, appetite and digestion, sleep, motor control, pain and pleasure, immune function, temperature, mood, and memory. It's also the system in which consumed cannabis product is processed, creating the high and other physiological effects associated with the various cannabinoids. It is perhaps the most important physiological system involved in establishing and maintaining human health.

The endocannabinoid system consists of three primary components:

>> **Cannabinoid receptors:** Located on the surface of cells, these receptors receive messages in the form of chemical molecules called cannabinoids. Imagine a cannabinoid as a key that fits into the cannabinoid receptor on a cell, triggering a biological response in the receiving cell; for example, Figure 2-2 shows the neuron at the top receiving a cannabinoid, which triggers it to

release neurotransmitters to a nearby neuron. Researchers have identified two cannabinoid receptors (also shown in Figure 2-2):

- **Cannabinoid receptor number 1 (CB1):** Located primarily in the brain and central nervous system and, to a lesser extent, in other tissues, CB1s receive THC and are indirectly affected by CBD.

- **Cannabinoid receptor number 2 (CB2):** Located primarily in the peripheral organs, especially cells associated with the immune system, CB2s receive CBN and are indirectly affected by CBD.

  REMEMBER

  CBD isn't a perfect fit with CB1 or CB2 receptors, but it has a powerful indirect impact on these receptors. How CBD interacts with CB1 and CB2 receptors is still being studied.

» **Endocannabinoids:** These small molecules are neurotransmitters (chemical messengers) that activate cannabinoid receptors. The two best known endocannabinoids are:

- **Anandamide (AEA)** is commonly referred to as the "bliss molecule" because it is thought to affect mood.

- **2-arachidonoylglycerol (2-AG)** plays an important role in the regulation of food intake and energy metabolism, anxiety and depression, addiction, immune system function, inflammation, and proliferation and invasion of certain types of cancer cells.

» **Metabolic enzymes:** These internal enzymes break down endocannabinoids after they're used. The metabolic enzymes that break down AEA and 2-AG are (respectively):

- Fatty acid amide hydrolase (FAAH)

- Monoacylglycerol lipase (MAGL)

REMEMBER

Cannabinoids come in three types:

» **Endogenous cannabinoids:** Also known as endocannabinoids, these neurotransmitters are produced naturally by the body. They affect brain areas that influence pleasure, memory, thinking, concentration, movement, coordination, and sensory and time perception.

» **Phytocannabinoids:** These cannabinoids, which include THC and CBD, are derived from plants.

» **Synthetic cannabinoids:** These cannabinoids are synthesized in a lab. They're generally used to help map the ECS. Some are also approved for different ailments outside the U.S.

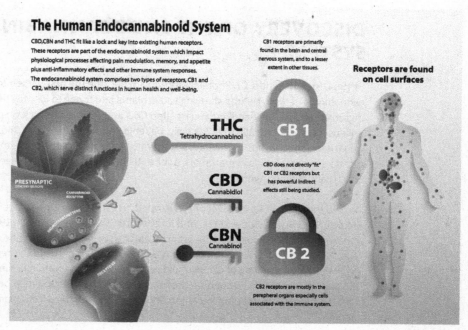

The Human Endocannabinoid System

CBD, CBN and THC fit like a lock and key into existing human receptors. These receptors are part of the endocannabinoid system which impact physiological processes affecting pain modulation, memory, and appetite plus anti-inflammatory effects and other immune system responses. The endocannabinoid system comprises two types of receptors, CB1 and CB2, which serve distinct functions in human health and well-being.

CB1 receptors are primarily found in the brain and central nervous system, and to a lesser extent in other tissues.

Receptors are found on cell surfaces

THC
Tetrahydrocannabinol

CB 1

CBD does not directly "fit" CB1 or CB2 receptors but has powerful indirect effects still being studied.

CBD
Cannabidiol

CBN
Cannabinol

CB 2

CB2 receptors are mostly in the peripheral organs especially cells associated with the immune system.

PRESYNAPTIC

CANNABINOID RECEPTOR

FIGURE 2-2: Cannabinoids enter receptors triggering the release or take-up of neurotransmitters.

Shutterstock.com

The effects of cannabis on the body through the endocannabinoid system are based on the shape of the cannabinoids and their receptors and the type of interaction the molecules have with the receptors. A cannabinoid is considered an agonist or antagonist depending on how it interacts with a receptor:

» **Agonist:** An *agonist* is chemical that binds to a receptor and activates it to produce a biological response. THC and CBN are CB1 and CB2 agonists.

» **Antagonist:** An *antagonist* is a substance that interferes with or inhibits the physiological response of a receptor. CBD is a CB1 and CB2 antagonist.

Getting high with tetrahydrocannabinol (THC)

THC, the most abundant and well-known cannabinoid in cannabis, is responsible for the psychoactive effects most people associate with cannabis. It has analgesic (relieves pain), *antiemetic* (reduces vomiting and nausea), *anti-proliferative* (inhibits the spread of cancer cells), antioxidant, antispasmodic, appetite stimulant, muscle relaxant, euphoriant, and *neuroprotective* (slows damage to the nervous system and brain) properties.

DISCOVERY OF THE ENDOCANNABINOID SYSTEM

In 1964, Israeli scientist Dr. Raphael Mechoulam became the first person to identify a cannabinoid — THC. He was studying sativa plants and trying to identify the active ingredients. Next, he identified and isolated CBD and started testing it on patients with epilepsy. While taking 200 mg CBD daily, patients had no seizures. In 1986, Mechoulam published *Cannabinoids as Therapeutics*, in which he discusses the many therapeutic effects of cannabinoids in mammals, but he still had no clue as to the mechanism by which cannabinoids worked.

Around the same time, Professor Allyn Howlett, a researcher at the St. Louis University Medical School, was studying THC and its effects on the human body. In 1988, she and her colleagues discovered the brain receptor to which THC binds. She named the receptor *cannabinoid receptor number 1* (CB1 receptor). Soon thereafter, researchers discovered a second type of cannabinoid receptor, CB2, and found an entire network of CB1 and CB2 receptors throughout the human body. The question then became "Why does the human body contain receptors for compounds derived from plants, particularly cannabis?"

Dr. Mechoulam and his colleagues believed they knew the answer to that question: The human body must produce its own cannabinoids, as well. This hypothesis led them, in 1992, to start searching for *endocannabinoids* (cannabinoids produced by the human body). After two years of research, they found a compound in the brain that acts on the cannabinoid receptors. They named the compound "anandamide" based on the Sanskrit word "ananda," which means supreme joy or bliss. In 1995, Mechoulam's team discovered a second endogenous cannabinoid, 2-arachidonoylglycerol (2-AG).

What's interesting about this story is that THC ultimately was the key that unlocked the door leading to a previously unknown chemical messaging system in the human body, a neurotransmitter network that regulates a broad spectrum of biological functions. Without cannabis and THC, the medical world would probably still be in the dark about this important messaging system.

THCa is the acidic precursor to THC. THCa converts to Δ9-THC when heated, as when cannabis is smoked. THCa is non-psychoactive and has many therapeutic uses. It's a natural insecticide and an analgesic (pain reliever), and it has anti-inflammatory, anti-insomnia, anti-spasmodic, anti-proliferative, antiemetic, and neuroprotective properties. It also has been shown to regulate the immune system while reducing inflammation.

Feeling better with cannabidiol (CBD) without getting high

Cannabidiol (CBD) is the main non-psychoactive cannabinoid in cannabis, and it has a wide range of therapeutic uses. Because of its many therapeutic uses and because it is non-psychoactive, it is often recommended for treating certain medical conditions in children, the elderly, and anyone who wants the medicinal benefits of cannabis without the high.

CBD has analgesic, antibacterial, antidepressant, antiemetic, anti-convulsant, anti-inflammatory, anti-ischemic (reduces the risk of artery blockage), antipsoriatic (treats psoriasis), anti-hyperalgesia, anti-proliferative, antipsychotic, anti-oxidant, antispasmodic, anxiolytic, bone stimulant, immunosuppressive, intestinal anti-prokinetic (reduces small intestine contractions), neuroprotective, neurogenic, and vasorelaxant (reduces vascular tension) properties. It may also be helpful in the prevention and treatment of diabetes, including insulin resistance, obesity, neuropathy, and the healing of certain skin conditions.

CBDa is found in elevated levels in specific cannabis strains. Like THCa, CBDa is an acidic precursor that converts to CBD when heated. CBDa is non-psychoactive and has antibacterial and anti-inflammatory properties and has also been shown to be antiemetic and anti-proliferative.

Reaping the sedative effects of cannabinol (CBN)

Cannabinol (CBN) is a mildly psychoactive cannabinoid that comes from the degradation of THC after an extended period of time due to exposure to oxygen and heat. (A fresh plant contains little or no CBN.) CBN has analgesic, antibacterial, anti-inflammatory, anti-insomnia, antiemetic, appetite stimulant, and bone stimulant properties. It's also effective in treating burns. CBN is only 10 percent as psychoactive as THC, but it can produce a very mild high.

Exploring the potential health benefits of cannabigerol (CBG)

Cannabigerol (CBG) is a non-psychoactive cannabinoid. It has analgesic, muscle relaxant, anti-erythemic (reduces redness is skin), antifungal, anti-depressant, anti-proliferative, anti-psoriatic, and anti-bacterial properties. As an antibacterial, it is a powerful weapon against the methicillin-resistant Staphylococcus aureus (MRSA) virus.

Discovering the potential health benefits of cannabigerol (CBG)

Tetrahydrocannabivarin (THCv) is less well known but similar to THC with some psychoactive properties in high doses. However, it is a powerful cannabinoid with some potential therapeutic value and unique effects that differ from those of THC. It is an appetite suppressant, stimulates bone growth, and may help with diabetes, Alzheimer's, and panic attacks in PTSD. It needs to be heated higher than THC to about 428°F when vaporizing.

Using terpenes to anticipate effects

In the not-so-distant past, consumers used plant strain to guide their product selection. Traditionally, sativas were considered more energizing and indicas more relaxing. However, relatively recently, the industry has moved to the use of terpenes (aromatic molecules) for product selection because they're more consistent identifiers for predicting the experience. Table 2-1 lists and describes the ten most common terpenes in cannabis.

TABLE 2-1   **Ten Common Terpenes in Cannabis**

Terpene	Aroma/flavor	Effects
Terpinolene	Floral with a smoky woodiness	Highly sedative, anti-microbial, anti-proliferative
D-Limonene	Citrus	Aids in the absorption of other terpenes through skin and mucous membranes, anti-anxiety, immunosuppressant, antidepressant, antibacterial, gastroprotective, kills breast cancer cells
Linalool	Floral and sweet citrus often found in lavender	Anti-anxiety, sedative, local anesthetic, analgesic, anti-convulsive
α-Pinene	Pine	Anti-inflammatory, bronchodilation, anti-microbial, focus and memory enhancement
β-Caryophyllene	Pepper, clove, spice	Anti-inflammatory, analgesic, anti-anxiety, antidepressant, antioxidant, anti-microbial, gastroprotective
Carene	Woody (cedar, pine)	Dries excess bodily fluid, including tears and saliva, may cause dry mouth and eye sensations
Geraniol	Floral (rose)	Mosquito repellant, protective against neuropathy

Terpene	Aroma/flavor	Effects
Humulene	Earthy, hoppy	Analgesic, anti-inflammatory, anti-bacterial, anti-proliferative, anorectic (appetite suppressant)
Terpineol	Floral (lilac)	Relaxation
Myrcene	Earthy, hoppy with tropical fruit	Sedative, analgesic, antibiotic, muscle relaxant

Exploring Cannabis Concentrates and Extracts

Although you can certainly consume cannabis whole (for example, by smoking bud), most products are concentrates or extracts or are made from concentrates or extracts. The line separating concentrates from extracts is beginning to blur, but the two differ in the following ways:

>> **Concentrate:** A *concentrate* includes only the most desirable components of the plant, including the cannabinoids and terpenes (in most cases) without the undesirable substances, such as the leaves and stems. Concentrates are generally made through mechanical processes; the use of carbon dioxide (CO_2) without heat or pressure; or processes that use ice, water, vegetable glycerin, vegetable oils, animal fats, isopropyl alcohol, or ethanol.

>> **Extract:** An *extract* is a concentrate made with CO_2 along with high heat and pressure or through the use of a hydrocarbon-based solvent (butane or propane) to extract chemicals from the plant material. (All extracts are concentrates, but concentrates aren't necessarily extracts.)

In the following sections, we list and describe the most common concentrates and extracts, along with products commonly made from concentrates and extracts.

REMEMBER

Cannabis products beyond smokable flower have always been available. As the industry has evolved and businesses have diversified, an even greater number of end products have become available in the legal market.

Concentrates

Concentrates include the following:

>> **Kief:** *Kief* is the fine amount of trichomes that may be left as a byproduct from flower. It consists of the resin glands — the sticky crystals that cover the

cannabis flower. These crystals are the primary source of the cannabinoids and terpenes that produce the desired effects. You can create your own kief (dry sift) using a three-chamber herb grinder; as you grind your cannabis in the top chamber, kief crystals pass through a screen into the bottom chamber. Kief is usually consumed by adding it to another cannabis product to increase its potency. It can also be pressed into a concentrate and consumed that way or be added to melted butter to create edibles.

>> **Bubble hash:** Bubble hash is a Kief product that can be pressed into a small flat cake. You can make your own bubble hash by mixing cannabis plant with ice water and then using a special filter to screen out the undesirable plant parts. What's left is your bubble hash.

>> **Rosin:** Rosin is the resinous sap from the bud. It's made by pressing cannabis flower between two very hot metal plates. The resulting rosin contains most of the flavor, aroma, terpenes, and cannabinoids from the original flower material.

>> **Cannabis oil:** Cannabis oil may be a concentrate or extract depending on how it's produced. If it's produced through CO_2 extraction under high pressure and at extremely low temperatures or with the use of ethanol (grain alcohol) or olive oil, it's an extract. The oil is then used in the manufacturing of multiple products including vape oils, tinctures, topicals, and edibles. Over time, cannabis oil can separate into crystallized THC and terpene liquid, and is sometimes sold in the industry as "sauce":

- **Crystals of THC:** Commonly consumed via dabbing (heating the product on a very hot surface and inhaling the resulting vapors), these crystals are highly concentrated forms of THC, but without the liquid they can be very harsh to consume.

- **Terpene liquid:** The liquid separated from the THC crystals contains far less THC but higher terpene levels.

>> **Tinctures:** Tinctures are alcohol-based (or mixed with other liquids like agave) cannabis concentrates. Many tinctures are *sublinguals* (taken underneath the tongue), which have the benefit of quickly being absorbed. These products are among the fastest acting consumables after inhalation. Tinctures are frequently produced with exclusive or very high CBD strains and tend to have a high ratio of CBD to THC.

Extracts

Common extracts include the following:

>> **Hashish:** *Hashish* is cannabis resin that appears as a sticky, black brick made through extraction with a hydrocarbon or fuel. It's not a legal U.S. dispensary product.

>> **Shatter:** *Shatter* (see Figure 2-3) is a semi-translucent extract created from dried and cured cannabis flower using a hydrocarbon extraction method. The extract is then poured in large sheets to set before being broken into small pieces, weighed, and sold. (See Figure 2-3.) Shatter is commonly used for *dabbing* — heating the product on a very hot surface and inhaling the resulting vapors. (See Chapter 6 for more about dabbing and other consumption methods.)

>> **Wax:** Sometimes referred to as "budder," wax is similar to shatter with the same starting material and extraction process. Then, it's whipped to create a chalkier consistency (see Figure 2-4). It's also used for dabbing.

>> **Live resin:** Live resin is created from fresh frozen cannabis flower that's not dried or cured. It's extracted through a hydrocarbon process and whipped like wax, but its starting material makes it softer with a higher terpene profile than shatter or wax, resulting in a more flavorful product. (See Figure 2-5.)

>> **Cannabis oil:** Cannabis oil is typically produced through CO_2 extraction, creating a concentrate. However, it can also be made with hydrocarbon solvents, such as butane or hexane, in which case the oil is an extract.

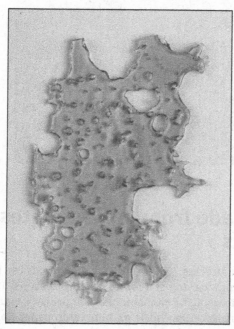

FIGURE 2-3:
Shatter.

Roxana Gonzalez/Shutterstock.com

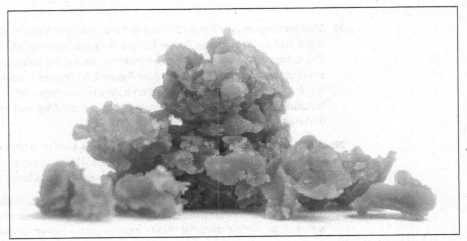

FIGURE 2-4:
Wax.

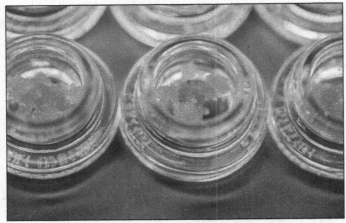

FIGURE 2-5:
Live resin.

Products made from concentrates and extracts

Through an extraction process, THC or other cannabinoids can be separated from the cannabis flower into varying states from liquid to solids. These usually have very high concentrations of the cannabinoid. The primary extraction processing methods used are: hydrocarbon such as butane/propane, CO_2 or ethanol. The desired end product dictates the process employed for extraction. Concentrates and extracts are commonly used to create a variety of consumable products, including the following:

- » **Sublingual sprays:** Some tinctures are developed into sublingual sprays. This is simply another delivery method for an oil based product. Like tinctures, these sprays tend to have a very high ratio of CBD to THC.

- » **Vape oils:** Cannabis oil is commonly sold as vape oil, which can be consumed via a vape pen or similar device.

- » **Cannabis liquor:** Interest in commercial products that blend alcohol and cannabis is growing. However, at this time, such products are not legal in the U.S. market. The cannabis flower is very similar to hops and many home growers mix with hops in a hot water extraction to create these products.

WARNING

Mixing alcohol and cannabis can create intense and unexpected effects. Consuming both products in a single experience is never recommended.

- » **Liquid/beverage:** Consuming cannabis in liquid form is very popular. Commercial producers are creating carbonated sodas and teas; flasks of small dose cannabis liquid; isolate powder mixes to be dissolved into beverages; and other emerging products.

- » **Edibles:** Edibles are part of the fastest growing consumption methods in cannabis. Products include items such as gummies, lollipops, chocolates including chocolate-covered coffee beans, baked goods, dried fruit, caramel corn, hard candies, mints, tablets, and pills.

- » **Cannabis butter:** Ground cannabis flower is sometimes mixed with traditional cow's milk butter to be used as an edible cannabis product or used in baking.

- » **Topicals:** Topical products are infused lotions and oils that are applied to a specific area of the body for direct effects. These are very commonly high CBD products meant to relieve localized pain or inflammation. They are produced from cannabis oil added to fats to create the lotions.

- » **Transdermals:** Transdermal patches are most commonly built on a plastic or cloth material as with other medicated patches. The oil is added along with solvents that dissolve as well as an isolate and a layer of glue. The layers of product diffuse into skin for localized relief or into bloodstream for more systemic delivery.

» Recognizing various restrictions

» Monitoring international efforts

» Flying below law enforcement's radar

» Keeping a cool head during police encounters

» Being a responsible parent

Chapter 3

Steering Clear of Legal Trouble

L egal marijuana is a relatively new reality, and you want to make certain you're staying on the right side of the law, but that can be more confusing than you may think.

Cannabis is currently still classified as a Schedule I drug in the U.S. and is federally illegal to sell, possess, or consume. However, two countries and numerous states in the U.S. have legalized cannabis to varying degrees. In the U.S. especially, the law gets confusing with each state enacting different rules and regulations, including whether cannabis is legal for both medical and adult recreational use, how and where you can buy it, and how much you can purchase and carry. Adding to the complexity is the fact that counties and municipalities within legal states can add their own rules or individually bar certain types of sales. Tax structures and delivery rules may differ from one county to the next, and consumption restrictions can be equally challenging to navigate.

In this chapter, we provide general guidance on federal, state, local, and international marijuana laws; call your attention to various restrictions you should be aware of; and steer you toward resources where you can find more detailed and current information. We also provide guidance on how to avoid encounters with law enforcement and how to respond in the event that such an encounter occurs. Finally, we offer insight on how to use responsibly for the safety of children.

Knowing the Laws: Federal, State, Local and International

The first precaution to take to steer clear of legal trouble with regard to cannabis is to know the law of the land. For example, in the United States, cannabis is illegal federally, legal for medical use in many states, and legal for both medical and adult recreational use in several states. On October 17, 2018, Canada become the second country and the first G7 member country to legalize recreational marijuana. In Quebec and Alberta, the legal age is 18; in the remainder of the country, the legal age is 19. Marijuana laws may also vary locally, so you need to be aware of where you are and know and obey the relevant laws and restrictions. Otherwise, you're likely to find yourself at an increased risk of being charged and possibly convicted of a crime.

In this section, we bring you up to speed on federal, state, local, and international marijuana laws in the hopes that by knowing the laws you'll be better equipped to avoid legal problems.

Keeping abreast of U.S. federal law and enforcement

The legal history of cannabis began in the early 1900s with state restrictions on its sale and use. Federal regulation didn't occur until President Franklin D. Roosevelt signed the Marihuana Tax Act of 1937, which required users to obtain a tax stamp for the purchase of marijuana. To obtain the tax stamp, users were required to provide details about the marijuana location and amount, thereby incriminating themselves. In 1970, the Supreme Court overturned the law, and Congress repealed it but simultaneously passed the Controlled Substances Act, designating marijuana an illegal substance.

REMEMBER

At the federal level, in the U.S., marijuana is illegal, period. Although law enforcement and prosecutors in states in which marijuana is legal aren't likely to enforce federal marijuana laws, they can still choose to do so.

WARNING

In particular, the following activities are federal crimes:

>> Transporting cannabis across any state line, even if it is going from one legalized state directly to another.

>> Flying with cannabis, because it enters into federal airspace. Some state governments have indicated that they will not be confiscating cannabis in an individual's possession if the amount is below the legal state limit at their airports. However, even in those locations flying with the product is a federal crime.

>> Possessing or using marijuana on federal land, including national parks and forests.

REMEMBER

Avoid online scams. Because federal law prohibits marijuana from being transported across state lines, no legitimate business will ship you any cannabis product that contains THC. Any online website, Facebook page, or other entity that promises to ship you cannabis with THC isn't legal. Even if the business or individual claims to be associated with a reputable dispensary, you're getting scammed as long as marijuana is federally illegal. However, hemp derived CBD products can be shipped legally across state lines.

THE COLE MEMORANDUM

During the Obama Administration (August 29, 2013), United States Deputy Attorney General James M. Cole issued a trio of memos including the Cole Memorandum to all United States Attorney Generals. The memo informed the state attorneys general that due to limited resources, the U.S. Department of Justice would not be enforcing federal marijuana prohibition in states that legalized and effectively regulated and enforced their own marijuana laws.

The memo directed the state attorneys general to "not focus federal resources in your states on individuals whose actions are in clear and unambiguous compliance with existing state laws providing for the medical use of marijuana." Instead, states were encouraged to address federal priorities; for example, "by implementing effective measures to prevent diversion of marijuana outside the regulated system and to other states, prohibiting access to marijuana by minors, and replacing an illicit marijuana trade that funds criminal enterprises with a tightly regulated market in which revenues are tracked and accounted for."

This memo was rescinded under the Trump administration in January 2018 by Attorney General Jeff Sessions. The impact of the rescission in individual states has yet to be determined, but it is a cause for concern because it indicates that the feds may be leaning toward greater enforcement of the federal prohibition on marijuana.

Getting up to speed on state laws

Although cannabis is federally illegal, each state has the right to legalize within its borders and set the rules and regulations for personal and commercial growth, production, transportation, sale, and use. States fall into one of the following three categories:

>> No laws legalizing marijuana

>> Marijuana legalized only for medical use

>> Marijuana legalized for both medical and adult recreational use

The easiest way to find out which category a state is in is to search online for "state marijuana laws map" and click one of the many links provided. You'll see a color-coded map.

REMEMBER

State marijuana laws change frequently, so access a map from a reliable source that has current information.

These color-coded maps provide only cursory information about which states have legalized marijuana for medical and/or adult recreational use. Specific rules and regulations are more complex and vary considerably from state to state. In the following sections, we highlight rules and regulations and give you a general idea of how they can vary from state to state.

REMEMBER

Carefully research the current law in any area you plan to purchase, possess, use, grow, gift, or sell marijuana before engaging in any of these activities. In the U.S., you should be familiar with federal, state, and local laws. You can find the information you need online. For example, searching for "Colorado marijuana laws" displays links to several sites with relevant information. Look for a link to sites that end in ".gov," which indicates a government sponsored site, such as www.colorado.gov/pacific/marijuana. Going to a government sponsored site ensures that you're getting accurate and current information.

Medical use

Most U.S. states have legalized marijuana for medical use, but you need to know more than whether medical use is legal or not in a particular state. You also need to be aware of the specific rules and regulations. For medical marijuana, rules and regulations typically stipulate the following:

PLAYING A ROLE IN LEGALIZING CANNABIS

With greater acceptance of marijuana and recognition of the value of the industry for all constituencies, more states are legalizing marijuana either for medical or both medical and adult recreational use. Some states put the question of legalization directly to the voters, typically in the form of a proposition, whereas others turn to state legislative bodies to make the decision.

As a citizen of your state, you can play a role in the decision process by contacting your governor and state and local representatives to let them know where you stand on this issue, voting for candidates who support your views, and casting your vote on any cannabis propositions included on your ballot.

» **Qualifying medical conditions:** Each state has a list of medical conditions that qualify a person to use medical marijuana. For example, in the state of Washington, qualifying conditions are cancer, intractable pain, glaucoma, Crohn's disease, hepatitis C, chronic renal failure, post-traumatic stress disorder, traumatic brain injury, and diseases, including anorexia, that result in nausea, vomiting, wasting, appetite loss, cramping, seizures, muscle spasms, or spasticity, when these symptoms are unrelieved by standard treatments or medications.

» **Quantity:** Most states limit or require the person's healthcare provider to specify a limit on the amount of marijuana the person is allowed to purchase or grow over a specified period of time. Limits may apply to the number of plants a person can grow or buy, the amount of marijuana infused product in solid or liquid form, and the amount of useable product derived from plants. Individuals who are recommended to have more plants are referred to by the industry as Extended Plant Count (EPC) patients.

» **Registry card requirements:** Medical marijuana users must submit a medical cannabis patient application and have it approved to obtain a medical marijuana registry card. Requirements vary among states but typically require that the person be a certain age and a resident of the state, have a qualifying medical condition, and have a signed physician certification. States may prohibit medical marijuana use for people in certain occupations, such as bus drivers, truck drivers, and law enforcement officers.

» **Ages:** States may stipulate certain age limits for those who use medical marijuana or for caregivers who dispense it. For example, in Colorado, medical marijuana users must be 18 years or older. Some patients under the age of 18 can receive permission for certain ailments under supervision of a parent or guardian.

- » **Caregivers:** Like users, caregivers are typically required to submit an application and have it approved prior to assisting someone in the medical marijuana program. States may allow caregivers to purchase and deliver medical marijuana to patients and perhaps even help patients grow their own.

- » **Commercial grows, production, transportation, and sales:** State laws governing the growth, production, transportation, and sales of medical marijuana are numerous and complex. If you're interested in entering the medical marijuana industry, we strongly recommend that you consult an attorney who specializes in this area.

- » **Home delivery:** States may or may not allow home delivery of medical marijuana. In states that do allow home delivery, limits may be placed on the amount delivered, the number of deliveries that can be made at one time, and so on.

- » **Taxes:** Medical marijuana typically has a lower sales tax rate than that for adult recreational marijuana. Even so, tax rates for medical marijuana vary from state to state. In several states medical marijuana is tax-exempt. However, cannabis businesses are still subject to the same federal income taxes regardless of whether they're medical, adult recreational, or both.

- » **Enforcement:** States also vary regarding penalties for breaking the law.

REMEMBER

A medical card may not be usable outside the state for which it's been issued. Because you're prohibited from traveling across state lines with cannabis, check in advance when travelling to ensure that you can purchase your medicine in the destination state.

Adult recreational use

Several U.S. states permit adult recreational use of marijuana, but that doesn't give you the right to consume as much marijuana you want anywhere you feel like it. State laws contain numerous rules and regulations to control adult recreational marijuana activities, such as the following:

- » **Age:** As with alcohol, states can specify minimum age requirements for buying, possessing, and using marijuana. For example, in Colorado, you must be 21 years or older to buy, have, or use retail marijuana, and sharing it with anyone under the age of 21 is illegal.

- » **Limits to buying:** State law may stipulate how old you must be to buy marijuana, where you can buy it from, and how much you can buy and carry with you at any one time.

- » **Limits to selling:** All states require that sellers be licensed; private sales are prohibited. State law may allow an adult user to give a limited amount of marijuana to another adult user, but not sell it, regardless of whether the product was purchased or homegrown.

>> **Carry limits:** State law may limit the amount of marijuana that you can have with you. For example, Colorado allows adults to carry up to 1 ounce of marijuana; possessing any more can result in legal charges and fines.

>> **Public use:** States typically prohibit or significantly restrict use of marijuana in any form in public places, such as sidewalks, parks, restaurants, and common areas of apartment buildings or condos. In addition, property owners may be permitted to ban the use and possession of marijuana on their premises, so if you rent an apartment or a motel room, you may be prohibited from consuming marijuana in it unless it is designated cannabis-friendly.

>> **Business regulations:** Every state in which marijuana is legal has numerous rules and regulations that apply to marijuana growers, producers, sellers, and distributors. These rules and regulations govern everything from verifying the identities of buyers to packing, labeling, and tracking products.

>> **Pregnancy considerations:** If you're pregnant, you shouldn't be consuming marijuana. Some hospitals test babies after birth for drugs. If a baby tests positive for THC at birth, the hospital may be required to report the test results to child protective services.

>> **Taxes:** States tend to tax adult recreational use marijuana at a relatively high rate. For example, Colorado collects a 15 percent marijuana excise tax plus a 10 percent sales tax on adult recreational marijuana.

>> **Enforcement:** States vary regarding penalties for breaking the law. For example, a state may have certain penalties if you're caught using marijuana in public and much stiffer penalties if you are caught using near a school.

See the later section "Knowing Your Limits" for additional details about restrictions.

Considering local laws too

In states where cannabis is legal, local municipalities can separately regulate its growth, production, and sale within their borders. They are also allowed to add taxes and fees to commercial efforts above and beyond those of the state. In some cases, municipalities can completely ban commercial endeavors. For example, Colorado Springs permits medical sales but has continued to ban adult recreational dispensaries. Penalties can vary significantly from one municipality to another.

WARNING

Don't rely solely on information about state rules and regulations. Research the municipality in which you plan to engage in any marijuana related activity before doing so. You may be able to find out what you need to know from the municipality's website or local law enforcement.

Knowing your employer's rules

Even if cannabis is legal in the state and municipality in which you live and work, your employer may prohibit it. Here's what you can expect in most states:

>> Some states where medical marijuana is legal have protections for medical marijuana users who are employees. In these states, employers are generally prohibited from discriminating against workers who have a medical marijuana card or qualified workers who have marijuana in their systems. However, employers can prohibit workers from using on the job or from being under the influence at work.

>> Other states where medical marijuana is legal do not provide protections for medical marijuana users, or they specifically allow employers to fire qualified employees for off-duty consumption.

>> In states where medical marijuana is legal, employers may be permitted to discriminate against medical marijuana users when seeking to comply with federal requirements, such as conditions for obtaining federal funding.

>> In states where recreational marijuana is legal, employers generally can enforce zero-tolerance workplace drug policies that also apply to marijuana. They can refuse to hire and can fire adult recreational users who test positive for marijuana in their systems, even if the use is outside work hours and the person isn't under the influence at work.

>> States vary in the degree to which they allow routine or random drug testing in the workplace. In most states, employers are allowed to routinely test workers. In other states, drug testing is permitted only when the employer has a good reason to do so, such as the employee appears intoxicated or is involved in a work-related accident that results in injury or property damage.

REMEMBER

Whether you're a medical marijuana or adult-recreational consumer, do your homework before consuming marijuana at work or even off-duty. Research state and local laws to find out what your employer is and is not allowed to do, and read your employee handbook to find out what your employer's drug policies are.

Researching international laws

REMEMBER

If you plan to travel outside of the U.S. and use cannabis at your destination, leave your stash at home and carefully research the laws that govern marijuana purchase, possession, and consumption at your planned destination.

BUSTING THE AMSTERDAM MYTH

Amsterdam is internationally renowned for its famed coffee shops, where tourists flock to smoke cannabis, and law enforcement tolerates it, but don't confuse tolerance with legality. Cannabis is illegal in the Netherlands; the government has simply decided to allocate more of its resources toward controlling hard drugs than soft drugs (such as marijuana).

Amsterdam has strict rules and social protocols regarding amounts of cannabis that can be purchased and in one's possession and restrictions on where it can be consumed — in coffeeshops. A *coffeeshop* is a public establishment that sells cannabis. If you want coffee, you go to a cafe or coffee house. If you want cannabis, you go to a coffeeshop.

However, even in Amsterdam, cannabis laws may be evolving, so before consuming cannabis there, be sure to check the current laws.

As of the writing of this book, marijuana is federally legal in only two countries: Uruguay and Canada, and in Canada, each province has its own rules and regulations. At the onset of legalization in Canada, the only products legal for sale nationally were flower, pre-rolled joints, and non-combustible oil extract. Rules, opportunities, and product selections will continue to evolve over time. For example, edibles are planned for the Canadian market in 2019.

With the legalization of adult recreational use in Canada, many of the world's nations will be watching to see how the process unfolds and its impact. You may see additional countries relaxing their laws or promoting full legalization in the near future.

Europe's legal system creates a more challenging environment for legalizing cannabis. Unlike the voter-initiated process in the U.S., cannabis legislation in Europe must be driven by the courts or legislators. As is the case in the U.S., medical marijuana is likely to come first followed by growing legislation across Europe. Italy may be first with measures currently moving through parliament in search of more support.

Some other countries and regions to watch include the following:

>> **Mexico:** Legislators have signaled the possibility of broad legalization.

>> **South and Central America:**

- Belize allows consumption on private property without designating medical or recreational use.

- Argentina, Chile, Columbia, and Panama have medical marijuana bills that have either passed or are in process.

- Costa Rica, Brazil, Peru, Ecuador, and Venezuela have some degree of *decriminalization* — cannabis is illegal, but the government doesn't prosecute minor offenses.

» **New Zealand:** Medical marijuana use is permitted, and a national referendum for adult recreational use is scheduled for 2020.

» **South Africa:** Adults can use and grow cannabis privately for personal adult use.

Knowing Your Limits

States and locales in which marijuana is legal have numerous rules and regulations in place to ensure product and public safety. Staying out of legal trouble with cannabis is often a matter of knowing and adhering to the limitations stipulated in the legislation.

In this section, we provide a different perspective on state and local laws by presenting them in terms of various limitations.

REMEMBER

Rules and regulations vary by jurisdiction and may change at any time, so do your homework to dig up the current details before engaging in any marijuana activities. If you have any doubts, consult a qualified attorney in the jurisdiction in which you plan on engaging in any marijuana related activities.

Age limits

As with alcohol, states have set age limits for marijuana use and for working in the industry. Although age limits may vary by jurisdiction, they generally contain the following brackets:

» **Adult recreational use:** In U.S. states in which marijuana is legal, you must be 21 years or older to purchase and use marijuana recreationally. In Canada, the legal age is 19 in most of the country and 18 in Quebec and Alberta.

WARNING

Giving or selling marijuana to a minor in the U.S. is a federal offense. In some jurisdictions, you're allowed to give a limited amount of marijuana to another adult. However, any mention of sharing or giving a product while you're purchasing it may require that the sales person void the sale. Exchanging funds for purchase inside a dispensary can also void the sale.

>> **Medical use:** In the U.S., a person must be 18 or older to acquire a state medical marijuana registry card. Some patients under the age of 18 can receive permission for medical use for certain ailments with parent or guardian supervision, but the parent or guardian must obtain a special registry card issued to caregivers.

>> **Working in the industry:** In most states, you must be at least 21 years old to work in the industry and pass a background check with fingerprinting as well as proof of state residency. Some states allow those 18 years and older to work in the industry.

Purchase limits

A purchase limit, sometimes referred to as a *carry weight* is the legal amount an individual can purchase in a day. While states and countries may have different rules, limits are generally as follows:

>> **Adult recreational:**

- 1 ounce of flower

- 8 grams of concentrate

- 800 mg of edibles

>> **Medical:**

- 2 ounces of flower

- Extended plant count (EPC) for additional amounts as recommended by a doctor

Grow limits

States in which marijuana is legal may allow persons over a certain age (typically 21 years) to grow their own cannabis plants. However, they often place limits on the number of plants that can be grown, processed, possessed, and transported. For example, as of the writing of this book, in Alaska, the grow limits are no more than six plants total of which no more than three can be mature. In Arizona, a patient or qualifying caregiver is allowed to cultivate no more than 12 plants and they must do so more than 25 miles from the nearest medical marijuana dispensary. In Connecticut, home cultivation is prohibited.

Dosing limits

States don't set dosing limits directly. By setting purchase and grow limits, they indirectly regulate the amount of marijuana any individual consumes. However, states and countries are able to set limits on edibles and sublingual products related to the total THC milligram content in packaged products. They may also require that individual doses in packaged products be separated. With products that are smoked, whether flower or concentrates, determining the THC content and separating doses is more difficult and less practical.

Driving limits

WARNING

High driving is dangerous driving, and driving high is considered driving under the influence, which is illegal. To steer clear of trouble, follow these rules:

>> Don't consume any form of marijuana in your car.

>> Don't drive high, regardless of whether you use cannabis for medical or recreational use. If you've been using or plan to use, order a ride or use a designated driver, as you would do with alcohol consumption.

>> Store any marijuana you may be transporting in a sealed container in the trunk or other storage area of your vehicle, not in any passenger area. Open container laws typically apply to cannabis as well.

>> Think twice about refusing to take a blood test for THC if you're stopped. You can have your driving privileges revoked regardless of whether you're convicted of a crime.

>> Keep in mind that penalties are generally far worse if you're driving under the influence with a child in your vehicle. You can be charged with child abuse!

Consumption locations

Public consumption is illegal, and many municipalities are diligent about enforcing those rules. When consuming cannabis, adhere to the following guidelines:

>> Consume only on private property, which may include the following:

- Private residences (your home or the home of a friend or relative)
- Rental properties that are expressly consumption friendly
- Hotels that are expressly consumption friendly

>> Do not consume on public property, such as the following:

- Parks (especially federal parks)
- Concert venues
- Car
- Hotel (unless listed as a consumption friendly location)
- Sidewalk
- Cannabis dispensaries (unless a specific area is set aside for doing so, which is allowed by law)

Your own personal consumption limits

Marijuana affects everyone differently and multiple variables impact the experience ranging from strain to consumption method to tolerance to environment. Knowing your own consumption limits is a practical way to stay out of legal trouble. As long as you remain in control of your own faculties, you're more likely to engage in behaviors that don't draw the attention of law enforcement, and if you do have an encounter with the police, you'll be better equipped to deal with the situation rationally.

See Chapter 8 for details about how to consume cannabis safely and identify your own personal consumption limits.

PROTESTING RESTRICTIONS ON CONSUMPTION LOCATIONS

The unofficial cannabis holiday known as 420 that takes place on April 20 of each year, has developed into a grass roots protest against the restrictions on public consumption. In legalized states, marijuana users often gather at various festivals to celebrate the legalization of marijuana and to protest restrictions on where cannabis can be consumed.

Although law enforcement agencies have a presence at these events, they generally don't arrest people for consuming in public. However, if participants disturb the peace or break other laws, they can be subject to charges for additional crimes, including those related to marijuana.

REMEMBER

Cannabis effects on an individual vary according to numerous factors, including the following:

>> Age

>> Gender

>> Elevation

>> Tolerance

>> Consumption method

>> Potency of product

>> Dose

>> Environment (specifically an individual's comfort level with their surroundings)

>> Product strain or terpene profile

>> Soluble fat content of recently ingested food (specifically, eating fatty foods before ingesting an edible marijuana product slows the absorption of THC into the body)

WARNING

Don't mix marijuana with other substances, such as alcohol.

REMEMBER

Start low and go slow. You can always consume more product if you're not experiencing the desired effect, but you can't remove product if you've consumed too much. Starting low and going slow is especially important when consuming edibles, which may require 30 minutes to two hours to take effect and up to four hours to produce the maximum effect. If you're impatient, you're likely to consume more product than necessary to achieve the desired effect and end up feeling very uncomfortable instead. Here are some general guidelines for starting low and going slow with edibles:

>> Start with 1–5 mg if you're a new consumer. (10 mg is a standard single dose of edibles, but micro-dose options are becoming more popular and offer individual dosing in 5 mg and less.)

>> Start with 5–10 mg if you're an occasional consumer.

>> Start with 10–15 grams if you're a frequent consumer.

>> Wait at least two hours before consuming an additional dose.

>> Have an experienced friend on hand to guide you through your initial consumption experiences or at least ask your budtender for guidance.

TIP

When you're first getting a feel for your tolerance, considering starting with a cannabis-infused beverage. Beverages tend to take effect much more quickly than edibles — within 45 minutes instead of up to two hours. That way, you can get a general idea of which dose is best for the desired effect without having to wait two hours between doses.

Avoiding Encounters with Law Enforcement

As Americans for Safe Access (ASA) advises, "The best law enforcement encounter is the encounter that never happens." Whether your state has legalized cannabis for medical or adult recreational use, growing, producing, transporting, purchasing, possessing, or using marijuana makes you a target of greater scrutiny by law enforcement. The best way to reduce your risk of being hassled, investigated, arrested, or charged with a crime is to fly below the radar as much as possible. Following are a few suggestions for avoiding uncomfortable encounters with law enforcement: •

>> If you consume marijuana for medicinal purposes, carry your medical marijuana registry card at all times.

>> Consume marijuana only on private property, preferably your home or the home of a friend or relative. If you're consuming via smoking, smoke inside with the windows closed. You want to avoid a situation in which a disapproving neighbor calls the police.

>> Keep a low profile. Arguments, loud music, barking dogs, physical altercations, and loud parties can also result in neighbors calling the police.

>> Don't consume marijuana in your car, regardless of whether it's parked or on the road. If you're stopped, and the officer gets a whiff of marijuana, you may be suspected of driving under the influence, and you increase your chances of having your car searched.

>> Carry only the amount of cannabis you need and that's within the carry limit in your jurisdiction. Keep the receipt with the product to prove compliance with the legal purchase and carry limit.

>> Store your cannabis products in glass jars or airtight plastic containers to reduce any odors that may be discernable. (Most dispensary containers are airtight to preserve the quality, so consider keeping that packaging.)

>> When transporting cannabis, keep it in your vehicle's trunk or other storage location in the back, not in the passenger areas. Also, make sure your vehicle is in good repair — for example, the headlights and taillights work — and drive safely. Traffic violations make you more susceptible to getting stopped.

>> Don't fly with cannabis, regardless of whether you have a medical marijuana registry card and regardless of whether you're flying in state. If you get caught, you may be subject to both state and federal criminal charges.

>> If you grow your own marijuana, growing indoors is best to avoid the scrutiny of neighbors and law enforcement. If you grow outdoors, make sure the area is secure and as private as possible. Compost or discard waste at a remote location, and keep the grow site location private.

>> Be discreet. Don't flaunt your marijuana activities. Limit your discussions to only trustworthy individuals on a need-to-know basis.

Responding Appropriately in Encounters with Law Enforcement

Even when you're very careful, encounters with law enforcement may be unavoidable. To make the best of a bad situation and avoid making the situation worse, follow these suggestions:

>> Remain calm.

>> Move slowly. Sudden movements may cause fear, which can trigger an overreaction on the part of the officer.

>> Be respectful and polite. Treating the officer with respect always leads to a better outcome.

>> Keep your hands where the officer can see them. For example, if you're stopped in your car, keep your hands near the top of the steering wheel. Don't reach in your pocket for a wallet or anything else unless instructed to do so.

>> Do what the officer tells you to do and only what the officer tells you to do that is within your legal rights. For example, don't reach inside the glove compartment of your car to retrieve your license and registration until told to do so.

>> Remain silent for the most part. Remember that anything you say can and will be used against you.

» If the officer starts asking questions or trying to engage you in conversation, ask whether you are being detained or arrested. If the officer says "no," then wait for him to finish what he's doing (such as writing a citation) and leave immediately. If the answer is "yes," then ask why you are being detained or arrested, and remember the officer's answer.

As soon as the officer informs you that you're free to go, go. Don't say a word. If an officer informs you that you're free to go, anything you say afterwards is considered voluntary.

» If the officer refuses to let you go or continues to try to engage you in conversation, say "I choose to remain silent. I want a lawyer."

» Don't consent to any searches. An officer can go through a bag you're carrying or pat you down to check for weapons but is not allowed to go through your pockets or search your home or vehicle without reasonable suspicion or a search warrant. If the officer asks to conduct a search or starts a search, simply say, "I do not consent to any searches." Don't try to stop the officer from conducting a search, because that can get you into more trouble.

Taking Responsibility as a Parent

Federal and state authorities are serious about preventing underage access to legal marijuana, and most responsible cannabis companies support this restriction. Numerous safety features are built into products to prevent children from being attracted to or being able to consume product, such as the following:

» Restrictions on animal shapes for edibles

» Childproof (and sometimes adult-proof) containers

» Strict ID checks in dispensaries

» Universal THC labels

Dispensaries and product manufacturers are also very limited in advertising. Most rules require proof that the print, radio, TV, or social vehicle has a 70 percent adult audience. In Canada, rules also include restrictions on any cartoon imagery that may be deemed enticing to children.

If you're a parent, the primary responsibility for keeping your kids out of your stash lies with you. Numerous products are available to help parents prevent unauthorized access to marijuana products, including pouches that lock for storing pharmaceutical medications, portable fireproof safes that lock with a key or combination, and even file storage boxes equipped with locks. The device doesn't have to be designed specifically for securing marijuana products, and it doesn't need to be expensive to be effective.

Plenty of programs and websites, some supported by the cannabis industry, provide age-appropriate and common sense curricula to parents and educators to help guide discussions about cannabis and maintain barriers to youth consumption. The Marijuana Education Initiative (MEI) provides exceptional guidance to parents and educators on how to help adolescents make informed decisions about marijuana. To explore MEI's educational resources, visit marijuana-education.com

REMEMBER

Although marijuana may be beneficial for helping with certain medical conditions in adults, it's generally harmful for children under the age of 18. Most brain development occurs during childhood and continues into the mid-20s. Any substances that have an effect on the brain, including marijuana, alcohol, cocaine, and opioids are harmful to children.

Chapter **4**

Tackling Cannabis Politics and Culture

annabis has a long history of use in many areas including medicine, textiles, religion, and even magic (in the ancient world). Perspectives about the plant, its uses, and its users have changed frequently around the world, especially over the last 100 years. In the United States, cannabis has often become a dividing line for culture — emblematic of certain counterculture groups from jazz musicians in the 1920s and '30s to the hippies in the '60s, with equal backlash from the establishment, which has traditionally seen its use as ranging from distracting to dangerous.

In the society of the early 2000s, cannabis is beginning to work its way into the mainstream. With the advent of legalization for first medical cannabis in 2009 followed by adult recreational legalization in 2012 in Colorado, a new fascination has developed around the plant and its use that is spanning all demographics.

This chapter brings you up to speed on current cannabis politics and culture, so you have a clearer sense of the prevailing perspectives and attitudes and where they seem to be heading.

Checking the Nation's Pulse

Legalization of cannabis for both medical and adult recreational use in the U.S. began as a movement with early activists coming from the more traditionally recognized user demographics of artists, musicians, and the stoner culture. However, growing acceptance along with expanding numbers of states legalizing use has begun to show that cannabis acceptance is a very big tent, encompassing people from every demographic of age, race, income, gender, location, and political party.

This section explores the factors that are driving people to change their attitudes about cannabis, examines the prevailing attitudes and perspectives, and encourages you to stay abreast of the ever-evolving social and political climate.

Acknowledging the drivers of change

Acceptance and use among the middle-America, middle-income, middle-aged white constituency has come mostly come from three drivers:

>> **Monetary impact to the community:** With amendment 64 in Colorado, voters approved adult recreational cannabis with an extremely high tax burden that directs funds to the state's rural education efforts through a grant program for school construction projects. Colorado was the first state to implement voter approved adult recreational cannabis sales, and the resulting state income from sales tax, excise taxes, and fees has provoked revenue-envy among other states across the country, forcing both politicians and voters to sit up and take notice. In any state where adult recreational cannabis use is legal, the taxes and fees are fairly steep.

>> **Reduction in stigma due to medical cannabis:** After a few states legalized medical cannabis use, more people started to accept its medicinal value. Increasingly, people are hearing from friends, relatives, and acquaintances who have had success using marijuana in many forms to help mitigate symptoms related to severe and chronic illness as well as more mundane aches and pains. Specifically, the use of marijuana to alleviate nausea and stimulate appetite in cancer patients, along with the support of physicians, has helped drive the narrative that marijuana can be used as medicine.

REMEMBER

In addition, statistics showing the drop in fatal opioid overdose in states where marijuana is legal have helped fuel the awareness of benefits to society. For example, in Denver alone, opioid deaths have dropped by six percent since marijuana was legalized.

>> **The rising tide of positive media coverage:** Traditional media outlets have begun to join the bloggers in their efforts to expose more people to the well-researched and substantiated facts about marijuana. As marijuana messaging becomes more positive in the press, it is beginning to alleviate fears and break down resistance to legalization.

Recognizing differences in attitudes about medical and recreational use

The difference in public perception regarding medical versus adult recreational cannabis use is reflected in how it's taxed — medical marijuana is taxed at a significantly lower rate. Medical use is gaining acceptance quickly as witnessed by the growing number of states that are legalizing it. Recreational use is still mired in the stigma but working to break through.

Growing numbers of scientific research studies demonstrating the value of cannabis for treating symptoms associated with many diseases, illnesses, and ailments are helping people recognize marijuana's medicinal value. Add to this the thousands of media articles, publications, blog posts, and positive word of mouth about medical usage, and the world begins to turn toward the positive perspective on at least one side of the industry.

Keeping pace with evolving attitudes

As perspectives related to medical cannabis change, sometimes at lightning speed, limited numbers of early adopters are turning into an avalanche of support. This has been translating to additional support for adult recreational use as people share their success stories through the press, social media, and word of mouth.

The dire warnings of societal destruction have failed to materialize, and even some ardent opponents have acknowledged the value of the industry and the benefits to individuals. Some dramatic pivots have occurred, even with constituencies that had virulently opposed cannabis, as they've hopped on the bandwagon. For example, former Speaker of the House, John Boehner went from staunch opposition to join the board of directors of a cannabis company!

As attitudes evolve, turn to social media and the Internet to follow the discussion and the evolving attitudes. With half the customer base under 35 years old, online and mobile interactions are leading the charge, and bloggers along with cannabis websites are a primary source of information.

Debunking Misconceptions of Cannabis and Users

Many of the anti-cannabis voices have harped on the myths of unintended consequences and unfounded allegations to drive fear of legalization. The largest misconception is rooted in the negative stereotype of the "stoner" culture. The reality is a much broader and inclusive demographic.

Many of today's cannabis dispensaries break the stereotypical image of the old "head shop." The background music isn't exclusively reggae or heavy metal, and you're much less likely these days to see the walls adorned with Jamaican flags and pictures of Bob Marley. The only black lights you're likely to see are those used by receptionists along with sophisticated ID scanners as they check for ID authenticity, age, or medical card compliance before allowing customers to enter secured "budrooms" for purchase. (A *budroom* is an area inside a dispensary where products are displayed and sold; it's often set up like a jewelry store, with products stored under glass.) Online sales also have high hurdles to protect against underage use.

Cannabis is becoming big business, and companies are building sophisticated marketing and branding designed to be welcoming and to appeal to all legal aged demographics. Market share based on price and exclusivity are creating brands that cater to upscale clientele with store space that can look like a high-end jewelry store or a tasteful yet hip hangout. Stores are as varied as the users who shop in them.

Clientele are breaking old molds too. In 2018, BDS Analytics' profiles of cannabis dispensary shoppers show that 40 percent of dispensary shoppers were age 21 to 34, and nearly one-fifth were age 55 or older. Four in ten had college degrees or higher education, and 63 percent were employed with an average annual income of $66.9K. Only 37 percent lived in the city, with the majority living in more suburban and rural areas. Seven in ten preferred inhalables as their method of cannabis consumption, and 34 percent purchased cannabis products at least once a week.

Many misconceptions about cannabis and its users fall into the category of myths of "unintended consequences" — the idea that legalization will result in vast increases in homelessness, crime, black market activity, overdose, impaired driving, addiction, and teen use. Science and research have debunked these myths:

>> Homelessness and crime have not increased due specifically to legalization of cannabis. After controlling for increased populations and traditional movement of people, the increases in homelessness are in line with those locations that have not legalized, and the levels are what are expected in those locations regardless of cannabis.

>> Statistics show that black market activity has actually decreased in areas with legal adult recreational use.

>> Due to a lack of receptors in specific areas of the brain for cannabis, people have no biological means to overdose on THC alone or to become biologically addicted (though emotional addiction or habitual use is as likely as with other substances and habits such as chocolate or exercise). No reported and confirmed deaths have been linked specifically to cannabis overconsumption alone.

>> Teen use has not increased in states with legalization. U.S. numbers show that teen marijuana use is currently holding at its lowest level in 20 years.

>> Impaired driving from marijuana alone is a fraction of the rate of impaired driving reported by law enforcement. In Colorado, statistics show that number to be close to six percent of all reports.

Examining Activism

The original effort to legalize marijuana began at the grassroots level by individuals with a great deal of passion and long odds to overcome years of fear and prejudice against cannabis. The focus was on marijuana as medicine and the value it offers to patients suffering symptoms of illness and diseases such as cancer and seizures.

Generations of Americans growing up since the Nixon era's War on Drugs and the "Just Say No" campaign of First Lady, Nancy Reagan, in the '80s had developed the perspective that equated marijuana with other Schedule I substances.

Yet these early activists were able to overcome steep hurdles, going directly to state constituencies with amendments on statewide ballots that succeeded to demonstrate the will of the people and the power of well-researched facts. As early adopter states demonstrated success with regulation, state revenue generation, economic drivers, and resident acceptance, more formalized groups began to organize.

In response, opposition groups became more active, as well, often heavily funded by industries that have seen marijuana as a threat to market share for their own products and bolstered by equally passionate individuals.

WHAT'S A SCHEDULE I SUBSTANCE?

The legal foundation of the U.S. government's war against drug abuse is The Controlled Substances Act, which is part of the Comprehensive Drug Abuse and Control Act of 1970. The U.S. Drug Enforcement Agency (DEA) has divided controlled substances into five categories called "schedules" based on each drug's safety, potential for addiction and abuse, and whether it has any legitimate medical use:

- Schedule I substances are deemed to have no accepted medical use and a high potential for abuse. They include heroin, LSD, marijuana (cannabis), ecstasy, methaqualone (commonly referred to by the brand name Quaalude, pronounced "Kway-lood"), and peyote.

- Schedule II substances are also considered dangerous and are deemed to have a high potential for psychological or physical dependence. They include cocaine, methamphetamine, methadone, hydromorphone, meperidine, oxycodone, fentanyl, Dexedrine, Adderall, and Ritalin.

- Schedule III substances carry a low to moderate potential for physical or psychological dependence. They include ketamine, anabolic steroids, testosterone, and products containing less than 15 milligrams of hydrocodone per dose or less than 90 milligrams of codeine per dose.

- Schedule IV substances are deemed to have a low potential for abuse and a low risk of dependence. They include Xanax, Soma, Darvon, Darvocet, Valium, Ativan, Talwin, and Ambien.

- Schedule V substances consist of products that contain limited concentrations of narcotics — typically cough suppressants, antidiarrheal medications, and analgesics.

However, as the tide has turned, the grassroots constituencies promoting cannabis have added professional trade organizations such as Colorado Leads and Cannabis Trade Federation. These organizations are working to secure the industry as a whole and further the march toward legitimacy through professionalism and promotion of industry standard practices as seen in many other established industries.

Tuning In to Cannabis Culture

Until relatively recently, the perception of the cannabis culture has been aligned fairly closely with the stoner culture as portrayed in popular movies such as Cheech and Chong's *Up in Smoke* and *Fast Times At Ridgemont High*, in which Sean Penn plays Jeff Spicoli, a failing high school student who routinely gets high before class, emerging from a VW van surrounded by clouds of smoke.

While these and other Hollywood comedies always portray a stereotype of the cannabis culture, the parody is mixed with the realities of Jamaican reggae culture and generations of real users consuming the illegal substance. An era of tacit acceptance began with the increased use among military personnel during deployment in Vietnam and returning to the U.S. with a newfound appreciation of the calming effects of cannabis and, in some cases, the counterculture that had formed around it.

Cannabis is an international substance that has been grown, sold, transported, and consumed around the world developing its own subcultures along the way and helping to shape the identity and perceptions of those locations. Amsterdam is a prime example. As the character Vincent, played by John Travolta in the cult classic *Pulp Fiction*, puts it:

> It breaks down like this: it's legal to buy it, it's legal to own it, and if you're the proprietor of a hash bar, it's legal to sell it. It's legal to carry it, but that doesn't really matter 'cause get a load of this, all right? If you get stopped by the cops in Amsterdam, it's illegal for them to search you. I mean, that's a right the cops in Amsterdam don't have.

Along the way to legalization, many high profile cultural icons, including Willie Nelson, Bill Maher, and Snoop Dogg, began acknowledging their own consumption publicly, making it more acceptable to talk about. The consumption question was even raised during the 1996 U.S. presidential race when then candidate Bill Clinton remarked that while a student in England in the 1960s, he had experimented with marijuana but had "not inhaled."

Today's cannabis culture is as individualized as the people who consume it in one way or another for their own personal reasons, whether as medicine for symptom relief, performance enhancement for athletes, adult recreational use for social activities, exploration of artistic appreciation, or relaxation. The culture is no longer defined by the Tetrahydrocannabinol (THC) for the "high" but includes other cannabinoids, such as CBD, and other benefits from the plant.

The culture has evolved to unapologetic and unabashed use by soccer moms and a growing number of professional athletes. Recent news stories showcase the increasing acceptance of cannabis use among high profile athletes with articles following NFL player Josh Gordon and his conflicts over consumption with the Cleveland Browns; New England Patriots coach Bill Belichick's perspectives on consumption by his players; ultrarunner Jenn Shelton, who was featured in the *New York Times* bestseller *Born to Run*; ultrarunners Avery Collins and Jeff Sperber, who have sung the praises of adding cannabis to their workouts or recovery regimen; as well as admissions from multiple retired athletes, including NBA player Matt Barnes, who has remarked that he consumed prior to each game.

But not everyone in the traditional cannabis culture is happy about the transition to mainstream that has come with legalization and the professionalization of the industry. A segment of the consumer population continues to lament the decline of the counterculture. However, even as cannabis becomes more mainstream, the industry is likely to continue to cater to the counterculture, as well, as evidenced by the industry's support of massive events such as the unofficial cannabis celebration holiday 4/20 on April 20th each year, which is focused on the mass civil disobedience of public consumption.

Regardless, one thing is clear, the cannabis industry, use, and culture are growing across the entire world with no signs of stopping, and this growth is driving a huge shift in cultural diversity among cannabis users.

2
Buying, Storing, and Using Cannabis

Choose a reputable cannabis dispensary and successfully navigate your way through your first shopping experience.

Discover the pros and cons of different cannabis consumption methods, including smoking, vaping, edibles, topical applications, tinctures, and pharmaceuticals.

Recognize the potential health and safety risks of cannabis consumption and discover ways to mitigate the risks.

Hone your skills and discern between high-quality and substandard cannabis products, so you'll be sure to get your money's worth.

Recognize common cannabis scams, so you won't get ripped off or end up in legal trouble.

Find out how to store your cannabis to keep it fresh and secure it to keep it safe.

Chapter **5**

Buying and Storing Cannabis

Before the cannabis legalization movement began to gain momentum and people could buy it legally in certain countries and certain states in the U.S., buying cannabis could be scary. Best-case scenario, you could buy from a friend who had a connection with someone who grew and sold high-quality product. Otherwise, you faced the prospect of buying a bag from a complete stranger or from a friend of a friend. The only assurance you had regarding the quality of the product was the person's word and how the product looked and smelled. You may have had no idea whether it had been "laced" with anything else or whether it was contaminated with pesticides, solvents, or other potential toxins.

Fortunately, buying cannabis in areas where it's legal is no longer a scary proposition. Cannabis legalization has transformed a former black market into a legitimate corporate industry with CEOs and retail locations, regulatory bodies, and Google reviews. The only frightening aspect of buying cannabis is the plethora of products and the new terminology.

In this chapter, we take you through the ins and outs of buying cannabis, where to get it, how to store it, and what to watch out for.

Evaluating Your Vendor Options: Where to Buy

As a consumer of any retail product, you always have to choose a retailer to buy from. You may have the option to buy a product from a local or online retailer, a seller on eBay or Craigslist, or someone at the local flea market. When choosing a retailer, you need to consider several factors, including the quality and selection of the products offered, prices and shipping costs, return policies, legality (whether the individual is selling stolen merchandise or knock-offs, for example), level of customer service; and so on.

The same is true when you're in the market for any cannabis products. One of the first choices you need to make is the person or business to buy from. You have several options, including legal dispensaries (for medical or adult recreational use), delivery services, and individuals or businesses that advertise and sell exclusively online but within state or province boundaries. You even have the option to buy it on the black market, although that would be illegal and is certainly a practice we don't condone.

REMEMBER

As in the U.S., when purchasing cannabis products in Canada you have the same options. And, even though it is federally legal, you may still have to wait until your province has its systems up and running with sales locations because, for now, a vendor you like in one province can't ship your preferred products across province lines if they don't have a license and distribution facility in your province.

In this section, we lead you through the process of exploring your options, so you can make well-informed choices. By choosing a reputable and reliable vendor, you take the first and most critical step toward ensuring that you're buying safe, quality cannabis products.

WARNING

Cannabis is currently a federally illegal Schedule I drug in the U.S. and is prohibited from being purchased legally, whether in a licensed dispensary or over the internet, and shipped illegally across state lines. Shipping cannabis across state lines constitutes drug trafficking. (See Chapter 3 for additional guidance on how to steer clear of legal trouble.)

Buying from a dispensary

We strongly recommend that you shop for and buy your cannabis from a reputable and licensed dispensary in an area in which cannabis is legal. While you may pay more at a dispensary, the benefits of shopping and buying at a dispensary are worth it:

>> **Cost:** You may actually pay less for products at a legal dispensary. Some black market dealers buy in a border town that's legal and charge more for it in a nearby state where it's not legal. By buying on the black market, you may be paying a premium and increasing your risk of being arrested and charged with a felony.

>> **Legality:** The peace of mind you feel dealing with a legal establishment is often enough to justify the possibility of having to pay a little more. You may think you're as safe as in the legal market when buying on the black market, but if you get caught or scammed or stuck with lousy or contaminated product, the costs can be considerably higher.

>> **Customer service:** A knowledgeable budtender at a reputable dispensary provides guidance to ensure an optimal experience for each customer, whose needs and desires may vary considerably. Licensed establishments also are more likely to respond positively to customer complaints.

>> **Product selection:** Most dispensaries, especially in well-established jurisdictions, carry a wide variety of products, edibles, lotions, tinctures, vape oils, concentrates, and strains of flower. Most dispensaries post a daily menu of the products and strains available.

>> **Quality assurance:** Many dispensaries have their own grow and production facilities to ensure product quality. If they obtain products from wholesalers, they do the work of carefully vetting those wholesalers, so you're sure to get safe, effective products.

TIP

Ask whether the dispensary has its own grow and production facilities. When evaluating products, ask whether it was grown and produced by the dispensary's operations or by a third-party grower or producer. The quality and freshness of a product is likely to be higher if a single company has control of all three operations — grow, production, and sales — although that's not necessarily the case.

See Chapter 6 for guidance on how to choose a reputable dispensary and how to navigate your first trip to a dispensary, so you feel more comfortable during your first visit.

Buying cannabis online or over the phone

In certain jurisdictions, you can order cannabis online or over the phone for pickup or delivery. In the U.S. your dispensary may have its own in-house delivery service or use a third-party service, similar to how some restaurants use delivery services such as Grubhub to deliver food. In Canada, you have the additional option of having cannabis delivered by Canadian Post.

REMEMBER

You must provide proof of age and identification if you're purchasing online or over the phone. The dispensary may require that you scan and send your ID and then present your ID for verification upon delivery.

The primary benefit of placing an order online or over the phone for pickup or delivery is convenience. Potential drawbacks include the following:

>> You can't physically inspect products before placing your order.

>> You're more likely to get pre-packaged items instead of packed-to-order.

>> You're at a greater risk of falling victim to a scam, unless you're ordering from a seller you know and trust.

WARNING

If you're considering placing an order online, take the following precautions:

>> Order only from a brick-and-mortar dispensary with which you've already established a relationship.

>> Don't order anything from a random website or Facebook page advertising products online. Doing so is an almost sure-fire way to lose your money.

>> Be very suspicious of any email messages you receive advertising cannabis products for sale. Don't click any links in such email messages.

>> Don't buy products containing THC from any out-of-state establishment or from any company outside the U.S. Shipping products that contain THC across the U.S. borders or across state lines is a federal offense. Any offer to ship across country borders or state lines is a huge red flag.

Note that CBD-only products made from hemp are federally legal, so they can be shipped across state lines.

REMEMBER

>> Get to know the dispensary, its staff, the products you like, and the store policies before placing an online order. This approach gives you a baseline to evaluate the quality of products and service delivered through the online experience.

>> Buy only from a dispensary that has reasonable return policies. When buying online, you don't have the opportunity to inspect the actual product before buying it, so you should have some recourse if the product you receive is unsatisfactory.

>> If you're having products shipped to you, have your dispensary ship the product in a way that requires your signature for delivery, to ensure that you receive the package and to provide you with the opportunity to reject the package if it's opened or damaged when it arrives.

Checking out cannabis "gifting" businesses

When a state or other jurisdiction legalizes cannabis for medical or adult recreational use, licensed dispensaries don't magically appear overnight. Consumers have to wait, sometimes several months, until dispensaries are licensed and brought into the system. In the meantime, individuals and businesses often take advantage of the gifting provisions in the law to make cannabis immediately available to consumers.

A *gifting provision* is a clause that permits an adult to give a limited amount of cannabis to another adult. Gifting provisions are on the books in most states and jurisdictions. Businesses and individuals often take advantage of this loophole to sell cannabis legally — a consumer will buy a legal item, such as a T-shirt, a sticker, a bottle of juice, a pair of socks, whatever, for an exorbitant price, with the understanding that the seller will "give" a certain amount of cannabis for free — wink, wink. In Massachusetts, a post on Craigslist advertised sandwich bags that cost up to $325 each; anyone reading the ad would know that each bag contained "free" marijuana.

We discourage anyone from buying cannabis from these gifting services for many of the same reasons we discourage people from buying cannabis on the black market:

>> This type of gifting undercuts licensed retailers, who are forced to comply with regulatory oversight and pay taxes.

>> Because gifting operations aren't subject to government oversight, consumers who buy from them are at a greater risk of getting scammed or receiving poor quality or contaminated products.

The hope among legislators and law enforcement is that as soon as legal cannabis businesses become available in a legal area, they'll push the gifting operations out of business because consumers generally prefer to buy lab-tested products from reputable sellers. However, even in areas with plenty of licensed cannabis dispensaries, these gifting operations seem to linger, and legislators and law enforcement are constantly looking for ways to shut them down.

Steering clear of the black market

One reason various states and jurisdictions legalize cannabis is to eliminate or at least curb the black market for cannabis, and for good reasons:

>> Cannabis sold on the black market isn't regulated or tested, which poses an increased risk to consumers of obtaining cannabis products that are poor quality or contain toxins and other potential harmful contaminants. Legal,

regulated dispensaries are required to test products for pests or contaminants as well as concentrations of THC, CBD, and other active ingredients.

» Black-market products aren't labeled with details about the cannabinoid concentrations and amounts, making it more difficult for consumers to estimate safe and effective doses. Legal products are required to be labeled with detailed information and must be stored in child-resistant containers.

» The quality of black market cannabis is questionable, with regard to flower in particular. Grow operations and the cultivation of quality cannabis plants are the very foundations of safe and effective products.

» Buying on the black market directly or indirectly supports the drug cartels, which increases the prevalence and seriousness of criminal activities in areas where the cartels operate.

If these reasons aren't enough to convince you to steer clear of cannabis on the black market, keep in mind that buying cannabis on the black market is illegal. Even if you're told that the product came from a legal source, purchasing from someone who brought it across state lines is still a felony. It's not worth the risk.

Making Two Key Decisions

Before you buy cannabis, you need to answer the following two questions:

» **What type of experience do you want?** Cannabis products contain a variety of cannabinoids, terpenes, and other ingredients in different combinations that produce different effects. In general, products that contain more THC make you feel high, whereas those with greater amounts of CBD mitigate much or all the high feeling of the THC and may be taken primarily for health reasons.

» **Which consumption method would you prefer?** Traditionally, consumers have smoked cannabis, and many still do. However, consumption methods have expanded considerably along with product options. You can now smoke cannabis in a variety of forms, including flower, hash, and resins; ingest it as an ingredient in edible products; inhale it through a vape pen or similar device; apply it topically to your skin as an ingredient in a cream, lotion, oil, or soap; take it sublingually (under your tongue) as an oil or tincture; and more.

TIP

Visit your local dispensary and consult with your budtender (or your doctor for medical marijuana) to explore cannabis products and consumption methods that are best for the desired experience. See Chapter 6 for details about choosing and visiting a cannabis dispensary and Chapter 7 for more detailed guidance about various consumption methods.

Getting Quality Product

Whenever you're in the market for consumer goods, you're likely to look for the best products you can afford or products that meet your needs at a reasonable price. Depending on the product and your standards, you may be willing to pay a little (or a lot) more for top shelf products.

In this section, we offer guidance for obtaining cannabis that meets or exceeds your quality standards.

WARNING

Don't assume that the product with the highest THC content is best. Potency isn't the only, or even the best, measure of quality! You can find a wide variety of products with a wide range of THC and CBD concentrations and ratios that differ significantly in terms of quality and price. The highest quality product is the one that most effectively delivers the desired experience to the greatest degree.

Buy from a reputable dispensary and be willing to pay more

The two most effective ways to ensure that you're getting quality products are these:

>> **Buy from a reputable dispensary.** Reputable dispensaries vet products for quality assurance and provide a variety of products at different prices that are likely to satisfy your needs and expectations.

>> **Be willing to pay more.** As with most consumer goods, when you're in the market for cannabis, you pretty much get what you pay for. If you have a bargain basement budget, you may be relegated to lower quality or, at the very least, inconsistent product. If you smoke low-quality flower, for example, you'll still feel the effects, but it may have a less appealing flavor, feel harsh on your throat and lungs, and leave you with a headache or other undesirable symptoms afterwards.

Check for third party testing

All products at a reputable dispensary are tested by a third party laboratory, but before you buy any cannabis product, read the label to verify that testing was performed. Third-party lab testing ensures safety and quality by identifying the following:

>> Potency (cannabinoid concentrations, amounts, and/or ratios)

>> Terpene profile, which affects the aroma

» Residual solvents (any chemical solvents, which are typically used in an extraction process to produce a concentrate, that remain in the product)

» Pesticides (to verify that a brand promoted as organic truly is)

» Mold or toxins

» Other potentially harmful contaminants

REMEMBER

Product labels typically contain very little information about third-party testing. You're likely to see a simple statement, such as "Third-party tested," which can have different meanings in different jurisdictions. If you're concerned or curious, ask the budtender for additional details about the third-party testing. You may be able to find out which lab performed the tests, what tests were performed, and the specific results of the testing.

Stick with trusted strains and brands

Within certain countries, states, or jurisdictions, certain cannabis brands earn a reputation for delivering consistently high-quality products to market. As you become a more experienced consumer, you'll begin to notice the dominant brands and identify the brands, strains, and specific products you like best.

While we don't want to limit your experience by discouraging you from trying different brands, strains, and products, you can ensure a more consistently satisfactory experience by sticking more closely to the strains and brands you trust and like. When you settle on a brand and specific strains and products that work for you, you will have a much easier time finding suitable products even when you're shopping at dispensaries other than your usual location. Other dispensaries are likely to carry the same brands.

REMEMBER

The costs and complexities of expanding into different states serve as an obstacle to many cannabis companies, so if you're shopping at a dispensary in another state, you may not find your favorite brands. Legalizing cannabis at the federal level would remove these obstacles.

Read the label

Dispensaries and regulators are very serious about packaging and labeling all cannabis products. By reading and understanding the label, you obtain nearly all the details you need to act as a well-informed consumer.

A label typically includes the following information:

>> **Strain name:** For example, Acapulco Gold, Bubba Kush, or Sour Diesel.

>> **Cultivator or Company:** The grower and/or producer.

>> **Strain:** Indica, sativa, or hybrid.

>> **Weight:** The total weight of the product, typically in grams.

>> **Warning information:** Whatever warning is required by state law.

>> **Nutritional information:** For edible products.

>> **Ingredient list:** Including all ingredients contained in the product.

>> **Cannabinoid concentrations and/or amounts:** Typically expressed in percentages of CBD, CBDa, CBG, CBN, THC, and THCa. (See Chapter 2 for more about cannabinoids.)

>> **Terpene concentrations:** Typically expressed in percentages of various terpenes, such as limonene, myrcene, linalool, and other terpenes.

>> **Lot number:** Very important in the event that a product recall is necessary.

>> **Date tested:** Indicates the date on which the product was tested by a third-party lab.

>> **Date harvested and/or date packaged:** Important for determining how fresh the product is.

>> **Use by date:** The last date on which the product should be used. Check this carefully to make sure you're not buying expired product.

Inspect the goods

When you're shopping for cannabis products, inspect products prior to making a purchase. With processed products, including edibles, vape oils, tinctures, and lotions, you can't tell much from inspecting the product beyond determining whether the packaging or the product is damaged. Finding satisfactory products is a matter of following your budtender's guidance along with your own trial and error.

When you're buying cannabis flower, however, inspecting the goods is one of the most effective ways to ensure you're getting a quality product. Cannabis is an agricultural crop, so you're looking for the harvest from healthy plants that have been properly harvested, trimmed, dried, and cured and then treated gently in their processing and transportation. Imagine shopping for apples or cantaloupe.

In the same way, you need to rely on your senses to evaluate the quality of the cannabis flower. Examine the following:

- **Bud structure:** Bud structure varies according to strain. High-quality indica buds are tightly packed and appear dense. You shouldn't be able to see the stem that runs through the center of the bud. High-quality sativa buds are less dense but have more of those red-orange follicle looking strands. When you get into hybrids, the buds can exhibit characteristics of both, so don't rely on just one deciding factor, use them all.

- **Color:** Specific colors vary among strains, but you're looking for buds with vibrant colors, mostly green. Colors will range from purple to yellow and they should look fresh but not overly moist. If the buds are overly brown and dry you may want to choose another strain or even another dispensary.

- **Trichomes:** Buds that contain high levels of THC are covered with trichomes, which appear as a layer of frost and are quite sticky. You won't be able to touch the bud to determine whether it's sticky, but you can gauge the trichome content by how frosty the bud looks.

REMEMBER

After harvesting the tall stalk of the cannabis plant, the buds are removed. In high-volume operations, this step is often performed with machinery that can be rough on the buds as they tumble and travel down rotating canisters. Trichomes are knocked off as the *nugs* (harvested buds) get tossed around. Trichomes can also be knocked off when handled carelessly in transporting buds to dispensaries or by dispensary personnel.

- **Aroma:** Your budtender should allow you to smell the product or a sample of it. The aroma should be strong and appealing. If you don't like the way the bud smells, you probably won't like the way it tastes. The aroma of the product is directly linked to the terpenes that have a significant impact on the overall experience.

TIP

- **Size:** Bud size can have an impact on price but you can be just as satisfied with a smaller *nug* (bud) from a wonderful plant. Some dispensaries sell their smaller nugs for less. In short, bigger isn't necessarily better.

- **Trim:** Very high quality buds are hand-trimmed to remove leaves and stems while keeping the bud intact and not dislodging the trichomes. You may pay more for the higher quality.

- **Seedless:** Seeds are generally undesirable in cannabis bud purchases. Grow operations go to extensive lengths to prevent plants from producing seeds, but you may come across a few over time. Steer clear of any flower that contains stems, leaves, or seeds, but if you come across a few seeds and the product was of particularly fine quality, consider the seeds a bonus item. You can save the seeds to grow your own plants, assuming it's legal to do so in your location.

>> **Absence of mold, powdery mildew, spider mites, and other insects:** Examine the bud and the container it's stored in for any signs of mold, mildew, or insects. The presence of any of these contaminants detracts from the quality of the flower and may even pose a health threat.

When you're shopping for flower, you're usually examining samples stored in jars. Most dispensaries have amounts pre-weighed in containers so you don't necessarily get your pick of the litter. However, examining the samples is still important because the product you receive is typically from the same batch as the sample. In some dispensaries, you're buying the product that's on display; you choose the flower you want, and the budtender weighs out the desired amount and packs it for you right then and there.

Avoiding Common Cannabis Scams

Cannabis is a huge and growing industry, and wherever you find plenty of money, you'll find crooks seeking to steal some of it. Most of the cannabis scams these days are directed at investors. The overwhelming desire to capitalize on the promising growth of the cannabis industry makes prospective investors easy marks for con artists. See Chapter 16 for guidance on how to invest wisely in cannabis companies.

Con artists often target consumers, as well. As long as you shop at licensed establishments, you don't need to worry about falling victim to common scams. However, you do need to be careful if you're thinking about placing an order online or over the phone for delivery. Avoid the temptation to place an order for cannabis online at just any random website or Facebook page. You probably wouldn't expect to order a car from Ford on a random Facebook page and have the company deliver it to you, so don't think you can order cannabis from just any online seller and have it delivered to your door, especially if you're in a jurisdiction in which cannabis hasn't yet been legalized.

To avoid falling victim to common cannabis scams that target consumers, take the following precautions:

>> If someone claims to be able to ship you any cannabis product that contains THC, especially over state lines, don't place an order. Shipping product over state lines is illegal and would make you party to the black market and federal drug trafficking.

>> If someone who claims to be associated with a reputable company offers to take your order and ship you product, look up the number or website of the reputable company and deal with it directly. Reputable companies are constantly having to field calls from consumers claiming that they ordered a

product online and never received it only to discover that the person placed the order with someone on a social site claiming to represent the company.

» If you stumble upon what looks to be the website of a reputable company, check the URL (page address carefully) and make sure it's the company's official website. Search for the company by name followed by "scam" to see if the company has been reported as fraudulent. Perform your due diligence.

» As explained in the earlier section "Buying cannabis online or over the phone," place orders online or over the phone only with brick-and-mortar establishments you've already developed a relationship with. Don't trust what you read and see only online.

Storing Your Cannabis

Different cannabis products (flower, edibles, concentrates, tinctures, and so on) have different storage requirements. If you simply purchased more cannabis at your dispensary than you plan to consume that day, follow the instructions on the packaging or those provided by your budtender for storing excess product. In general, keep the product in its original packaging (assuming it's airtight) and store it in a cool, dark place out of the reach of children and other critters.

If you need to store substantial amounts of flower for extended periods of time, follow these guidelines:

» Store in a cool, dry place out of direct sunlight. Cool means between 77 and 86 degrees Fahrenheit. Dry means relative humidity of between 59 and 63 percent. You can use a thermometer to measure temperature and a hygrometer to measure humidity.

» Don't store in a refrigerator or freezer. In a refrigerator, temperature and humidity fluctuations make cannabis more susceptible to mold and mildew. In a freezer, the trichomes tend to become brittle and fall off when handled.

» Store in glass, metal, or wood containers. Plastic bags and containers are susceptible to developing a static charge that attracts the trichomes. Plastic is okay for short-term storage.

» Vacuum-seal your jars or other containers to remove excess air. Too much air can cause oxidation, which degrades the quality of the cannabis.

REMEMBER

Keep your product out the reach of children. See Chapter 8 for additional guidance on how to prevent underage access to cannabis.

» Navigating through your first visit to a cannabis dispensary

» Figuring out how to get a medical marijuana card in your state

Chapter **6**

Choosing and Visiting a Cannabis Dispensary

One of the key benefits of legalizing cannabis is that you can now buy it at safe, legal, regulated marijuana dispensaries. Prior to legalization, cannabis has been available only on the black market, where its origin, quality, and safety are often suspect. Purchasing through a state-regulated dispensary, you know exactly what you're getting and getting what you paid for. Equally important is the fact that licensed dispensaries are the only place where you can purchase cannabis legally (at least according to state laws), which makes the dispensary the hub of all cannabis sales.

The problem is that not all cannabis dispensaries are created equal. Some may not be in compliance with state rules, others may have unqualified personnel or non-child-resistant packaging, and some may be less concerned about their customers and the community in which they operate than others. While cannabis is legal, you still need to be careful about where you buy it to ensure that you're getting the best products and the best advice.

This chapter is all about laying the groundwork for buying quality marijuana product legally. We lead you through the process of choosing a reliable and legal pace to shop, help you navigate your first visit to a cannabis dispensary, and lead you through the steps involved in obtaining a medical marijuana card.

Choosing a Cannabis Dispensary

Cannabis dispensaries all have different personalities and attitudes. This includes the atmosphere, clientele, sales staff, products, quality, policies, locations, and the prices. While a visit to a random dispensary for those who know what they're looking for is perfectly reasonable, we advise people with less expertise to choose a dispensary with as much care as they choose their products.

TIP

You can check out most dispensaries online to get a feel for what they offer and their general atmosphere. To find locations near you, simply google "marijuana dispensaries near me" or use one of the many available marijuana dispensary maps or locators online, such as www.leafly.com/finder.

Some states, including Colorado, Oregon, and Washington, have established brands with multiple locations, as well as "mom and pop" shops sprinkled liberally around municipalities that allow cannabis sales. Larger brands offer the comfort of an established company that stands behind its products, which may make the shopping experience less intimidating for new consumers. If you want to support local businesses, a mom-and-pop shop may be the better fit.

REMEMBER

In states that recently legalized marijuana, you're likely to find fewer well-known brands because expansion into other states is an expensive proposition.

After finding a few promising candidates, you're ready to narrow your list. In the following sections, we present factors you should consider when deciding which cannabis dispensary is right for you.

Comparing medical and recreational dispensaries

One of the first considerations to make is whether to shop at a medical or recreational dispensary. Actually, they're exactly alike, as is the plant from which the products are derived. However, the products and the packaging, dose, and legal purchase limits differ.

First identify the legal marijuana status of the state in which you want to purchase (see Chapter 3 for details). Does the state allow only medical marijuana or adult recreational use, as well? If you're looking for a dispensary in a medical-only state, you don't have a choice, but you do need a medical marijuana card, as explained in the later section "Getting a Medical Marijuana Card." If you do have a choice, you'll find this section helpful in making your decision.

REMEMBER

Dispensaries for both medical and recreational marijuana may carry a variety of flower/bud, concentrates or infused products from their own plants or from other dispensaries, as well as other brands. Products may have varying THC potencies or ratios that include CBD to THC. You're likely to find a variety of products, including the following:

>> Flower/bud

>> Concentrates

>> Edibles

>> Sublingual and topical sprays

>> Lotions

>> Tinctures

>> Transdermal patches

WARNING

Cannabis is currently a federally illegal Schedule I drug and is prohibited from being purchased legally, whether in a licensed dispensary or over the internet, and shipped across state lines. Shipping cannabis across state lines constitutes drug trafficking. (See Chapter 3 for more legal guidelines.)

Getting the scoop on medical marijuana dispensaries

Obtaining a medical marijuana card and shopping at a medical marijuana dispensary offer two big benefits over buying marijuana for adult recreational use:

>> Medical marijuana is usually less expensive because most states tax it at a lower rate than they do marijuana for adult recreational use.

>> You can usually buy medical marijuana in larger quantities.

The drawback is the necessity and expense of a doctor's visit to obtain a recommendation necessary to register for the medical card.

The total amount that may be legally purchased in a single day for each individual varies by state and is determined by a physician recommendation called a "plant count." The standard plant count is 6, which refers to the legal number of plants a patient can grow in his own home for personal use. Some patients receive an "extended plant count" recommendation to support their individual needs.

Patients who want to purchase their products from a medical dispensary are limited to the amount equivalent to their plant count. Most patients "sign over" their plant count to a dispensary to grow and produce the products for them, but they can switch their plant counts to a different dispensary, usually after 30 days. Dispensaries can grow only the number of medical plants signed over to them by their patients.

TIP

While you don't need to become a member of a cannabis dispensary to obtain medical marijuana, some dispensaries offer discounts to patients who sign over their plant counts or become members. Of course, cost shouldn't be the primary factor for choosing one dispensary over another, but it can be the deciding factor when choosing between the top two dispensaries on your list.

Dispensaries that serve both medical and recreational consumers may have a single *budroom* — the area inside a dispensary where products are displayed and sold. However, if the dispensary wants to serve medical marijuana users between the ages of 18 and 20, separate budrooms for medical and recreational sales are required. A medical-only budroom provides privacy by allowing only a few patients at a time, all holding medical marijuana registry documentation and proof of identity.

Getting a feel for recreational dispensaries

Adult recreational use dispensaries don't require membership. Any adult over 21 years of age can purchase a product from a legal dispensary as long as they can provide a valid picture ID, such as a state-issued driver's license or a U.S. passport. (In Canada, the legal age is 19 years.)

When purchasing from a recreational dispensary, be aware of the following rules:

>> You can purchase products for personal use only. Any discussion of sharing the products, purchasing for another individual, or gifting the product may cause the budtender to cancel the sale immediately. (A *budtender* is a customer service rep at a cannabis dispensary.)

TIP

You can legally "gift" the product to any adult over the age of 21 within the state after leaving the dispensary. Just don't mention it when you're inside the dispensary.

>> You can purchase only limited quantities as specified by state law.

>> You're not allowed to share or pool money inside the facility to purchase a product.

>> Any discussion about taking the product out of state results in cancellation of the sale.

>> No sampling of product is allowed.

>> No consumption of product inside of or within 15 feet of the dispensary.

>> Dispensaries may not complete a sale after legal hours by even a second and may cancel transactions in process if they're not concluded at the stroke of close or may not allow new sales to begin within a certain timeframe near closing to avoid non-compliance.

WARNING

State purchase and consumption rules may vary, so brush up on state and local laws before heading to the dispensary. See Chapter 3 for federal, state, and local marijuana law basics.

REMEMBER

Rules and regulations vary from state to state but may include a restriction that limits product sales to a minimum THC content, in which case you can't buy CBD-only products in that state's dispensaries.

Finding a reliable and legal place to shop

Whether you're in the market for medical or adult recreational marijuana, you want to be sure that the dispensary is licensed and reliable and that you feel comfortable and confident shopping there and making a purchase. Performing your due diligence as a savvy consumer helps to ensure your safety and the quality of the products you buy, as well as the overall experience.

In the following sections, we provide guidance on how to evaluate different cannabis dispensaries based on several factors, including reputation, product quality, consistency, and variety along with the store's overall environment and the staff's knowledge.

TIP

Vertically integrated companies — those that grow, manufacture, and sell their own product — are generally more reliable because they control their entire supply chain. Products from third-party vendors must still meet all state requirements, but the dispensary must ensure that the vendors they work with have complied with these rules.

Making sure the dispensary is legit

The first order of business is to weed out any dispensaries on your list that may not be licensed. One approach is to search an online registry that lists only legitimate dispensaries, such as www.leafly.com/finder. Leafly also has a search tool for finding doctors who evaluate patients and offer recommendations or authorizations to patients — www.leafly.com/doctors.

Many states also provide online tools for checking whether a dispensary has a state license. For example, the California Cannabis Portal Check a License page at cannabis.ca.gov/check_a_license provides access to lists of licensed retailers, distributors, cultivators, manufacturers, and more. In Oregon, you can visit `www.oregon.gov/olcc/marijuana/pages/default.aspx` to find several links to lists of licensed retailers, including a link to an interactive map of recreational cannabis retailers and laboratories. Use your favorite online search tool to search for something like "check marijuana dispensary license" followed by the name of your state to see whether your state provides such information. Stick with your state's official website, which ends in .gov.

Also check the dispensary's website and its reputation. Search the web for the dispensary by name and visit its website to determine whether it appears professional. Your search is likely to return links to various online reviews of the dispensary, as well, for example, on Yelp or Google Reviews.

TIP

You can also determine whether a dispensary is legit by using good old-fashioned common sense. Visit the dispensary, as explained in the next section, to see if it looks like a legitimate business. If it's in a run-down area of town, has a hand-painted sign out front and a dilapidated parking lot, you may want to drive right past it. If you go inside and the dispensary looks more like a garage than a bona-fide business, you may want to cross it off your list.

WARNING

Don't try to buy THC products on the internet from social media "dispensaries," such as those listed on Facebook or Twitter, for shipment via the U.S. postal service either in or out of state, even if individuals claim to be part of an established company. These online sales are scams.

Visiting and evaluating different dispensaries

The single best approach to evaluating different dispensaries is to visit them. During your visit, evaluate the following:

>> **Location:** Obviously, you want a dispensary that's convenient — near your home, work, or gathering place. However, this factor contains less weight than other factors in this list.

REMEMBER

If you're visiting from out of town and have limited transportation, location may be a key consideration. You won't have time to shop around. However, prior to arriving at your destination, scope out online what's available in the area, visit the websites of those dispensaries, and check out their reviews.

>> **Atmosphere:** Is the dispensary clean and well-organized? Are the product displays attractive? Do you feel welcome and comfortable or unwelcome and awkward?

>> **Staff:** Does the staff seem friendly, engaged, and knowledgeable? Strike up a conversation with the budtender. Let him know what you're looking for and the experience you expect and listen to his recommendations. Is the budtender able to connect with you on *your* level and explain product choices clearly?

- » **Product quality:** You probably can't evaluate product quality until you purchase and consume products, but be sure to check reviews online (and offline from friends and acquaintances). Product quality is determined in the grow room and manufacturing facility, in which you'll probably never set foot, but well-run establishments with good reputations typically sell quality product. (See Chapter 5 for more about evaluating product quality.)

- » **Variety:** Does the dispensary carry a variety of products with different ratios of cannabinoids and terpenes? More importantly, does it carry a variety of products that meet your needs/wants? A dispensary that carries a wide variety of products is more likely to meet your current and future needs.

- » **Cost:** As you visit different dispensaries, compare the costs of similar products, but don't make cost the sole determining factor of where to shop. Paying a little more for quality products and service and for peace of mind is often best. You just want to make sure you're not getting ripped off.

TIP

Don't feel compelled to make a purchase simply because you entered the store and peppered the staff with questions. You're giving them the opportunity to prove themselves to you and earn your business.

Inspecting the packaging

Responsible dispensaries must comply with all rules and regulations stipulated by state laws. Part of that is ensuring that packaging of all products adheres to those regulations.

To evaluate packaging, check for the following:

- » Every package should display the universal THC symbol.

- » All packages should be child-resistant. Ask the budtender to show you how they lock and open.

- » Labels should specify the strain or plant classification such as sativa, indica, or hybrid.

- » Every package should contain a product expiration date.

- » Dosage information should be included on the package in adult recreational products.

- » Flower should have strain and potency listed.

REMEMBER

Rules regarding pre-packaging or changing packages after the product arrives at the store vary across states. For example, some states may not allow a store to open a package of flower to weigh out a smaller amount.

Looking for socially responsible messaging

As with the use of other psychoactive substances, cannabis consumption should be treated with awareness and responsible participation. Some cannabis companies have been taking the lead in this arena above and beyond any regulatory rules and requirements to provide information to patients, customers, and the general public regarding some of those issues such as:

>> Directions not to drive while impaired.

>> Instructions on legal carry-weight limits in the state.

>> Rules regarding legal consumption locations.

>> Directions about consumption effects to ensure a positive experience and deter over consumption.

>> Barriers to product access by minors.

>> Parental responsibility to prevent access to minors.

Some dispensaries, provide customers with an exit card that contains guidance on how to buy and use cannabis legally and safely, as shown in Figure 6-1.

REMEMBER

Standard within the industry is the phrase "Start low and go slow." One of the most important messages to look for is the focus on ensuring a positive experience, and that begins with a slow start.

Checking for community involvement

Being a good corporate citizen has become a hallmark of socially responsible and reputable companies across all industries, including the cannabis industry. Dispensaries should be participating in their local communities beyond the tax dollars that come to states and municipalities. To gauge a dispensary's community involvement, ask the following two questions:

>> Do you donate funds to local nonprofits? If so, which ones?

>> Do the leaders and staff members donate service hours to local charities?

Comparing purchase/delivery/ pickup options

Depending on where you're shopping, you may have a variety of options for purchase and delivery:

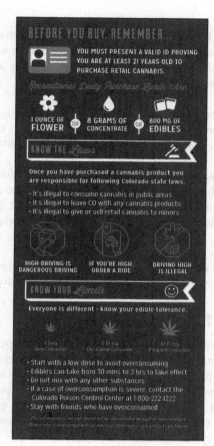

FIGURE 6-1:
Cannabis
dispensary
exit card.

» Buying in person at a dispensary.

» Ordering over the phone or online and picking up your order.

» Ordering over the phone or online and having the product delivered to you. Home delivery is currently an option only in Oregon, California, and Nevada. Colorado, Washington state, Alaska, and Washington, D.C. prohibit it.

In the following sections, we explain these three options in greater detail.

Buying at the dispensary

The advantage to purchasing cannabis flower in a dispensary is the ability to check out the product before buying it. Your budtender can open jars of the current batch of available strains, allowing you to see and smell them, but no touching — only the budtender is permitted to handle the jar. You may not be able to see and smell the actual flower you buy because the state may require that it be weighed and sealed beforehand, but at the least you can get a sense of what you're buying by seeing and smelling the display samples. Daily menus with the available strains should be posted or available as a handout.

Laws prohibit anyone from opening non-flower products including edibles, salves, tinctures, lotions, and concentrates before the sale is complete. However, a dispensary may provide samples of edibles without cannabinoids that you can taste.

Additionally, access to and advice from a knowledgeable budtender are two of the biggest advantages to purchasing your cannabis products in the store. The sales teams should be well trained to answer your questions about products, rules, effects, strains, potency, and use. Take advantage of their knowledge and ask all the questions you have.

REMEMBER

Any budtender unwilling to take the time to answer each and every question isn't deserving of your business, regardless of whether others are waiting in line.

Ordering products for pickup

When you're comfortable with your regular dispensary and the products you like, ordering ahead can save you time and perhaps a little money, as well. Some dispensaries offer loyalty programs with discounts for ordering ahead. These programs are usually accessible through a website or online portal. They may require that you place your order a certain number of days in advance, so they have time to prepare the order, and/or pick up the product within a certain number of days after placing your order to ensure it's fresh.

TIP

Bring cash or a debit card (if accepted by your dispensary). Some locations can process a debit card transaction as an ATM withdrawal; they typically round up to the nearest dollar and return the change in cash. Other locations may have an ATM inside the budroom. Current laws forbid credit card payments. Don't forget to tip your budtender if they've done a good job and you see a tip jar.

Having your cannabis delivered

Having your cannabis delivered is the ultimate in convenience and especially helpful if you're a medical patient with difficulty getting to your dispensary. Just be sure you're comfortable with the dispensary and the products before opting for home delivery.

Prior to arranging home delivery, make sure you understand the process and any pertinent rules or regulations. Contact your dispensary and ask the following questions:

» What's your payment policy? Do I need to pay in advance or in person? State law may dictate the dispensary's payment policy.

» Will the product be delivered by a third party or by dispensary staff? Integrated dispensary delivery is best, because if an issue arises, you can resolve it with the dispensary. If you use a delivery service, you have two parties that may be responsible — the dispensary and the delivery service.

» What form of ID do I need to provide, and how do I get it to you? You may need to provide identification in person.

» Can I refuse the product if any of the packaging is open or damaged? If so, what process do I need to follow? If the dispensary prohibits you from refusing an open or damaged package, scratch it off your list.

» Is product guaranteed? If so, what is your return policy and procedure? Dispensaries should be able to work with you if a product such as a vape pen is defective, but once a container of flower is open even a dispensary with a liberal return policy may be reluctant to accept the return.

Canada allows home delivery through a delivery service or the Canadian Post. Certain verification rules and payment processes are required to ensure that product isn't delivered to minors.

Visiting a Cannabis Dispensary

Visiting a cannabis dispensary for the first time may cause considerable anxiety. Knowing what to expect can help to alleviate some of that tension and make you feel less awkward. In this section, we let you know what to expect.

REMEMBER

Most importantly, dispensary staff should treat you with respect regardless of your cannabis knowledge and experience. You should feel comfortable asking as many questions as you have without feeling rushed, and you shouldn't feel pressured to make a purchase if you don't like the experience, the staff, or the products. You have plenty of dispensaries from which to choose, so if one isn't working for you, take your business elsewhere.

Knowing what to expect

Your first visit to a cannabis dispensary depends a great deal on the store's location, appearance, layout, products, product displays, and staff. However, the process you follow from the time you step into the dispensary to the time you exit with product in hand is pretty standard.

Upon entering through the front door, you find yourself in a vestibule or foyer that's sort of like a waiting room in a doctor's office. A receptionist, sitting at a desk behind what looks like a bank teller window, greets you, requests to see your identification, verifies and scans it, and then enters your information into the dispensary's point-of-sale (POS) system. Being entered into the system typically reserves your place in line to see the next available budtender. You may have to spend some time in the waiting room, or the receptionist may buzz you in immediately, unlocking the door to the budroom.

As you enter some budrooms, you'll see numerous waist-high glass counters, like those at jewelry stores, displaying various products. You may also see, along the walls, glass display cabinets and/or signage, such as product menus, rules and regulations, safe-consumption tips, and socially responsible messaging. The glass counters and cabinets are great, because they allow you to browse at your convenience. Some dispensaries have different types of products at each counter or cabinet; for example, flower may be on display at one counter, edibles at another, and vape oils at still another. Other dispensaries may have several counters each with identical products and its very own dedicated budtender to serve customers. The budroom may also contain a designated area for customers to wait in line for the next available budtender.

When it's your turn, the budtender gestures you to join him at the counter, or he approaches and greets you and then initiates a discussion as to how he can help you. The budtender should be highly trained in general cannabis knowledge, available products, potency and dosing, and state and local laws. He may check your ID again to re-verify your age and identity and match it to your customer information in the POS queue, a step that initiates a compliant transaction.

The budtender asks a series of questions to evaluate your needs, desires, and expectations, so he can better guide your product selection. He then presents you with suitable products, and you choose the ones you want to buy. The time you spend shopping with the budtender will probably feel like a routine visit to a typical retailer where jewelry, electronics, or appliances are sold. The one big difference is that as you choose cannabis products, the budtender checks to be sure your order doesn't exceed state and local purchase limits. (See the next section for details about interacting with your budtender.)

When you're done shopping, assuming you've chosen one or more products to purchase, the budtender goes back through the items you chose to confirm the purchase and registration through the POS system. He scans all items, tells you the total due, and explains the various payment options — cash, debit, or credit (possibly in Canada where cannabis is now federally legal). After you pay, your payment is registered via the POS system.

REMEMBER

Due to current banking restrictions, in the U.S. payment must be made in cash, although some dispensaries accept debit cards.

After payment is processed, the POS system prints "sale" stickers associated with each individual unit purchased. Each sticker includes the product name, weight, potency, location license, date of sale, and any regulatory requirements. The budtender places each sticker on its corresponding product in a place that doesn't cover any prior labeling. He then prints your receipt and places the products and receipt in an opaque exit bag and hands you the bag. At this point you're good to go.

Sizing up the budtender

A *budtender* is a cannabis sales rep. At this time, no universal education certifications are required for this role within the U.S., outside of the state badging system that allows an individual to work in any capacity within the industry.

Your dispensary should provide suitable training that enables its budtenders to meet the following criteria:

>> Be well versed in all the rules and regulations regarding purchase and consumption in the state and municipality in which the dispensary operates.

>> Know the different products the dispensary carries and be able to direct customers based on their desired experience or need.

>> Be knowledgeable about cannabis in general.

>> Be willing to take the time to answer all customer questions.

>> Be polite and meet the same standards of customer service you would expect in any other retail experience.

>> Not claim to be a medical professional unless they actually are and are legally qualified to offer medical advice.

>> Operate compliantly with all rules and regulations, even if that means not completing your sale if a rule is broken in the process. For example, in Colorado a budtender cannot legally proceed with a sale in the store if

- Your ID is invalid or expired.

- You exchange money or discuss paying back another person funds borrowed for the purchase.

- You discuss sharing or gifting a medical or recreational product, even to another adult.

- You discuss traveling across state lines with the product or otherwise removing it from the state.

- You appear impaired by alcohol or other psychotropic substances.

Getting a Medical Marijuana Card

Access to legal medical marijuana requires a state-issued medical marijuana card. Each state has its own list of qualifying medical conditions for which medical marijuana use has been approved. Visit www.leafly.com/news/health/ qualifying-conditions-for-medical-marijuana-by-state to view the list of qualifying medical conditions for your state. Because marijuana is illegal at the federal level, you won't find a list of qualifying conditions in the U.S. Canada's list of qualifying medical conditions includes the following:

» Palliative care

» Chemotherapy-induced nausea and vomiting

» Wasting syndrome and loss of appetite in AIDS or cancer patients

» Multiple sclerosis, amyotrophic lateral sclerosis, and spinal cord injury and disease

» Epilepsy

» Pain

» Arthritis and musculoskeletal disorders

» Movement disorders including dystonia, Huntington's disease, Parkinson's disease, Tourette's syndrome, and spinocerebellar ataxias

» Glaucoma

» Asthma

» Hypertension

» Stress and psychiatric disorders including anxiety, depression, sleep disorders, post-traumatic stress disorder (PTSD), alcohol and opioid withdrawal symptoms, schizophrenia, and psychosis

» Alzheimer's disease and dementia

» Inflammation

>> Gastrointestinal system disorders including irritable bowel syndrome, inflammatory bowel disease, hepatitis

>> Diseases of the pancreas including diabetes, pancreatitis, and metabolic syndrome/obesity

If you have or suspect that you may have one of the qualifying medical conditions listed for your state, consult a doctor. You can consult your doctor (if he's able to submit certification documents with the state) or another physician who specializes in evaluating patients and providing recommendations or authorizations for medical marijuana use. To find a doctor with more experience providing recommendations and authorizations, visit www.leafly.com/doctors.

After you've visited a doctor and received confirmation of your qualifying diagnosis, your physician will need to submit certification to your state. You will then need to apply via your state's online form and pay a fee. Check with your own state's regulatory or government body that oversees cannabis for specific information on applying for yourself or as a registered caregiver or parent/guardian of a minor.

You should be able to follow the progress of your form and find out what's required for renewal on the state's website.

» Deciding whether to smoke or vape

» Consuming cannabis via edibles and drinks

» Exploring topical applications

» Considering cannabis tinctures and pharmaceuticals

Chapter 7

Consuming Cannabis

Traditionally people consumed marijuana by smoking it or baking their own marijuana brownies or cookies. Those methods are still very popular these days, but with the commercialization of marijuana and advances in technology, options have multiplied. Now, many consumers vape cannabis. Some who use cannabis for arthritis or localized pain prefer to use a topical application, such as a lotion. Others may relax at the end of the day by consuming an edible or a steaming cup of cannabis tea, similar to how alcohol users may have a cocktail or a glass of wine.

In this chapter, we take you on a tour of the various modes of cannabis consumption and point out some of the benefits and drawbacks of each along the way. We cover everything from smoking and vaping to edibles, topicals, tinctures, and pharmaceuticals, along with additional methods you may have never imagined. Through this approach, we provide you with a menu of consumption methods from which to choose and instructions for how to consume using the various methods.

REMEMBER

Your choice of consumption method and products are personal decisions and may change with your mood or needs or the situation (the occasion, the setting, the people you're with, and so on). Explore options you find interesting and be open to new information to make well-informed choices.

Going Old School: Smoking or Vaping

Inhaling cannabis smoke or vapor is a highly popular form of consumption. Smoking involves burning marijuana plant matter (typically flower/bud) and inhaling the smoke. Vaping involves heating a high-potency cannabis oil (or cannabis flower) to vaporize the active ingredients and then inhaling the vapor.

WARNING

Cannabis vape pens are similar to those used for vaping nicotine products, but the two device types aren't interchangeable — don't attempt to use or modify a nicotine device to vape cannabis.

Both methods — smoking and vaping — share the benefit of quick delivery. You begin to feel the effects soon after you inhale, because the active ingredients enter the lungs where they're quickly transferred to the bloodstream. Due to the speed at which the cannabis takes effect, smoking and vaping are especially popular among medical marijuana consumers who don't want to wait for relief.

In this section, we describe each option in greater detail, highlight the pros and cons of each, and present various methods of smoking and vaping.

Smoking cannabis

Prior to smoking cannabis, you must grind or break up the flower using your fingers, a grinder, scissors, or some other method. Breaking up the flower makes it easier to pack into the smoking receptacle and ensures a steadier burn through enhanced air flow.

TIP

Grinders vary. A one-chamber grinder has a top and bottom with teeth that shred the cannabis. A two-chamber grinder is equipped with a screen at the bottom of the top chamber that allows *kief* to fall through to the bottom chamber. (Kief is the resinous trichomes that contain high concentrations of cannabinoids and terpenes. Some consumers like to save it and use it as a concentrate or add it to a bowl or joint.) Ask the budtender at your local cannabis dispensary to recommend a grinder.

Here's how to break up your flower using your fingers and a one-chamber grinder:

1. **Remove the top lid from the grinder.**

2. **Use your fingers to break the larger buds into smaller pieces and place them between the grinder's teeth, as shown in Figure 7-1.**

3. **Replace the lid and twist it back and forth several times to allow the teeth to shred the cannabis.**

   You want your cannabis broken down, like pipe tobacco, not finely ground.

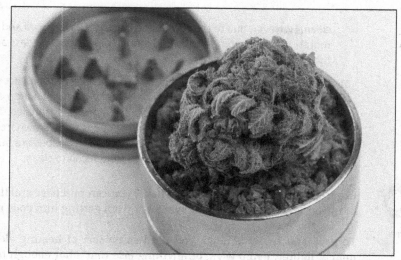

FIGURE 7-1:
Load small
pieces of bud
into your
grinder.

4. **Remove the lid and tap the cannabis out onto a clean, dry surface, such as a piece of paper.**

You may have to tap several times to loosen any pieces of bud stuck between the grinder's teeth.

After breaking up your cannabis bud, you can pack it into a variety of different smoking receptacles, such as a pipe, or use it to roll your own joints, as explained in the following sections.

Smoking with a pipe

A pipe is a traditional tool for smoking cannabis. It simply requires a bowl in which to place the product and another opening to inhale the smoke. Most pipes are similar to those used for smoking tobacco, but pipes for smoking cannabis are typically made from different materials, such as glass or metal, and they tend to have a smaller bowl. Many cannabis pipes also have an extra hole through the bowl called a *carb* that you can cover and release to control air flow. A pipe can be made out of almost any material as long as it's not flammable and doesn't emit any gasses that can harm the lungs.

Although pipes come in a variety of shapes and sizes, they're typically broken down into the following categories:

>> **Hand pipes (dry pipes):** Small enough to fit in the palm of your hand, a hand pipe is typically made of glass and typically used by casual smokers. Hand pipes are inexpensive, portable, discreet, easy to use, and relatively easy to

clean. However, due to the short distance between the bowl and the user's mouth, the smoke tends to be hot, though pipes made of glass and metal cool the smoke to some degree.

>> **Water pipes:** Often referred to as *bongs* or *bubblers* (for smaller versions), water pipes have a chamber filled with water (or a combination of water and ice) through which the smoke passes before being inhaled. The water cools the smoke and traps any ash that happens to be drawn from the bowl, enhancing the smoking experience. However, water pipes are bulkier, so they're not discrete, and they may be more difficult to clean.

TIP

Regardless of the type of pipe you have, you can purchase small screens to place in the bottom of the bowl to prevent ash from getting into your mouth or lungs.

To pack and smoke a bowl, you need some sort of heating element, such as a match, lighter, hemp wick, or anything else that's hot enough to ignite the cannabis. Then, take the following steps:

1. **Place your cannabis in the bowl, and pack it down loosely at the bottom and somewhat more tightly at the top.**

   A denser top layer maintains a steady burn or "cherry," while the looser bottom layer enhances air flow.

2. **If the pipe has a carb, hold your finger or thumb over the carb while you light up to increase air flow through the cannabis.**

3. **Fire up your heating element (match, lighter, whatever), hold it near the cannabis at the top of the bowl, and draw the smoke into your mouth as if you were smoking a cigar.**

4. **When you're just about done taking a puff, release the carb, so you draw any remaining smoke from the stem.**

   This step is referred to as "clearing the bowl."

5. **Remove your mouth from the pipe while inhaling the smoke, along with fresh air, deep into your lungs.**

TIP

   If you're sharing a bowl with others, *corner the bowl* — instead of lighting the center of the bowl, hold the heating element near the rim of the pipe, so you ignite the cannabis in only your corner of the bowl. This allows others in your smoking circle to get a quality hit.

6. **Hold your breath for one or two seconds, and then slowly exhale.**

   Holding your breath longer than a few seconds doesn't increase the effect much more and can make you feel uncomfortable.

Clean your pipe occasionally. If you use a water pipe, change the water daily and clean the bowl weekly. If you use a hand pipe, clean it at least once a week. You can buy pipe cleaner solution at your local dispensary. Some people use nail polish (acetone) or isopropyl alcohol and coarse salt, but we recommend using nonflammable and less potentially harmful products.

Rolling your own joints (or smoking pre-rolls)

The familiar joint resembles a cigarette and can be personally rolled or purchased as a pre-rolled product in many dispensaries. Pre-rolled joints are also referred to as *cones* because of their shape and the fact that many companies purchase the paper pre-formed into cones that can be easily filled. When a joint is rolled in cigar paper made from tobacco plants, it's called a *blunt*. When the joint is filled with a mix of tobacco (typically five to ten percent) and cannabis, it's called a *spliff*.

When shopping for pre-rolled joints, ask about the product used in the joint. Joints made from ground flower are generally more consistent in terms of quality than those made from shake or trim. (*Shake* refers to the remnants that fall off the flower when it's stored, moved, or handled; it's not necessarily poor quality. *Trim*, on the other hand, is leaf removed from the plant during processing, and it's often used in poor-quality cannabis.)

Joints can also come with additional products to enhance flavor or potency; for example, *caviar* is a joint made from bud that's first dipped in cannabis oil then rolled in kief.

To roll your own joint, take the following steps:

1. **Grind your cannabis as explained earlier.**

2. **Obtain a crutch/filter.**

   A crutch goes in one end of the joint to keep the cannabis from getting into your mouth and prevent you from burning your lips. You can buy crutches at a dispensary or make your own.

   To make a crutch, take a thin piece of cardboard (from an index card, thin business card, or magazine subscription card, for example), trim it to about 1-by-2 inches, make four or five narrow but loose accordion folds (about 1/16 inch) on one of the short sides, and then roll the accordion folds into the remaining cardboard. You should end up with a cylindrical tube with an M shape in the middle formed by the accordion folds (see Figure 7-2).

3. **Place your crutch at one end of your rolling paper (glue end up) and hold the paper and crutch in one hand, as shown in Figure 7-3.**

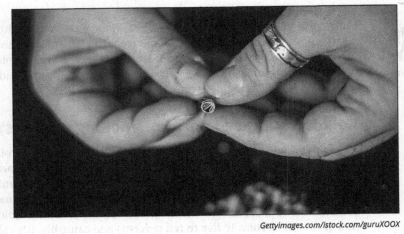

FIGURE 7-2:
A rolled crutch.

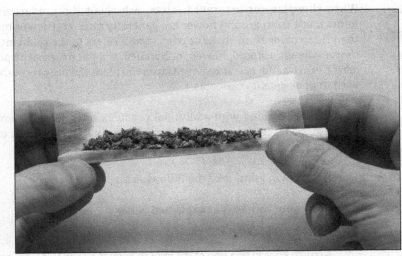

FIGURE 7-3:
Hold the crutch
and rolling paper
in one hand
while adding
the cannabis.

4. Using your other hand, place about one half to one gram of ground cannabis into the fold of the rolling paper.

5. Pack the joint by rolling the joint back and forth between your thumbs and fingertips, as shown in Figure 7-4.

6. Starting at the crutch end, roll the unglued edge of the paper up, tuck it down into the roll, and continue rolling until you reach the edge with the glue (see Figure 7-5).

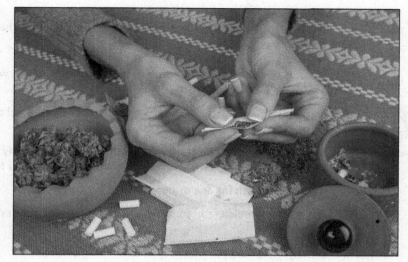

FIGURE 7-4:
Roll the joint
back and forth
between your
thumbs and
fingers.

Gettyimages.com/istock.com/Olaf Speier

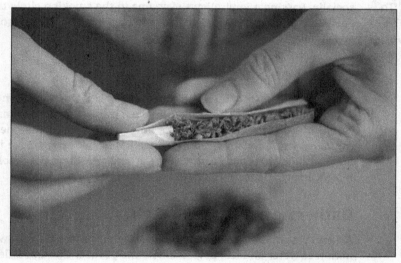

FIGURE 7-5:
Tuck and roll.

Gettyimages.com/istock.com/Oleg Malyshev

7. **Lick edge with the glue to moisten it slightly, and then tack it down.**

8. **Use a pen or similarly shaped object to pack down the cannabis at the
   end opposite that of the crutch and then twist the end of the rolling
   paper to create a seal.**

Smoking a joint may seem like a no-brainer, but following the right technique ensures a more enjoyable experience:

1. **Draw the smoke into your mouth first, as you would if you were smoking a cigar.**

   Don't draw the smoke directly into your lungs, because the heat of the smoke will burn.

WARNING

2. **As you remove the joint from your mouth, breathe in slowly and deeply to draw the smoke, along with plenty of fresh air, into your lungs.**

3. **Hold your breath for one or two seconds.**

   This is not a "how long can you hold your breath" contest. One or two seconds is sufficient.

4. **Exhale slowly and steadily.**

REMEMBER

One of the best features of a joint is that it provides a means for enjoying cannabis socially. Passing a joint allows everyone in the smoking circle to have an equally enjoyable experience. When you're passing a pipe, the last person may get little if any smoke.

Using a one-hitter

If you're smoking by yourself, a *one-hitter* (or *chillum*) may be an attractive option. A one-hitter looks like a hollowed-out cigarette with a stem. To pack it with cannabis, you repeatedly push the empty tube end of the one-hitter into your cannabis with a twisting motion. Once it's loaded, you smoke it like a cigarette, but you hold the flame just at the tip, and you draw the smoke first into your mouth and then into your lungs.

Gathering around a hookah

A *hookah* is similar to a bong in that the smoke passes through water (or a combination of water and ice) as you inhale the product through a flexible hose with a nozzle. However, a hookah may have numerous hoses and nozzles attached to it (for communal smoking), and instead of loading the bowl with cannabis and lighting it, one or more hot coals are placed on aluminum foil with holes poked in it just above the bowl of cannabis. When you inhale, the heat from the coals is drawn down through the cannabis.

The big drawback is that hookahs are designed for smoking *shisha* (wet tobacco), not for smoking a dried herb such as cannabis, which burns a lot faster. The quick burn often ruins the flavor and produces smoke faster than it can be inhaled, thus wasting product. To overcome this limitation, the cannabis is often placed between two layers of shisha, but if you're not a fan of smoking tobacco, this solution may not appeal to you. Another drawback is that a hookah is difficult to clean. You need to change the water and clean the hoses, nozzles, stems, and shafts after every few sessions.

Checking out homemade devices

Cannabis culture wouldn't be complete without homemade devices for smoking weed. Perhaps the most famous is the apple pipe (see Figure 7-6).

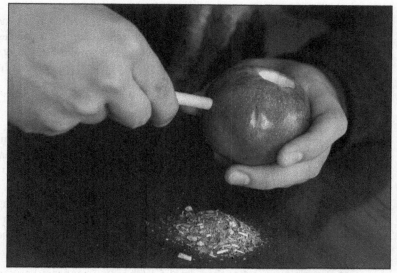

FIGURE 7-6:
An apple pipe.

Fotos593/Shutterstock.com

To create your own apple pipe, take the following steps:

1. **Remove the stem from the apple.**

   This area serves as the bowl in which you pack your cannabis. For a larger bowl, you can cut or scoop out this area, but don't make it so deep that you're getting into the area with the seeds.

2. **Poke a small hole straight down into the apple where the stem was.**

   You can use a toothpick, but poke it deep enough so it reaches down into where the seeds are.

3. **Poke five more small holes around the area where the stem was.**

   Go deep enough to reach the area containing the seeds.

4. **(Optional) Poke a small hole straight up from the bottom of the apple to create a carb.**

5. **Bore a hole from the side of the apple into its core (you can use a drill or the body of a pen, without the cartridge, or a similar object to bore the hole).**

The top of the apple serves as your bowl. Pack your cannabis into this bowl-shaped area and light it while drawing from the hole on the side of the apple. You can insert the body of a pen or a similar hollow cylindrical object into the hole to serve as the stem of your pipe, as long as it fits snugly into the hole.

Creative consumers have created pipes out of everything from soda cans to empty paper towel roles (to create pipes called *steamrollers*). All you need is a part that serves as the bowl and a hole to draw out the smoke. Search online for "home-made marijuana pipes" to check out some of the more creative innovations.

Vaping cannabis

No doubt, you're familiar with the concept of vaping as an alternative to smoking cigarettes, but vaping has also become a popular method for consuming cannabis. Vaping cannabis offers several benefits, including the following:

>> **Vaping can be portable and discreet.** Pens and other small vaporizers are easy to carry and use without attracting a lot of attention. In addition, because plant matter is not being combusted, you don't have the lingering smell of smoke.

>> **Vapor is smoother than smoke.** With many vaporizers, you can control the temperature, so you don't feel a burning sensation in your throat or lungs as is common with smoking.

>> **Vaping is convenient.** You load the oil or oil cartridge and press a button to produce the vapor. You don't have to grind or load cannabis or light anything. With some vaporizers, you don't even have to press a button; the heating element is activated when you begin to puff.

>> **Your lungs will thank you.** Vapor is gentler than smoke on the lungs and doesn't contain the toxins and tar contained in smoke from combusted plant material.

>> **Like smoking, the effect is nearly immediate.** You don't have to wait to feel the effect of the cannabis as you do with edibles.

>> **Vaping is efficient.** Vape oil and equipment convert more than 45 percent of the available THC from dry plant matter, whereas combustion methods (smoking) yield only about 25 percent.

>> **You have more control over dosing.** With consistent vape oil and a high-quality vaporizer, you can more accurately estimate the amount of THC, CBD, and other ingredients you're ingesting.

Of course, vaping also has some drawbacks, including the following:

>> **Vaping is expensive.** Quality vaporizers aren't cheap, plus you must replace the heating element regularly and perhaps replace the battery, assuming it's replaceable.

>> **Batteries run low.** If you're using a vaporizer that runs solely on battery power and the charge is depleted, you can't vape until you replace or recharge the batteries. (Some vaporizers don't use batteries or allow you to continue to vape when the battery is being recharged.)

>> **The high is different.** Some people describe the high from vaping as weaker than that from smoking. Others describe the high as cleaner. You may prefer one over the other.

If you're in the market for a vaporizer, you have several considerations to make, such as the following:

>> **Loose leaf or oil?** Most vaporizers use high-potency cannabis oil, while others use loose-leaf cannabis, such as you would use in a pipe or joint. If you like to smoke and want to sample a greater variety of cannabis, you may lean toward a loose-leaf (flower) vaporizer. If you're looking for high-efficiency and a cleaner high, an oil vaporizer may be the better choice.

REMEMBER

Cannabis vape oils come in a variety of strains, blends or THC/CBD ratios. However, the variety may not match that of flower/bud. Also keep in mind that the potency of oils can be much higher than the original plant matter from which it is derived.

>> **Conduction or convection?** A loose-leaf vaporizer heats by conduction or convection. With conduction, the cannabis must be in contact with the heating element — similar to the way a pan must be in contact with the heating element on a stove. With convection, the vaporizer heats the cannabis with hot air, which generally results in more uniform vaporization of the cannabis. With oil vaporizers, you don't have this option.

>> **Disposable or refillable?** Some oil vaporizers are disposable, others enable you to reload with pre-filled oil cartridges, and others contain a refillable chamber into which you pour the oil. All loose-leaf vaporizers are refillable, equipped with a chamber into which you pack your ground cannabis.

>> **Portability:** Vaporizers come in various shapes and sizes, from desktop models down to vaporizers that are the size of pens or thumb drives. The smaller models are more portable and discrete, while the larger models are more powerful and may be more suitable to vaping in groups.

>> **Battery power, life, and recharge time:** For vaporizers that run on battery power, consider the power rating, how long the device is expected to run between charges, how long it takes to charge, and whether you can use the device (plugged into an outlet) while it's charging. Loose-leaf vaporizers have an on/off switch, so they use power continuously when they're turned on, whereas oil vaporizers use power on demand, which is more efficient.

>> **Adjustable heat settings:** Some vaporizers have only one heat setting, whereas others allow you to adjust the heat setting. The ability to adjust heat settings is a nice feature, because it allows you to control the production of vapor and reduce the heat if the vapor is too hot.

>> **Heating element composition:** Traditional oil vaporizers rely on a cotton wick to hold the cannabis oil while it's being heated. When the wick gets burnt (as it does over time), the burnt flavor transfers to the vapor, and the wick becomes less efficient. Newer ceramic (c-cell) vaporizers are sturdier and more efficient. They can also function at higher temperatures to produce more vapor.

>> **Other bells and whistles:** Fancier (and more expensive models) may include additional features, such as breath activation, so you don't have to press a button. With some models, you can adjust the heat setting using an app on your smart phone or even lock the device to prevent access to minors. As the technology evolves, you're likely to see products with more options.

REMEMBER

While some brands of vaporizers look similar to tobacco vaporizers, the two products have distinct differences, and the refillable pods are not compatible with tobacco vape pens or with other marijuana vape batteries.

Dabbing

Dabbing is another way to inhale cannabis. This method uses a solid form of marijuana concentrate such as wax, shatter, or live resin, which can be very potent and produce an intense high.

Dab rigs are frequently made of glass and look like a water pipe, although they may or may not use water to filter and cool the smoke (see Figure 7-7).

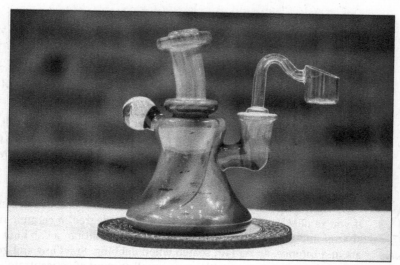

FIGURE 7-7:
A sample dab rig.

To dab, you need the following equipment and supplies:

>> **Cannabis concentrate:** Wax, shatter, or live resin. See Chapter 2 for more about different concentrates and Chapter 13 for instructions on how to create concentrates.

>> **Dab rig:** A *dab rig* (or *oil rig*) is similar to a water pipe, but instead of a connector for a bowl, it contains a male or female glass joint for holding the nail (described farther down in this list).

>> **Dab mat:** Set your dab rig and other equipment and supplies on a *dab mat* or *dab rag* — a soft, non-flammable surface that protects the rig from breaking if it tips over and protects the table or other underlying surface from burns and stains.

>> **Nail:** The *nail* is a metal, glass, or ceramic "tray" that fits inside the glass joint. When dabbing, you heat the nail and place a small amount of cannabis concentrate on the head of the nail to vaporize it.

We recommend using a titanium, quartz, or composite nail and avoiding glass nails, which can shatter when overheated.

You also have a choice between domed and domeless nails. A domed nail has a removable enclosure that contains the smoke. A domeless nail sort of has a built-in dome surrounding a central cylinder through which the smoke passes. A domeless nail generally takes longer to heat, but you don't have to place a dome over it after heating it. Another option is an electric nail, which doesn't require the use of a torch to heat.

>> **Dome:** The *dome* is a collar that rests on the rim of the joint and surrounds the nail to keep the smoke contained. The top is open to allow airflow.

>> **Dabber:** A *dabber* is a wand, typically made of metal, glass, or ceramic, for picking up the cannabis concentrate and placing it on the head of the nail. A dabber looks like an instrument you'd see in a dentist's office.

>> **Torch:** You need a propane or butane blow torch to heat the nail. A chef's torch, commonly used to caramelize sugar atop crème brulee, is perfect. You can buy a suitable torch online or at your dispensary, a hardware store, or any store that carries high-end kitchenware.

WARNING

Dabbing is generally safe, but be careful. The torch and nail become very hot, and if you're dabbing with a glass or (to a lesser degree) a ceramic nail, the nail can shatter and send chards toward your face. In addition, a dab high can be immediate and intense, so remain seated when dabbing. Start low and go slow your first two or three times; start with a very small amount of concentrate — the equivalent of a few crumbs or a tiny drop of liquid.

To dab, follow these steps:

1. **Set aside the amount of concentrate you want to use, so you can quickly and easily pick it up with your dabber later.**

You may even want to place it on the tip of your dabber.

2. **Place the nail in the joint and be sure it's properly seated.**

3. **Use your torch to heat the nail until it starts to glow red.**

If you're using an electronic nail, follow the instructions that came with it.

4. **If you're using a domed nail, place the dome onto the joint, so it surrounds the nail, being careful not to touch the hot nail.**

5. **Let the nail cool for 15 to 45 seconds depending on the material — a titanium nail is cool enough in about 15 seconds, whereas you may need to allow a quartz nail to cool for up to 45 seconds.**

Experiment with the wait time and the temperature of the nail to personalize the experience. You don't want the nail so hot that it combusts (burns) the concentrate, but you want it hot enough to vaporize the concentrate.

6. **Use your dabber to pick up the desired amount of concentrate.**

7. **Place your mouth on the mouthpiece. While inhaling slowly, use the dabber to transfer the concentrate to the nail(see Figure 7-8).**

Where to place the concentrate varies according to the nail used. With domed nails, you generally place your dab on the very top of the nail. With domeless nails, you generally place the dab in the collar surrounding the center core.

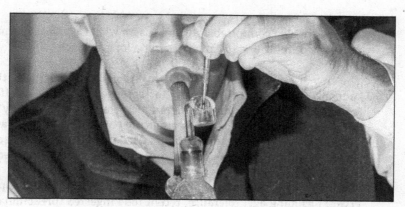

FIGURE 7-8:
Dabbing.

Mitch M/Shutterstock.com

TIP

When placing the dab on the nail, rotate the tip of the dabber to make sure all concentrate is transferred to the nail.

8. **Continue inhaling until you've breathed in all the smoke from the pipe and then remove your mouth from the mouthpiece while continuing to inhale.**

9. **Hold your breath for a second or two and then exhale slowly.**

Eating and Drinking Cannabis: Edibles

Edibles are one of the fastest growing segments of cannabis consumption methods. While the concept of mixing marijuana and food has been around for as long as the pot brownie, commercial products have expanded the offerings for almost every taste and preference. Edibles are discreet, cost effective, portable, and come in a wide variety of product types, including the following:

» Gummies, hard candies, and lollipops

» Chocolates

» Baked goods, such as brownies and cookies

» Butter

» Hot cocoa

» Tea

» Soda

» Juice

» Alcoholic beverages

Edibles are also comfortable for new users who are exploring marijuana for the first time or returning to cannabis after a long absence.

The only drawback to edibles is the time required to experience the effects of the cannabis. You don't get the nearly instantaneous and intense effect that you get from smoking, vaping, or dabbing. In fact, you may not feel any effect for a half hour to an hour as the cannabis gradually enters your system, and you may not feel the full effect for two to four hours. Medical patients and those who are accustomed to smoking, vaping, or dabbing, may be disappointed by edibles.

Numerous factors affect the speed at which cannabis (edibles specifically) takes effect, including age, tolerance, recent food ingested (predominantly fat-soluble content will increase effect), altitude, and environment. Starting low and going slow is particular important with edibles and for novice consumers. When you consume an edible and don't feel any different within 15 to 30 minutes, you may be tempted to consume more, which increases your risk of taking too much and having an uncomfortable experience.

REMEMBER

Start low and go slow. When shopping for cannabis edibles, consult your budtender and read the labels carefully to obtain the following information:

>> **CBD-to-THC ratio:** Cannabidiol (CBD) is the non-psychotropic, and tetrahydrocannabinol (THC) is the psychotropic component of cannabis. Edibles may blend the two in various ratios, such as 1:1, 5:1, 10:1, 20:1, and even 50:1. The higher the CBD ratio, the less psychotropic effect or "high" is felt. At 20:1, even a first-time user would likely feel nothing at all but still reap the health benefits of CBD. Yet, even a small amount of THC added to CBD drives the CBD molecules into the CB1 receptors in the body, thereby intensifying the effects of the CBD.

>> **Total milligrams:** Total milligrams of CBD, THC, or both in the entire package.

>> **Milligrams per serving:** Number of milligrams of CBD, THC, or both in each serving when purchasing recreationally.

>> **Serving size:** Many packages divide the product into servings, such as gummies or squares of chocolate to help with dosing. Each serving contains a specific amount of CBD and/or THC. Some states require product manufacturers to provide individual servings in adult recreational purchases.

>> **Strain:** The label may include the strain(s) of cannabis used to create the product.

>> **Other ingredients:** Some edibles blend the cannabis with other ingredients, such as magnolia, green tea, or caffeine, to intensify the effects, add flavor, or deliver a unique experience.

Using Topical and Transdermal Products

If you're looking for localized relief for pain, sore muscles, tension, or inflammation without the high you get from inhalants or edibles, you may want to consider topical or transdermal cannabis products. *Topicals* are cannabis-infused lotions, oils, and creams that you rub or spray on the skin (they also include salts you can add to bath water). *Transdermals* are patches that stick to the skin. Topicals deliver cannabinoids only to the network of CB2 receptors, so they're not intoxicating. Transdermal patches, on the other hand, can deliver cannabinoids into the bloodstream, so they can make you high, although the high isn't likely to be very intense.

In addition to providing pain relief, topicals and transdermals may be helpful in treating muscle cramps, headaches, itchy skin, and inflammatory skin conditions, such as psoriasis and dermatitis.

REMEMBER

Creams and lotions for arthritis, injury recovery, and localized pain can provide relief to substitute for over-the-counter pain medication as well as prescription medication (even opioids). Studies show substantial reductions in overdose deaths from opioids in some cities after legalization of recreational marijuana.

Although the selection of cannabis topicals and transdermal products is vast, the following list presents a range of options:

>> **Salves:** For intense localized pain relief, salves are a great option. They're easy to apply, absorb quickly, and leave little mess.

>> **Lotions:** For more generalized, less intense pain and to moisturize your skin in the process, consider a lotion.

>> **Oils:** Oils are great for massage and for fast pain relief for feet and joints. However, they can be messy, leaving an oily residue.

>> **Lubricants:** Cannabis-infused lubricants can enhance the sexual experience for both males and females.

>> **Lip balms:** For chapped lips, consider cannabis-infused lip balms, that not only heal chapped lips but can alleviate the pain.

>> **Bath salts:** For whole-body relief and to relax before heading to bed, consider cannabis-infused bath salts or a bath bomb.

>> **Transdermal patches:** Transdermal patches are great for localized pain and to gradually release cannabinoids into the bloodstream (timed-release).

Topicals may be blended with other ingredients, such as cayenne pepper, wintergreen, peppermint, menthol, or clove to boost their effectiveness or enhance the overall experience.

REMEMBER

Even if a topical contains THC (the psychoactive cannabinoid), it won't make you high, because it doesn't enter into the bloodstream. However, cannabinoids in a transdermal patch may enter the bloodstream.

Using Cannabis Tinctures or Pills

Tinctures are liquid products that can be added to food or drinks, as well as taken sublingually (under the tongue). They're available from a multitude of vendors in differing strengths as well as ratios and with other blended herbs, and they're easy to make at home (see Chapter 13). Sublingual delivery is the fastest acting delivery method after smoking. You should begin to feel the effects within approximately ten minutes. If you add the tincture to your food or drink, you can expect the same delayed reaction characteristic of edibles.

Sublingual consumption is most common and enables you to easily control the dose. The tincture comes in a spray bottle or a bottle with an eye dropper. You simply apply the desired number of drops or sprays under your tongue, hold it in your mouth for a few seconds, and then swallow. You should start to feel the effects within ten minutes and reach your peak in about 90 minutes. Because tinctures taken sublingually take effect much more quickly than edibles, you can more quickly figure out which dose is ideal for you.

Many product manufacturers are also creating THC and/or CBD products in pill form. These products are more generalized and have more overall health benefits than do topical products.

FINDING YOUR BRAND IN ANOTHER STATE

Because marijuana is federally illegal, cannabis can't be transported over state lines, so if you travel to another state, you may have trouble finding your favorite brands of products.

For a company to sell its brand in another state, it must set up a grow operation, MIP facility, and retail facilities in that state or partner with an established company in that state, license its recipes to that company, and provide the packaging. Either option makes it difficult and expensive for companies to expand into other states.

Taking Pharmaceutical Preparations

Even if you live in a state in which medical marijuana is not legal, you may be able to benefit from the medical effects of cannabis by taking it in prescription form. A few prescription medications contain cannabinoids and may be legal in certain states where cannabis is still illegal:

» **Dronabinol (Marinol):** Dronabinol is a manufactured form of cannabis used to treat loss of appetite and resulting weight loss in people with AIDS and severe nausea and vomiting caused by chemotherapy used to treat cancer.

» **Sativex:** Sativex is a peppermint flavored whole-cannabis-plant mouth spray approved as a botanical drug in the United Kingdom in 2010 to alleviate neuropathic pain, spasticity, overactive bladder, and other symptoms of multiple sclerosis. Sativex is not legal in the U.S., so it's not allowed to be shipped to the U.S.

» **Epidiolex:** Epidiolex is a prescription form of cannabidiol (CBD) and the first cannabinoid medication approved by the U.S. Food and Drug Administration (FDA). It has been approved for the treatment of seizures associated with Lennox-Gastaut syndrome and Dravet syndrome — two rare and sever forms of childhood onset epilepsy.

Chapter **8**

Using Cannabis Safely and Responsibly

C annabis is an herb that some research has shown to be valuable and powerful enough to provide symptom relief for people with a wide range of medical conditions. Anything that's powerful enough to relieve symptoms has the potential to cause adverse side effects in some individuals.

For many, cannabis can be a valuable component to their health, wellness, or recreation when used safely and responsibly. In this chapter, we call your attention to the possible health and safety risks and offer guidance on how to consume responsibly to mitigate those risks. Here you discover how to find the right dose for the desired experience without overdoing it, how to avoid and deal with the possibility of overconsumption, and how to prevent potential negative impacts on underage individuals.

Recognizing the Health and Safety Risks

Although we generally sing the praises of cannabis throughout this book, it does pose certain risks to the health and safety of some consumers and others, especially if the consumer fails to use responsibly. In this section, we list and describe some of the more common short-term (transitory) and long-term adverse effects of cannabis to call your attention to the potential downside of using or abusing it.

REMEMBER

Cannabis flower and other products contain different concentrations of different *cannabinoids* — the primary active ingredients in cannabis. Tetrahydrocannabinol (THC) is the psychoactive component that produces the euphoric high. Cannabidiol (CBD) doesn't produce an intoxicating effect but can make you drowsy and lower your blood pressure, so it's not risk-free.

Checking out undesirable transitory effects

Cannabis consumption can produce a number of undesirable effects that arise particularly when the concentration of THC is high and the consumer consumes too much. These effects are transitory; that is, they go away over time, assuming the person stops consuming for several hours. Undesirable transitory side effects include the following:

>> **Impaired motor control:** Slowed reflexes and impaired physical coordination negatively impact your ability to drive or operate machinery.

>> **Impaired memory and cognition:** Your ability to learn or remember, to think or communicate clearly, or to make decisions may be diminished. These adverse side effects could negatively impact a consumer's performance at school or at work and compromise their problem-solving and communication skills.

>> **Altered perception of time:** Cannabis can make you feel as though time has slowed down. You may like or dislike this feeling, but it can pose a safety risk if you're crossing the street, driving, operating machinery, or even cooking. Of course, it may also make you feel as though you've accomplished more in less time.

>> **Anxiety or paranoia:** Although cannabis is generally associated with a calm sense of bliss, it can increase anxiety to the point of paranoia or even delusional thinking (distorted thoughts or emotions) or psychosis (a break with reality). Whether cannabis calms or creates anxiety can be related to the person, the product, the dose, the person's state of mind, or a combination of factors.

>> **Light headedness or fainting:** Cannabis may cause a temporary drop in blood pressure (if you're susceptible) that can make you feel lightheaded or dizzy or may cause you to faint.

>> **Increased heart rate:** Cannabis can raise a person's heart rate for up to three hours after the effect kicks in, which may increase the chance of heart attack in those with pre-existing vulnerabilities. If you're older or have a history or family history of cardiovascular issues, you should be aware of this fact.

Another transitory issue to consider is the fact that THC remains in the body (in fat-soluble tissue) long after it has been consumed, which increases the potential of failing a drug test. While testing is improving, current tests are unable to differentiate residual from recent-use THC. Typically, THC is detectible in bodily fluids for up to 30 days, but for daily heavy users, that period may extend to more than 90 days!

Looking ahead to potential long-term complications

Long-term health problems related to cannabis are typically associated with continuous heavy usage over months or years. Possible adverse long-term side effects include the following:

>> **Breathing difficulties:** If you choose smoking as your method of consuming cannabis, you're at an increased risk of having respiratory issues, including bronchitis, lung infections, wheezing, and coughing. As with tobacco, the combustion of cannabis plant material produces tar and other toxins, carcinogens, and irritants that are unhealthy for the lungs.

REMEMBER

You can avoid this particular long-term side effect by not smoking cannabis. As explained in Chapter 7, plenty of consumption methods are available that don't involve smoke. Vaping cannabis oil can deliver many of the benefits of smoking without subjecting your lungs to smoke, and edibles bypass your lungs entirely!

>> **Psychiatric issues:** Long-term cannabis use has been linked to increased risks of anxiety, depression, and psychosis. It also may increase the risk of schizophrenia in people who are predisposed to that condition.

>> **Cannabinoid hyperemesis syndrome (CHS):** CHS is a condition in which continuous heavy consumers experience regular cycles of severe nausea, vomiting, and dehydration. These symptoms typically subside when the consumer stops using cannabis, so it's both a transitory and long-term effect.

Continuous heavy consumption of cannabis also has the potential to cause problems beyond health issues, including increased absences and poorer performance at work or school, relationship issues, and decreased satisfaction with life in general for some individuals.

REMEMBER

To reduce the risk of long-term adverse effects, consume in moderation — both in frequency and amount — especially if you're a recreational user (as with other substances). That way, you can reap the benefits of cannabis while avoiding many of the most serious adverse effects.

Making Dosing Decisions

If you're a cannabis novice, you're probably wondering, "How much should I take?" The answer to that question is simple: Take as little as possible to produce the desired effect and avoid potential adverse side effects.

Unfortunately, that answer provides little to no practical guidance for new cannabis users. The truth is that we can't provide specific guidelines because the variables are so numerous. Products differ. Consumers differ. Situations differ. What's too much for one consumer is not enough for another. Some people achieve the experience they want with *microdosing* — taking a small dose (1–5 mg daily) of a non- or slightly intoxicating cannabis product to enhance overall health and productivity without getting high. Others achieve optimal results with megadoses of up to 2,000 mg daily without experiencing adverse side effects.

REMEMBER

More isn't necessarily better, although it can be. Increasing the dose up to a certain point initially produces stronger effects, but beyond that point, the desired effects may become weaker with an increase in adverse side effects. However, increasing the dose beyond the point at which it produces the desired effects may, in some cases, produce additional desirable effects.

The best approach is to follow the age-old wisdom of starting low and going slow and experimenting with products that have different concentrations and ratios of cannabinoids and different terpenes until you find *your* sweet spot.

In the following sections, we provide additional guidance by helping you define the experience you desire and evaluate some of the key factors that typically impact the experience. Our hope is that by following our guidance, you can find your sweet spot faster and reduce the amount of trial and error — although trial and error can make the experience more enjoyable as well.

Defining your desired experience

People consume cannabis for different reasons. Some take it for pain relief or seizure prevention. Others take it at parties to relax and remove some of their inhibitions. Some take it to boost their productivity or enhance their athletic performance. And many certainly take it to feel the buzz.

REMEMBER

To determine the optimal dose of cannabis for you, first define your desired experience. The experience you want can certainly change over time, and it may change based on the situation. For example, after a long, hectic day at work, you may want to use cannabis to relax, whereas pain relief may be your goal if you've suffered a physical injury.

After identifying your desired experience, you'll find it easier to match the product, amount, and delivery method to best hit that target. If the desired effect is an uplifting experience in a social setting with friends, smoking flower may be the best choice. If relaxation at the end of a busy day is the outcome, similar to a glass of wine with dinner, perhaps a soothing cannabis tea or bath would be best to deliver the desired result.

Considering the chemical composition of products

Whether you're smoking flower/bud, vaping oil, consuming edibles or tinctures, or using a cannabis lotion, consider the chemical composition of the products. Different blends of cannabinoids, terpenes, herbs, and other ingredients produce very different effects that can vary among individuals.

Knowing your strains

Numerous strains (breeds) of cannabis plants exist, but they all originate from two primary strains: indica (sometimes referred to as "in da couch" for its sedative properties) and sativa (a more stimulating strain). See Chapter 2 for more about the different strains. Table 8-1 compares the general effects from these two major strains.

Indica and sativa are only two of many strains. These two primary strains have been cross bred to create numerous hybrids with colorful names, such as Blue Dream, Pineapple Express, AK-47, Chernobyl, and Tangerine Dream. To add to the variety, these strains come in numerous *phenotypes* — variations resulting from the interaction of the plant's genotype (nature) and environment (nurture).

TABLE 8-1 **Indica and Sativa Compared**

Strain	Qualities
Indica	Nighttime use
	Metal relaxation (sedative)
	Muscle relaxation
	Decreased nausea
	Pain relief
	Appetite stimulation
Sativa	Daytime use
	Stimulant (improved focus and creativity)
	Anti-anxiety
	Anti-depressant
	Chronic-pain relief

TIP

To find out more about the various strains and phenotypes and their effects, check out the Cannabis Strain Explorer at Leafly: www.leafly.com/explore. For a specific recommendation, describe the effect you desire to your budtender, who can suggest various strains that are likely to do the trick.

REMEMBER

Evaluating products by strain is only one way, and not necessarily the best way, to determine whether a product will deliver the desired effects. You may find that cannabinoid concentrations and ratios and terpene profiles, as discussed in the following two sections, provide a better indication of the effect a product is likely to have. However, strains provide a quick and easy way to reference and talk about different products, especially if you've discovered certain strains you really like.

Checking out cannabinoid ratios and amounts

Cannabinoids are the primary active ingredients in all cannabis products, so the ratios and quantities of the different cannabinoids provide a fairly accurate indication of what you can expect from any given product. Although cannabis contains about 100 cannabinoids (by some estimates), only two (THC and CBD) are responsible for delivering a majority of the benefits (and any adverse effects) and only two others are notable at this time:

>> **Tetrahydrocannabinol (THC):** THC takes most of the credit for producing the euphoric high associated with cannabis. It's strongly psychoactive, meaning it changes brain function, which can result in alterations in mood, memory, perception, thinking, and behavior.

>> **Cannabidiol (CBD):** CBD can help alleviate symptoms of certain medical conditions, such as pain, inflammation, and anxiety, without the intoxicating effects associated with THC. In fact, CBD tends to modulate the psychoactive effects of THC.

>> **Cannabinol (CBN):** When THC oxidizes, it converts to CBN, which decreases the concentration of THC. CBN is a fairly strong sedative that provides other potential benefits. It can be helpful as a sleep aid, pain reliever, antibacterial, anti-inflammatory, anti-convulsive, and appetite stimulant and has been shown to promote bone growth.

>> **Cannabigerol (CBG):** CBG is a precursor (building block) of THC and CBD. Like CBD, it's not intoxicating, and it may help with a host of medical conditions, including glaucoma, inflammatory bowel disease, Huntington's disease, cancer, bacterial infections, cachexia (muscle wasting), and bladder dysfunction.

REMEMBER

See Chapter 2 for additional details about the different cannabinoids.

When shopping for cannabis products, examine the amount of each cannabinoid in the product and their ratios. The CBD-to-THC ratio is particularly important and should be included on the packaging of any cannabis product. Ratios can be broken down into the following three categories:

>> **THC dominant:** High THC and low to no CBD produces the intoxicating, euphoric high associated with cannabis. However, higher ratios of THC have a greater potential to produce the adverse side effects described in the earlier section "Recognizing the Health and Safety Risks."

>> **Balanced:** Balanced blends of CBD and THC are psychoactive, but less so than THC-dominant products. The CBD tends to lessen the intoxicating effect of the THC, and the two cannabinoids may work synergistically to enhance the overall experience.

>> **CBD dominant:** High CBD and low to no THC products are primarily for those who seek the medicinal benefits of CBD without the intoxicating effects of THC. However, even if you're consuming cannabis purely for medicinal purposes, a little THC added to the CBD can improve its effectiveness.

REMEMBER

Ratios tell you nothing about the *amount* of each cannabinoid in a product. Also check the amount per serving if you're purchasing adult recreational products and the total amount of each cannabinoid (typically in milligrams) in the entire package. When dosing, pay particular attention to the amount of THC, because consuming too much may increase the risk of adverse effects. High doses of CBD are unlikely to produce any serious adverse effects.

Taking a spin on the terpene wheel

Terpenes are the volatile aromatic compounds that give different strains and even individual plants their unique aromas (see Chapter 2). (Terpenes are part of products and natural substances not exclusive to cannabis.) Combining different terpenes with different cannabinoids produces what's referred to as an *entourage effect* — the synergy of all ingredients in a cannabis product that produce the unique experience associated with that product. Think of the combination in terms of wine: CBD and THC content is like a wine's alcohol content, but each wine has its own aroma, flavor, acidity, and texture, which are comparable to the characteristics of terpenes.

Table 8-2 lists and describes the eight most prevalent terpenes in cannabis.

TABLE 8-2	Common Terpenes		
Terpene	Aroma	Found in	Benefits
Caryophyllene (CYE)	Pepper, spicy, woody, cloves	Black pepper, cinnamon, cloves	Anti-inflammatory Pain reliever Protects cells lining the digestive tract
Humulene (HUM)	Earthy, woody	Basil, cloves, coriander, hops	Appetite suppressant
Limonene (LME)	Lemon	Citrus fruits	Mood elevation Stress relief Reduces acid reflux Anti-anxiety
Linalool (LNL)	Floral	Lavender	Calming Sedating Anesthetic Anti-convulsant Pain reliever Anti-anxiety
Myrcene (MYR)	Earthy, herbal, cloves	Mango, lemongrass, thyme, hops	Calming Sedating Enhances THC's psychoactivity Muscle relaxant

Terpene	Aroma	Found in	Benefits
Ocimene (OCM)	Sweet, herbal, woody	Basil, pepper, parsley, mint, mangoes, orchids	Antiviral
			Antifungal
			Antiseptic
			Decongestant
			Antibacterial
Terpinolene (TPE)	Floral, herbal, pine	Lilac, lime blossoms	Calming
			Sedating
α-Pinene (PNE)	Pine	Pine needs, rosemary, basil, parsley, dill	Mental alertness
			Memory retention
			Anti-inflammatory
			Anti-bacterial

TIP

Terpene characteristics and benefits are often presented in the form of a terpene wheel. You can find numerous terpene wheels online by searching for "terpene wheel."

Sampling other ingredients

Cannabis is commonly combined with other ingredients to intensify the effects of the cannabis or of the other ingredients and enhance the consumer experience. Other ingredients commonly added to cannabis products include tobacco, coffee, tea, chocolate, alcohol, herbs, and spices.

Comparing methods of consumption

How you consume cannabis can have a tremendous impact on the way it affects you, including the speed and intensity of your response and the overall sensation. In Chapter 7, we describe a variety of ways to consume cannabis. Table 8-3 lists your options and presents pros and cons of each to provide you with a quick reference guide for choosing a method that's most conducive to the desired effect in any given situation.

REMEMBER

Some people have a favorite consumption method they rely on exclusively. Others like to switch it up or use different methods for different purposes or in different situations; for example, smoking socially and vaping when alone.

TABLE 8-3 **Comparing Consumption Methods**

Consumption Method	Pros	Cons
Smoking	Fastest acting	Irritates the lungs
	Intense sensation	Smell lingers
	Lots of variety	Not discreet
	Great for social situations	Somewhat complicated
Vaping	Discreet	May be more expensive than smoking
	Portable	Less variety (than smoking)
	Easier on the lungs than smoking	Less intense onset
	Smoother hits	
	Easy to use	
	Fast acting	
Edibles	Discreet	Slow acting
	Long-lasting	Highest calorie option
	Easy to use	Difficulty taking enough without taking too much
	Strong effect on both mind and body	
Topicals	Discreet	Non-intoxicating
	Localized	
	Non-intoxicating	
Transdermal patches	Discreet	Expensive
	Localized and full body	Weak or non-intoxicating
	Timed release	
Tinctures and pills	Discreet	Slower acting than smoking or vaping
	Easy dosing	
	Faster acting than edibles	
	Easy to use	

Accounting for other medications or substances used

While some medication may have little to no known interaction with marijuana, others are well known to intensify its effects, and many can have unintended consequences based on the type of cannabis and an individual's health. For example, some strains or blends can increase a person's blood pressure raising the risk of heart attack or stroke in vulnerable individuals.

WARNING

Don't mix marijuana with alcohol or other psychoactive substances. If you have a history or family history of any medical conditions or you take any medications (prescription or over-the-counter) or supplements, consult your physician before using cannabis.

Examining your body's biochemistry

Two people who consume the same cannabis at the same dose in the same way at the same place and time can have a vastly different experience. These differences can be attributed primarily to variations in their biology and chemical makeup (and perhaps in their emotional state or mind-set, as well). Factors that may impact your biochemistry and thereby influence the experience you have include the following:

» **Age:** Many users report that their experience with cannabis has changed over time; for example, cannabis that once helped them relax now makes them feel anxious, or cannabis that once made them paranoid now makes them feel more creative.

» **Gender:** Cannabis appears to affect men and women differently, although the research in this area is limited. For example, in small doses, cannabis seems to increase sexual desire in women, whereas in men, smoking or vaping cannabis reduces sexual desire and sperm production.

» **Recent meals:** Whether you've eaten anything before consuming cannabis and what you've eaten can impact its effects, especially with edibles. Consuming cannabis on an empty stomach increases the rate at which it is absorbed, thus increasing the potential risk of anxiety and paranoia. Certain foods may intensify the effects, whereas others modulate the effects; for example, mangoes are thought to intensify the high, whereas lemon is thought to lessen it.

» **Body composition:** Your height and weight, or more accurately your ratio of muscle mass to fat-soluble tissue may impact the onset time and the intensity and duration of the effects. THC binds to fat, which is why meals can impact the effects of cannabis. Your body's makeup may also have an impact. It may also be involved in determining how long THC may be identified in your body through testing.

» **Altitude:** The effects of high altitude together with the effects of the cannabis itself can make you *feel* higher, so if you're consuming at a high-altitude location, particularly a location you're unaccustomed to, start lower and go slower to find your sweet spot. This is a recognizable effect with alcohol, as well.

- » **Genetic disposition:** Genes (heredity) play a major role in how any given individual responds to cannabis. Just as amphetamines (stimulants) tend to calm people who have attention deficit hyperactivity disorder (ADHD), a cannabis strain that makes one person anxious may have a calming effect on another.

- » **Consumption frequency (tolerance):** Regular heavy cannabis users build up a tolerance for it. Over time, you may find that you need higher doses to experience the same effects.

- » **Susceptibility to certain mental health conditions:** Certain people are more susceptible to certain mental health conditions (such as anxiety, depression, and psychosis) than others, so they may be more prone to experiencing adverse effects, especially at high doses.

Considering the environment or setting and your mood or mind-set

Just as a restaurant's ambience, the people you're dining with, and the person who's serving you all impact your enjoyment of your meal at a restaurant, the environment, the people you're with, and your own mood or mind-set influence your overall cannabis experience. Of course, if the cannabis doesn't suit your tastes, you're not going to have the greatest experience, but assuming it's the right product, and you're in an enjoyable setting with great people and are in a good place yourself, you can expect to have a delightful experience. On the other hand, if you're in an uncomfortable situation with unfamiliar people and are feeling uptight, you may have a terrible experience, even if you're consuming the right product.

REMEMBER

Start lower and go slower in unfamiliar situations with unfamiliar people or when trying any cannabis products you haven't used in the past. Also, if you know you're going to be consuming in an unfamiliar setting or with strangers, avoid trying any new products. If possible, bring your own product — one you've used in familiar and comfortable surroundings — so you're better able to anticipate your response to it.

Keeping Safety in Mind

With rights come responsibilities. Even in areas where cannabis is legal, you're expected and legally obligated to consume responsibly for the health and safety of yourself and others. Being a responsible consumer means no mixing cannabis with other drugs, medications, or psychoactive substances; using in moderation; making rational decisions; and staying home or using a designated driver when you're high or plan to become high. In this section, we provide additional guidance on how to consume cannabis responsibly.

Using cannabis in moderation

Moderation is the key to reaping the greatest benefits from cannabis and avoiding the worst of its potential adverse effects. Moderate use can also save you a good deal of money! As a general rule, moderation means taking the smallest amount necessary to achieve the desired effect. Here are some general guidelines for any given session (*sesh*):

>> 1–5 mg for beginning users

>> 5–10 mg for occasional users

>> 10–20 mg for frequent users

>> For medical use consult your doctor or other qualified healthcare provider

Making rational decisions

High doses of cannabis products with high concentrations of THC can impair your judgment, so you must decide to use your good judgment in dosing *before* becoming so intoxicated that you can no longer make rational decisions related to consumption and other important matters.

WARNING Don't consume marijuana to the point of becoming irrational. When your mental faculties are impaired, you're at a greater risk of making bad choices, such as driving under the influence, mixing alcohol with cannabis, and trusting the wrong people.

Committing to no impaired driving

WARNING Don't drive under the influence of marijuana, regardless of whether *you* think you're high. Stay home or plan ahead for transportation, for example, by choosing a designated driver or another means to get around. Driving under the influence of marijuana is both dangerous and illegal. (See Chapter 3 for more about steering clear of legal trouble when using cannabis.)

Dealing with Overconsumption

Cannabis is meant to be used for health and/or enjoyment. Overconsumption is neither healthy nor enjoyable. You want to find your sweet spot — the point at which you experience the maximum benefits of cannabis with little or no adverse effects. Overdo it, and you may pay the price by suffering one or more of the following consequences:

>> Rapid heart rate

>> Panic attack

>> Delusions or hallucinations

>> Confusion

>> Paranoia

>> Nausea or vomiting

>> Dry mouth

These symptoms are rarely, if ever, life threatening and typically subside a few hours after consumption stops, but they can ruin an otherwise enjoyable cannabis experience. In the following sections, we offer guidance on how to avoid and respond to an episode of overconsumption. But first, we draw the distinction between overconsumption and overdose.

Remember that overconsumption of THC, the psychotropic cannabinoid in marijuana, is not lethal. There has been no confirmed case of fatal THC consumption without any other substance involved.

Distinguishing overconsumption from overdose

The terms "over consumption" and "overdose" are not interchangeable. In the case of cannabis, humans can't overdose on THC because of human biology and the limited number of CB1 receptors in the brain, specifically in the medulla oblongata. In other words, physically overdosing on THC is impossible, and it's not even a concern with CBD because CBD isn't a psychoactive substance.

However, overconsumption of THC can occur, and, although it is not fatal on its own, it can be an awful and upsetting experience. The effects wear off in a few hours and hopefully convince the individual to avoid overconsuming in the future. As William Blake once wrote, "The road of excess leads to the palace of wisdom."

Avoiding overconsumption

Avoiding overconsumption is much more pleasant than recovering from it. Here are a few overconsumption avoidance tips:

>> Be especially careful when you're first starting out or are returning from a long absence from the product. You may not have a good feel for your tolerance level, and newer products may have higher amounts of THC than you were accustomed to in the past.

>> Avoid products with high concentrations of THC at first. Consider starting with more balanced products, such as those with a CBD-to-THC ratio of 1-to-1, and working up or down from there.

>> Start with a small dose, and avoid taking any more THC until that dose has had a chance to take effect, which can be as long as two hours for edibles.

>> Try smoking, vaping, or tinctures first to gauge your tolerance and get a feel for the ideal dose for you. The cannabis kicks in more quickly, so you don't have to wait so long to find the right dose. After identifying the dose that's right for you, you'll be better able to estimate accurate doses of other products.

It is best to make smart choices in consuming cannabis, especially when consuming for the first time or after a long absence from the product. Begin with a small dose and be committed to waiting for full effect before adding more THC.

Responding to overconsumption

Although avoiding overconsumption is the best course of action, overconsumption happens even to experienced users. If you or a fellow consumer experience this uncomfortable mishap, here are some suggestions on how to respond:

>> Stop consuming.

>> Remain calm. Those who really suffer the consequences of overconsumption are the ones who freak out. It's not the end of the world, and as long as you have not mixed substances, you can be confident that the experience will not be fatal on its own.

>> In an emergency situation, call 911 or have a sober friend take you to the emergency room. Emergency situations with cannabis-only use are uncommon, but they're more common when the cannabis is combined with other psychoactive substances, legal or illegal.

» Don't go it alone. Have someone who's sober (and preferably experienced with overconsumption) stay with you until the adverse effects subside.

» Take a fast-acting CBD-only product, which may help to prevent the side effects from worsening. CBD changes the shape of the THC molecules and keeps them from attaching to the CB1 receptors in the brain.

» Sniff some black pepper, but don't snort it. You can crack a couple peppercorns with your molars, roll the pieces around in your mouth, and then spit them out. Black pepper has terpenes that seem to have a similar effect as CBD. Sniffing a lemon may also help.

» Lie down in a quiet room or with some calming music. Sleep it off, if possible.

» Drink plenty of water.

» Eat a little something (not more brownie!).

Within a few hours of stopping consumption, the symptoms should start to subside, and within 24 hours you'll start to feel like your old self.

Considering Underage Development

The growing trend toward legalizing marijuana has increased its acceptance and availability among adults. This trend has also raised the concern (and fear) among many people that cannabis will become more accessible to and popular among under-aged individuals. Such concerns are certainly valid. The science shows that consuming marijuana under the age of 21 can negatively impact brain development and IQ. In addition, decision making and experience are not fully developed in minors, placing them at a greater risk of making poor choices regarding cannabis consumption.

REMEMBER

However, these concerns must be placed in the proper context. State agencies are reporting record low teen marijuana consumption across the U.S., without major increases in states with legalization.

As with alcohol, prescription medications, and other substances that are potentially harmful to minors, those who use cannabis have a responsibility to keep these substances out of the hands of minors. Parents and educators also have a responsibility to provide age-appropriate guidance on the potential benefits and adverse effects of marijuana, so young people are equipped to make good choices when they come of age.

Following are some guidelines to keep children safe while preparing them to make good decisions when they can legally consume cannabis:

>> Don't use cannabis if you're pregnant or breastfeeding unless advised to do so by and under the careful supervision of a doctor or other qualified healthcare provider. Cannabis consumption may negatively impact the health of the fetus or infant.

>> Use the same safeguards you would use with alcohol and medications to prevent/discourage access to cannabis stored in your home. This can range from setting rules and boundaries to keeping your cannabis under lock and key.

>> Model the desired consumption habits and behaviors you would like to see your children develop when they come of age.

>> When educating children about marijuana, avoid the hype and the hysteria. Base your talks on credible, scientific information and research.

>> Adhere to the age restrictions and guidelines established in your jurisdiction. Prohibit minors from using marijuana recreationally, and allow minors to use it medically only under the direction and supervision of a doctor or other qualified healthcare provider.

WARNING

Unless you're a parent or guardian permitted by law to provide cannabis to a minor who has a medical marijuana registry card, giving or selling cannabis to minors or helping them buy it is a federal offense. Don't do it.

3

Reaping the Potential Benefits of Medical Marijuana

Discover the potential benefits of cannabis for symptom relief for a long list of medical conditions — from acne and arthritis to sexual dysfunction and stress.

Find general guidance for choosing the right cannabis product(s) for possible symptom relief associated with specific medical conditions.

Recognize potential adverse side effects, so you can tell when the cannabis may be making you sick.

Discover how to use cannabis to provide potential symptom relief for common medical conditions in pets (with the guidance of your veterinarian, of course!).

Explore products, delivery methods, and dosing challenges for your pets, so you can maximize the benefits while minimizing any adverse reactions.

Chapter 9

Using Marijuana for Medicinal Purposes

People have been using cannabis medicinally for centuries to relieve symptoms of a wide range of health conditions, and now doctors are beginning to recommend cannabis to patients with certain conditions in states where medical marijuana is legal. Cannabis is thought to have several medicinal properties that make it potentially useful in symptom relief:

» Analgesic (relieves pain)

» Anti-angiogenic and anti-proliferative (preventing the spread of cancer cells)

» Antibacterial

» Anticonvulsant

» Antiemetic (relieves nausea and vomiting)

» Anti-inflammatory

» Antioxidant

» Appetite stimulant

» Bronchodilator

>> Immunomodulatory (helps to regulate immune system function)

>> Neuroprotective (protects nerve cells, including brain cells)

In this chapter, we present a number of health conditions whose symptoms cannabis may be helpful in relieving, along with general guidelines on strains or CBD-to-THC ratios that may be more appropriate for each condition. To present a balanced view, we also call your attention to possible adverse side effects associated with cannabis.

WARNING

The information in this chapter is not a replacement for professional medical advice. Consult your doctor for diagnosis and treatment options and use cannabis medicinally only under the direction and direct supervision of your doctor. Don't try to self-medicate.

REMEMBER

A physician in the U.S. is not allowed to "prescribe" cannabis or provide a sample as they can for a pharmaceutical, but only recommend that a patient consider it as an option. While health insurance covers some FDA-approved drugs derived from cannabis and produced by the pharmaceutical industry, coverage depends on your individual plan. Insurance companies are skeptical of paying for medical marijuana and are waiting for more clinical research, so if you choose to use cannabis expect to have to pay out-of-pocket.

Understanding the Current and Ongoing Status of Medical Marijuana

Cannabis has gained increasing acceptance due in large part to the discoveries surrounding its use in providing potential symptom relief for individuals suffering from illness, injury, and various disease states. Traditional scientific research has been taking place, but slowly, and for those suffering too slowly to wait for relief.

Much of our understanding of what works in some situations and for some patients is anecdotal. Patients first exploring the possibility of cannabis use for relief often rely heavily on the budtender at their nearby medical dispensary. Physicians themselves often lament the fact that they're not certain how to direct their patients regarding strain, consumption method, amount, potency, frequency, or ratios of CBD to THC. A growing number of medical conferences are trying to address this lack of understanding.

MOMENTUM IS BUILDING

Israel is generally acknowledged as the world leader in cannabis research. In the 1960s Raphael Mechoulam discovered the cannabinoid THC and the endocannabinoid system and he continues to play an important role in moving the science forward, identifying new discoveries, and helping millions around the world to benefit from cannabis.

The Netherlands, Uruguay, the Czech Republic, Canada, Spain, and the UK are also actively researching cannabinoids and cannabis. Both Uruguay and Canada have federal legalization of adult recreational marijuana. Scientists in the U.S. are also involved in active research, and those in legalized states are striving to do more. However, legally in the U.S. cannabis for research can only be procured from the University of Mississippi, and researchers acknowledge that the potency and quality of the product is nowhere near the levels available from commercial vendors and dispensaries, which further limits their ability to conduct applicable research.

Some scientists are working around these legal barriers by asking test subjects to purchase their own products, and in some cases such as at the University of Colorado at Boulder, researchers are bringing the lab to the subjects in a van to comply with government rules yet still do valuable work.

With a world of scientists eager to reveal the truth about the potential medicinal properties of cannabis and its potential clinical benefits, we can all look forward to a growing body of more reliable evidence.

As scientific evidence builds from more reliable clinical studies, more people around the world are turning to cannabis as a potentially viable alternative to synthetic medications. Research leaders in the area are making great strides and moving the body of work forward regardless of the legal challenges.

Choosing Medical Marijuana Products

REMEMBER

Medical and adult recreational marijuana are the same. The only differences between the two are how they're taxed, where they're sold, and limitations on the amount a consumer is able to purchase or possess at one time. Another difference is related to the various factors you should consider when shopping for medical marijuana products, including the following factors:

>> **Speed of onset:** You may want to opt for faster-acting consumption methods, such as smoking, vaping, or taking a tincture sublingually, instead of edibles, which take much longer to produce the full effect.

- >> **Effectiveness and duration of relief:** Edibles and tinctures may be more effective than products that are smoked or vaped because the body may absorb more of the cannabinoids and terpenes. Edibles and tinctures may also provide longer-lasting relief because they take longer to eliminate from the body.

- >> **Cannabinoid content:** Different cannabinoids affect different cannabinoid receptors (See Chapter 2), so some cannabinoids may be more effective for certain illnesses than others. For example, CBG may be more effective in treating fungal infections, whereas CBD, CBC, CBN, and THC are more closely associated with pain relief. (See Figure 9-1.) Products with different terpene profiles may also contribute to the overall effectiveness of a product. (Terpenes are the aromatic substances in cannabis and other plants.) When choosing a product, be sure to match its cannabinoid and terpene profiles to the type of relief you're seeking.

- >> **CBD-to-THC ratio:** If you're looking for the potential medical benefits without the intoxicating effects, consider products with higher CBD-to-THC ratios, such as 1:1 or even up to 50:1. You can even find CBD-only products, but having a little bit of THC may be beneficial, because some evidence suggests that the two cannabinoids work synergistically to enhance the effects of one another.

THC is the psychoactive component of cannabis; it produces the intoxicating effect. You can buy products that contain THC only at a dispensary. CBD is not psychoactive. Hemp-derived CBD-only products are federally legal and may be sold online and shipped over state lines, but they may be illegal in some jurisdictions.

- >> **Localized or systemic relief:** If you're looking for localized relief, for example of pain and inflammation, a lotion or cream may provide the relief you need without making you high. On the other hand, if you're looking for whole-body relief or your symptoms are internal, smoking, vaping, edibles, sublinguals or transdermal patches may be the better choice.

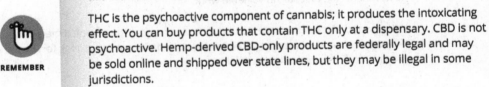

You may not always be able to select a specific strain or the precise cannabinoid and terpene profiles for your needs, but by understanding the basics of which cannabinoids and terpenes are generally best for the condition(s) you have, you can more effectively consult with your budtender to find one or more suitable products in stock. Don't be shy; your budtender has probably heard it all and may have some suggestions as well as anecdotal experience from consulting with another patient with similar issues.

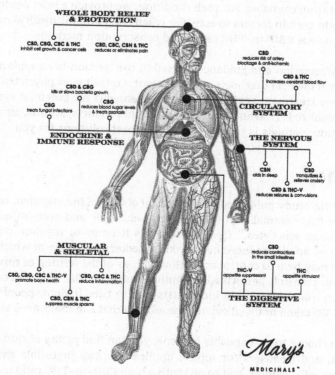

CANNABIS MAN

WHOLE BODY RELIEF & PROTECTION

CBD, CBG, CBC & THC
inhibit cell growth & cancer cells

CBD, CBC, CBN & THC
reduces or eliminates pain

CBD
reduces risk of artery blockage & anti-ischemic

CBD & THC
increases cerebral blood flow

CIRCULATORY SYSTEM

CBD & CBG
kills or slows bacteria growth

CBG
treats fungal infections

CBG
reduces blood sugar levels & treats psoriasis

ENDOCRINE & IMMUNE RESPONSE

THE NERVOUS SYSTEM

CBN
aids in sleep

CBD
tranquilizes & relieves anxiety

CBD & THC-V
reduces seizures & convulsions

MUSCULAR & SKELETAL

CBD, CBG, CBC & THC-V
promote bone health

CBD, CBC & THC
reduce inflammation

CBD, CBN & THC
suppress muscle spasms

CBD
reduces contractions in the small intestines

THC-V
appetite suppressant

THC
appetite stimulant

THE DIGESTIVE SYSTEM

Mary's
MEDICINALS™

Photo courtesy of MM Technology Holdings, LLC.

FIGURE 9-1:
Match the cannabinoids to your needs.

Seeking Symptom Relief for Specific Conditions

Because researchers are still gathering data on most of the conditions below, the medical community has not officially recommended the use of cannabis to treat or cure medical conditions. As of the writing of this book, most evidence that supports the use of cannabis in providing symptomatic relief for any of the medical conditions covered in this section is anecdotal (stories from patients or doctors). To decide whether cannabis may be helpful to you, discuss your treatment options with your physician.

In this section, we present some of the ailments and medical conditions that may benefit from cannabis. For each condition, we provide a brief description of it and highlight certain factors to consider when shopping for medical marijuana products, such as CBD-to-THC ratios and consumption methods.

WARNING

The information and guidance offered in this section is no replacement for professional medical diagnosis and treatment. Consult your physician before starting any new treatment regime. Also, using cannabis for potential symptom relief is individualized. Trial and error with different products, strains, amounts, and consumption methods is required to find the best solutions for you.

Acne

In a 2014 study published in the *Journal of Clinical Investigation*, researchers concluded that "cannabidiol (CBD) exerts sebostatic and anti-inflammatory effects on human sebocytes." (*Sebostatic* means it helps to regulate the production of *sebum* — an oil produced by the skin.) Reducing the rate at which sebum is produced may help to control acne. However, as of the writing of this book, we could find no research performed on human subjects. The only evidence from actual human trials comes from individuals who've tried it. Some people also claim that that CBD taken orally alleviates the anxiety that can make acne worse.

If you choose to try cannabis for acne, you can find plenty of skin creams, lotions, soaps, and cleansers for topical application. Any ingestible cannabis products (flower, oils, edibles, and so on) with a high CBD-to-THC ratio may help calm the anxiety that may exacerbate acne breakouts for some individuals. Topical lotions may also reduce inflammation and reduce the appearance or height of a pimple.

WARNING

While CBD isn't likely to cause skin irritation or adverse reactions, other ingredients in a product may do so. Be sure to read the label and avoid any products that contain substances you're allergic or sensitive to.

Addiction

Research is heating up around the possibility of using cannabis to treat addictions to more dangerous substances, including cocaine and crack, heroin and other opioids, and alcohol. In a 2018 study published in the journal *Addiction*, researchers found that "State-wide medical cannabis legalization appears to have been associated with reductions in both prescriptions and dosages of Schedule III (but not Schedule II) opioids received by Medicaid enrollees in the United States."

In another study published in 2014 in the *Journal of the American Medical Association* (*JAMA*), researchers concluded that "Medical cannabis laws are associated with significantly lower state-level opioid overdose mortality rates." Case in point, a few years after adult recreational legalization, Denver reported a six percent drop in opioid overdose deaths. Other studies have shown that CBD has successfully broken the cycle of addiction from alcohol and cocaine in rats.

To be fair, one study found that early onset and long-term cannabis use "increase the severity of cocaine withdrawal during detoxification."

REMEMBER

Those prone to addiction may be wise to stick with hemp-derived CBD products that document zero levels of THC content. CBD is generally cited as the cannabinoid that may be most helpful for weaning people off potentially more dangerous and addictive substances.

REMEMBER

Due to the lack of receptors in the brain, specifically the medulla oblongata, you will not become physically addicted to cannabis itself. However, you can become addicted to the emotional experience or the routine of consuming cannabis.

Alzheimer's

Alzheimer's disease (AD) affects nearly 30 million people around the world and is the leading cause of dementia. Several pre-clinical studies suggest that the endocannabinoid system protects against certain pathological events associated with the onset and development of AD, including inflammation, oxidative stress, and *excitotoxicity* (a process that damages neurons). A number of clinical trials have shown that THC slows production and reduces the buildup of amyloid beta proteins in the brain, which are believed to be a leading cause of AD. One study published in the *Journal of Alzheimer's Disease* concluded, "Adding medical cannabis oil (MCO) containing THC as an add-on to pharmacotherapy is safe and a promising treatment option." Other benefits may include appetite enhancement and reductions in anxiety for patients.

WARNING

While certain cannabinoids may help to manage some of the behavioral symptoms of Alzheimer's and dementia (for example, agitation and aggression), heavy, long-term use of cannabis may be associated with diminished memory and thinking. In addition, as of the writing of this book, no evidence shows that cannabis can help prevent the onset of Alzheimer's or dementia.

If you or a loved one suffers from Alzheimer's or other forms of dementia, consult a doctor who specializes in this area and has experience recommending cannabis to patients who suffer from these conditions. Combining cannabis with other medications and getting the right ratios and concentrations of cannabinoids are crucial. Otherwise, adding cannabis to the mix can cause more harm than good.

While THC is most commonly cited as the cannabinoid that may be most beneficial, a whole-plant product that contains a combination of CBD and THC may be best. For patients who aren't comfortable smoking cannabis, edibles or transdermal patches may be two of the more attractive consumption methods.

Amyotrophic lateral sclerosis (ALS)

Also known as Lou Gehrig's disease, *amyotrophic lateral sclerosis* is a neurodegenerative disease that affects nerve cells in the brain and spinal column mostly involved in voluntary muscle movement. Evidence of the benefits of cannabis in helping to alleviate symptoms of ALS are mixed:

>> Some pre-clinical evidence shows a possible connection between the endocannabinoid system (ECS) and disease progression. Under certain conditions, elevating cannabinoid levels has been reported to "modestly delay disease progression and prolong survival in these animal models."

>> Some ALS patients have reported that consuming cannabis decreased muscle cramps and *fasciculations* (spontaneous muscle contractions involving a small number of muscle fibers just below the skin).

>> In one small four-week study, "doses of 2.5 to 10 mg per day of dronabinol (a synthetic form of THC) were associated with improvements in sleep and appetite, but not cramps or fasciculations."

>> A two-week study of patients taking 10 mg daily of dronabinol showed no improvement in sleep, appetite, cramps, or fasciculations."

Although the current, very limited research doesn't show any clear benefits of using cannabis in the treatment of ALS, clinical trials have shown that "dronabinol was well-tolerated with few reported side effects in this patient population at the tested dosages."

Cannabis' antioxidant, anti-inflammatory and neuroprotective properties may have some potential to slow the progression of ALS It can improve cellular energy and help prevent cell death as well as reduce saliva, improve sleep, increase appetite, reduce pain, and relax muscles.

Due to the need for the "entourage effect" provided by the whole plant, cannabis products that include terpenes, CBD, and THC may be most valuable. However, smoking may exacerbate some ALS symptoms, so edibles, tinctures, and transdermal patches may be better options for some patients. Sativa strains with high-energy terpenes should probably be avoided and indicas preferred.

Anxiety

According to the Anxiety and Depression Association of America, nearly 40 million people in the U.S. (approximately 18 percent of the population) suffer from anxiety disorders. Certain studies have shown that medical cannabis may be helpful in relieving anxiety:

>> In 2017, researchers at the University of Illinois at Chicago and the University of Chicago reported that low levels of THC (about 7.5 mg) reduces stress while slightly larger doses (in the range of about 12.5 mg) actually increased anxiety.

>> Early studies show that certain components of cannabis, particularly CBD, may be useful in managing the level of the neurotransmitter GABA in the brain. Benzodiazepines, a class of prescription medications commonly used to reduce anxiety, also target GABA but are potentially more dangerous than cannabis.

WARNING

If you're using cannabis to alleviate anxiety, do so only as directed by your doctor. Proper dosing is crucial for reducing anxiety and not worsening it. Avoid high-potency THC products. Although THC may be helpful in alleviating anxiety, high doses may exacerbate it. Consider leaning more toward products that have a higher CBD-to-THC ratio and higher levels of myrcene in their terpene profiles.

Appetite loss

Cannabis has a strong reputation among consumers for increasing appetite (giving them "the munchies"). Plenty of scientific evidence supports the effectiveness of cannabis in stimulating appetite and combating weight loss and malnutrition, which weaken the body when it's trying to combat illness. These properties make cannabis potentially useful for certain patients with AIDS, cancer, anorexia, and other disorders, and for those receiving medical treatments, such as chemotherapy, that result in undesired weight loss. Specifically, medical cannabis has been shown to increase levels of ghrelin and leptin — two hormones that play a key role in regulating hunger — without significantly changing insulin levels. In one study, AIDS patients gained an average of 10 pounds after a year of being on dronabinol — a synthetic form of THC.

For medical use, products that contain THC and cannabinol (CBN) may be the best choices. Both may stimulate appetite and CBN may do so with little to no psychoactive (intoxicating effect). CBN forms over time when THC breaks down. Though you can simply allow your cannabis to age and dry, a growing number of CBN-specific products are on the market. Mary's Medicinals (www.marysmedicinals.com) has a family of CBN products — CBN Transdermal Patch, CBN Transdermal Gel Pen (a patented product), CBN Distillate Vape, CBN PAX Pod and 1:1 CBN:CBD Sublingual Tincture.

Rapid onset of effects when smoking often makes this the preferred consumption method of patients looking for quick relief. However, other applications such as the transdermal patch may offer longer term relief in a time-released form that's more convenient. Consult your doctor and budtender to evaluate your options.

Arthritis

According to the Arthritis Society, about two thirds of Canadians who use cannabis for medical purposes do so to help manage arthritis symptoms, which makes sense — cannabis has analgesic, anti-inflammatory, and immunomodulatory properties. (*Rheumatoid arthritis* an autoimmune disorder in which the immune system attacks the joints. *Osteoarthritis*, which is much more common, results from the erosion of cartilage over time.) According to the Arthritis Foundation, severe arthritis can result in chronic pain, an inability to perform daily activities, and permanent adverse changes in the joints. Some types of arthritis may also negatively affect the heart, eyes, lungs, kidneys, and skin.

Cannabis has anti-inflammation and pain reduction properties that have been demonstrated to have strong positive effects for arthritis suffers. Several studies also reveal a link between the endocannabinoid system (ECS) and bone growth, which points to the potential of using cannabis to promote bone health or at least prevent bone loss.

REMEMBER

Most arthritis suffers find that direct application of cannabis-infused salves and lotions to affected joints works best. Products should be high in CBD but also contain some THC to drive the CBD effects into the molecules and improve effectiveness. Topical products such as lotions even with small amounts of THC won't get you high.

Asthma

Asthma is a chronic disease in which the airways narrow and swell and produce excess mucus, which makes breathing difficult and may result in a tightening of the chest, coughing, wheezing, and shortness of breath. Cannabis has anti-inflammatory and anti-spasmodic properties, which may offer some relief to asthma sufferers. Unlike cigarette smoke, which constricts the bronchial passageways, cannabis, whether smoked or vaped, expands them, potentially relieving many of the symptoms associated with the condition. CBD and other components of cannabis may also help to alleviate anxiety, which is often associated with asthma attacks.

REMEMBER

In one large study published in the *Journal of the American Medical Association*, researchers concluded that "Occasional and low cumulative marijuana use was not associated with adverse effects on pulmonary (lung) function." However, if you have asthma, you may be wise to consume cannabis using methods other than smoking it, such as vaping. A vaporizer that sends warm air across the cannabis is extremely efficient because it doesn't burn the product and would not include any smoke as an irritant for those during an attack. Edibles, in particular warm cannabis teas, may provide symptom relief as well.

Attention deficit hyperactivity disorder (ADHD)

The National Institute of Mental Health (NIMH) describes attention-deficit/hyperactivity disorder (ADHD) as "a brain disorder marked by an ongoing pattern of inattention and/or hyperactivity-impulsivity that interferes with functioning or development."

Cannabis may provide relief to those living with ADHD because it raises dopamine levels in the brain. Some studies have shown that products with a 1:1 CBD-to-THC ratio improved behavior and cognition in ADHD patients. It may also help with anxiety and depression found in some people suffering with ADHD. The consumption method of choice varies depending on personal preferences and perhaps the need for discretion.

WARNING

Don't play doctor with your children. If your child is diagnosed with ADHD or you suspect that your child has the condition, consult your child's doctor to discuss your concerns and treatment options.

Autism spectrum disorders

Condition: According to the National Institute of Mental Health, autism spectrum disorder (ASD) is "a developmental disorder that affects communication and behavior." It's commonly considered a "developmental disorder" because symptoms generally appear in the first two years of life.

Most of the data supporting the use of cannabis in treating ASD is anecdotal evidence from parents claiming to successfully manage their child's symptoms with cannabis. Some initial studies in Israel have indicated that THC binding to the CB2 receptor and the management of neuro-inflammation through the endocannabinoid system have shown therapeutic value for autism. However, very few research studies are underway due to the fact that most autism spectrum disorders appear in early childhood and therefore test subjects would be children.

WARNING

If your child has been diagnosed as having an ASD, consult your child's doctor for treatment options. If your child's doctor recommends a trial of cannabis, be sure to discuss which strains, blends, and consumption methods may be most appropriate. A strain such as *Charlotte's Web strain*, which is high in CBD and has little to no THC may be most appropriate. (For more about Charlotte's Web strain, see the later section "Epilepsy.")

Autoimmune disorders

According to the National Institute of Allergy and Infectious Disease (NIAID), "More than 80 diseases occur as a result of the immune system attacking the body's own organs, tissues, and cells. Some of the more common autoimmune diseases include type 1 diabetes, rheumatoid arthritis, systemic lupus erythematosus, and inflammatory bowel disease."

Some studies suggest that cannabis may help to regulate the immune system and to reduce inflammation, which, if true, would likely make it effective in alleviating symptoms of autoimmune disorders and possibly reducing the resulting damage to organs, tissues and cells.

According to a report published in The National Center for Biotechnology Information from the U.S. National Library of Medicine, National Institute of Health, "The fact that both CB1 and CB2 receptors have been found on immune cells suggests that cannabinoids play an important role in the regulation of the immune system. Recent studies demonstrated that administration of THC into mice triggered marked apoptosis [cell death] in T cells and dendritic cells, resulting in immuno-suppression. In addition, several studies showed that cannabinoids downregulate cytokine and chemokine production and, in some models, upregulate T-regulatory cells (Tregs) as a mechanism to suppress inflammatory responses."

Both CBD and THC have anti-inflammatory properties that may be valuable in combatting symptoms of a variety of autoimmune disorders. Products that contain non-psychoactive cannabinoids THCa and CBDa can also be useful. The goal is to harness the power of the endocannabinoid system in down-regulating a hyperactive immune system to restore homeostasis (a healthy balance).

REMEMBER

Consulting a doctor who specializes in treating autoimmune disorders is essential to identify and treat the underlying cause(s) of any autoimmune disorder, which may include imbalances in gut microbes, exposure to mold or other environmental toxins, nutritional deficiencies, genetic susceptibilities, and more. Don't settle for symptomatic relief. Find a doctor who won't stop until he identifies the root cause(s).

Bipolar disorder

Bipolar disorder, also referred to as "manic depression," is a brain disorder that causes unusual shifts in mood, energy, activity levels, and the ability to carry out day-to-day tasks. Because cannabis, especially the THC in it, affects the brain and impacts mood, it may stabilize or destabilize mood and affect the brain in other positive or negative ways. Further complications may result from drug interactions between cannabis and pharmaceutical medications used to treat the condition.

WARNING

The one thing experts seem to agree on is that high-potency THC is contraindicated for people with bipolar disorder, because it increases the risk of triggering acute anxiety and paranoia in people who are more susceptible to those conditions.

Also, if you've been diagnosed as having bipolar disorder and you consume cannabis medicinally or recreationally, let your doctors know. They need to account for your cannabis use when prescribing medication, offering other medical advice, and providing therapy. For more about bipolar disorder, check out *Bipolar Disorder For Dummies*, by Candida Fink, MD.

Cachexia (Wasting)

Cachexia is physical weakness, wasting, and malnutrition usually associated with chronic disease, such as HIV/AIDS, cancer, chronic renal failure, and multiple sclerosis, and certain cancer treatments such as chemotherapy. Cachexia patients suffer from a severe lack of appetite and have challenges battling loss of muscle mass even if they're able to take in enough calories through food. They may experience nausea, fatigue, depression, lethargy, and a diminished quality of life.

Cannabis has *antiemetic* (anti-nausea) and appetite stimulant properties that make it possibly effective in treating cachexia. Specifically, THC and CBN.

For medical use, products that contain THC and cannabinol (CBN) may be the best choices. Both may stimulate appetite. CBN may do so with little to no psychoactive (intoxicating effect). CBN forms over time when THC breaks down. Though you can simply allow your cannabis to age and dry, a growing number of CBN-specific products are on the market. Mary's Medicinals (www.marysmedicinals.com) has a family of CBN products — CBN Transdermal Patch, CBN Transdermal Gel Pen (a patented product), CBN Distillate Vape, CBN PAX Pod and 1:1 CBN:CBD Sublingual Tincture.

Rapid onset of effects when smoking often makes this the preferred consumption method of patients looking for quick relief. However, other applications such as the transdermal patch may offer longer term relief in a time-released form that's more convenient. Consult your doctor and budtender to evaluate your options.

Cancer

Cancer is any disease in which abnormal cells divide without control and can invade nearby tissues and spread to other parts of the body through the blood and lymph systems (as in malignant forms of cancer).

Many cancer patients have reported finding relief in cannabis, both in supporting tumor reductions as well as battling adverse side effects from various medical treatments. THC can help relieve pain and nausea, reduce inflammation, and act as an antioxidant. Cannabinoids and terpenes, especially when blended with other botanical herbs, may also help patients relax and sleep.

Some evidence suggests that cannabis plays a role in killing cancer cells. More precisely, certain cannabinoids serve as messengers to trigger the body's natural cell signaling pathways that cause certain cells to kill themselves — a process referred to as *programmed cell death (PCD)* or *apoptosis*. PCD is the body's way of eliminating old and damaged cells. As a result, cannabis may help reduce tumor sizes, support other therapies in that effect, and help reduce metastasis of cancer cells to other areas of the body. In tumors, CBD has the ability to interfere with cellular communication as well as initiate apoptosis. Some research shows CBD helps to shut down cellular growth receptors in genes involved in aggressive metastasis.

WARNING

Cannabis hasn't been proven to be a miracle cure for cancer, despite the anecdotal evidence you can find online and the excitement over treatments such as Rick Simpson Oil (RSO). Discuss all treatment options with your oncologist, and if cannabis is recommended, ensure your products are produced cleanly and lab tested from reputable, legal dispensaries.

Some research suggests that a combination of THC and CBD may be most effective for controlling or reversing tumor growth, but no clear guidance is offered for specific CBD-to-THC ratios or terpene profiles. Your choice of strain, cannabinoids, and terpenes depends on the nature of the cancer and the symptoms you're experiencing; for example, pain, nausea, or insomnia.

Consider whole-plant products such as flower that you can vape to benefit from the *entourage effect* (the synergy of all the chemical compounds in the cannabis working together). Avoid smoking cannabis, though, because the combustion process releases tar and other carcinogens. Vape oil, transdermal patches, sublingual tinctures, and edibles are all options to consider. Lotions and salves may be more appropriate for skin cancers. Also, check the terpene wheel in Chapter 2, which can direct you in your selection beyond the strains of indica, sativa or hybrid for a more catered effect. Strains high in limonene are uplifting and have worked well for cancer patients.

Cannabinoid hyperemesis syndrome (CHS)

Daily, long-term cannabis users are at an increased risk of developing *cannabinoid hyperemesis syndrome (CHS)* — a rare condition that leads to repeated and severe bouts of vomiting. Cannabis typically reduces nausea and vomiting, but in some high frequency, long-term users, it has the opposite effect.

WARNING

If you're experiencing constant and repeated vomiting, stop consuming cannabis and seek medical attention immediately. Inform your doctor of how much and how frequently you consume cannabis and how long you've been doing so. Your condition may or may not be related to your cannabis consumption, but your doctor needs to know as much as possible to make an accurate diagnosis and provide the best treatment possible.

If you're diagnosed as having CHS, you'll probably need to stop all cannabis consumption for some period of time to recover. If you're using cannabis to combat symptoms of another disease state, discuss other options to manage symptoms and how long you'll need to abstain from cannabis.

Celiac disease and gluten sensitivity

Celiac disease is a serious autoimmune disorder in which the immune system reacts to *gluten* — a protein in wheat, barley, and rye. Symptoms include weight loss, vomiting, abdominal bloating, and persistent diarrhea or constipation. It affects about 1 in 100 people worldwide and about three million in the U.S. Far more people, about 18 million in the U.S. alone, have gluten sensitivity — a related condition that's less severe. People with celiac disease are advised to adopt a gluten-free diet. Even tiny amounts of gluten can trigger reactions in sensitive individuals. (Check out *Celiac Disease For Dummies*, by Ian Blumer and Sheila Crowe, for details.)

Cannabis can't cure celiac disease or gluten sensitivity, but it may help to alleviate some of the symptoms, including nausea, loss of appetite, vomiting, inflammation, and pain. It may also help to modulate immune system function and reduce the severity of muscle spasms.

REMEMBER

If you have symptoms of celiac disease or gluten sensitivity, consult your doctor or gastroenterologist. Don't merely try using cannabis, because it may mask the symptoms without addressing the underlying causes. In addition, although you may encounter anecdotal evidence from people claiming that cannabis "cured" their celiac disease, no solid scientific evidence supports these claims, and it's highly doubtful that cannabis can cure a hereditary illness.

If your doctor recommends cannabis, find out which strains are recommended. Whole-plant products or those that contain a higher CBD-to-THC ratio may be most appropriate.

WARNING

If you choose to consume edible cannabis in commercial products, check the ingredients listed to be sure the product is specifically labeled "gluten-free." To avoid the possibility of ingesting even a small amount of gluten, stick with whole plant products. Concentrates, including vape oils and transdermal patches, are very likely to be gluten-free unless the plant that produces them also makes products with gluten, which is highly unlikely. On the other hand, topical creams, salves, and lotions may contain gluten, so be sure to read the labels carefully.

Depression

Depression (major depressive disorder or clinical depression) is a common but serious mood disorder characterized by persistently depressed mood or loss of interest in activities the person previously found enjoyable. Symptoms may impact how you feel, think, and handle daily activities, such as sleeping, eating, and working. To be diagnosed with depression, symptoms must be present for at least two weeks.

Cannabis products that contain different chemical profiles (mixtures of cannabinoids and terpenes) may be more helpful for some symptoms of depression than others. For example, products that have higher levels of the terpenes limonene seem to be better for boosting mood. Products higher in pinene may be better for combating fatigue. Products with higher CBD-to-THC ratios may be more appropriate for curbing anxiety. If insomnia is a problem, products that are higher in CBD and myrcene may be the better choice.

WARNING

Avoid high-potency THC products, which may increase the risk of anxiety and paranoia, especially if you have any family history of bipolar disorder or schizophrenia. Begin with products that have higher CBD-to-THC ratios, and check terpene profiles. Limonene has an uplifting effect, pinene may help with memory retention, and myrcene tends to help with relaxation and sleep. Sativa strains that have a high percentage of CBD may be most helpful for boosting mood and energy while mitigating the risk of anxiety and paranoia.

Diabetes

Diabetes is a disease in which blood glucose (sugar) is too high. *Type 1 diabetes* is a genetic condition in which the pancreas doesn't produce *insulin* — the hormone that controls blood sugar levels. *Type 2 diabetes* (insulin resistance) is a condition in which the body doesn't use insulin properly, and the pancreas can't produce enough insulin to overcome the effects of that resistance. If not properly managed, diabetes can lead to vision loss, kidney damage, and other serious medical conditions. (Check out *Diabetes For Dummies*, by Alan L. Rubin, for details.)

While research is limited and conclusions are mixed, some evidence suggests that various properties of cannabis may help with the prevention and treatment of diabetes in certain individuals. Cannabis may help in the following ways:

>> **Modulate the immune system:** Type 1 diabetes is an autoimmune disease, in which the body attacks and destroys the insulin-producing cells of the pancreas. THC may regulate the autoimmune response so that less insulin medication is needed to regulate blood sugar. Also, CBD may reduce the occurrence and delay the onset diabetes.

>> **Reduce inflammation:** Diabetes is associated with inflammation. Reducing inflammation may help to stabilize blood sugar levels.

>> **Open blood vessels:** Cannabis is a mild vasodilator that opens blood vessels, which explains why consumers may have bloodshot eyes when using cannabis and why heartrate tends to increase. The good news is that cannabis opens blood vessels and improves circulation.

>> **Facilitate weight management:** CBD may restore balance in the endocannabinoid system, making it easier for people to lose weight. Weight loss for those who are overweight can help prevent the onset of diabetes or even help toward reversing type 2 diabetes.

>> **Prevent nerve damage:** Cannabis has neuroprotective properties that may help to prevent nerve damage associated with diabetes.

>> **Improve sleep:** The calming effect of certain strains of cannabis may help to alleviate "restless leg syndrome" and help those with diabetes sleep better.

WARNING

Avoid products that cause munchies for you personally. Binging on junk food won't help your body regulate blood sugar, so stay away from strains like: Goo, Monster Cookies, Maui Bubble Gift, Sonoma Coma, Platinum Purple Kush, Orange Skunk, Gigabud, Caramelo, Pure Kush, and Diablo. This may require personal experimentation.

However, strains high in THCv have shown an ability to lower appetite, regulate blood sugar levels, and reduce insulin resistance. The most noted high THCv strain is Doug's Varin at 24.3 percent THCv. Explain to your budtender that you want a strain that won't give you the munchies, and stress the *V* in THCv as it is a lesser known cannabinoid. THCv is more of an appetite suppressant. Like THC, however, it has psychoactive properties.

TIP

High CBD strains generally have a lower impact on your desire to raid the fridge, and they minimize psychotropic effects.

Eating disorders

According to The National Institute of Mental Health (NIMH), *eating disorders* are "serious and often fatal illnesses that cause severe disturbances to a person's eating behaviors. Obsessions with food, body weight, and shape may also signal an eating disorder. Common eating disorders include anorexia nervosa, bulimia nervosa, and binge-eating disorder."

Though cannabis, especially those strains that may trigger increased appetite, can be helpful for those in recovery, much of the underlying causes of eating disorders are based in societal and early life experiences. Cannabis can help with anxiety, which may support other therapeutic interventions. In addition, a small number of studies suggest that underlying imbalances within the endocannabinoid system are prominent across eating disorders, which suggest that cannabis may have some therapeutic value by restoring homeostasis.

WARNING

If you have an eating disorder, consult a doctor or therapist to discuss treatment options. Don't try to self-medicate with cannabis or any other substances. Some doctors or therapists may be more open to and experienced with using cannabis as part of the treatment plan for patients with eating disorders.

Epilepsy

Epilepsy is a chronic disorder of the brain characterized by recurrent *seizures* — brief episodes of involuntary movement that may involve the entire body (generalized) or a part of it (partial), and are sometimes accompanied by loss of consciousness and control of bowel or bladder function. Seizures vary from the briefest lapses of attention or muscle jerks to severe and prolonged convulsions. They can also vary in frequency, from less than one per year to several per day.

REMEMBER

One seizure doesn't signify epilepsy (up to 10 percent of people worldwide have one seizure during their lifetime). Epilepsy is defined as having two or more unprovoked seizures in one's lifetime.

Recently, the FDA approved the use of Epidiolex (a hemp-derived CBD drug) to treat seizures for people two years of age and older with Dravet syndrome or Lennox-Gastaut syndrome (LGS). This is the first approved treatment for Dravet syndrome. Much anecdotal evidence and advocacy along with some research has resulted in the wide acceptance of CBD in treating seizures in children. The *Charlotte's Web* strain has been used by numerous children suffering with seizures to lower the frequency and severity of those episodes.

REMEMBER

High CBD strains such as Charlotte's Web, with very low THC are the best choices for seizure symptom relief, especially in children where THC is determined to present a potential danger to brain development in those under the age of 21 years. You can look at hemp-derived CBD-only products to ensure only minimal THC content, though whole-plant products may yet prove to be most effective.

Fibromyalgia

Condition: According to the Mayo Clinic, "Fibromyalgia is a disorder characterized by widespread musculoskeletal pain accompanied by fatigue, sleep, memory, and mood issues. Researchers believe that fibromyalgia amplifies painful sensations by affecting the way the brain processes pain signals." No cure is available for fibromyalgia, but certain medications along with regular exercise, relaxation, and stress management may help to alleviate symptoms.

The analgesic (pain relieving) and anti-inflammatory properties of cannabis may help mitigate pain and tension for some fibromyalgia sufferers. Cannabis products that enhance relaxation and sleep may also be helpful in improving the amount and quality of restorative sleep and rest.

Because fibromyalgia symptoms are so variable, you need a highly personalized cannabis mix for potential symptom relief. Each day is different, and severity of symptoms may be based on events from the day before. High CBD strains or even hemp-derived products can be a good fit during the day to leave you with a clear head. Heavier THC products and strains may be better in the evening to improve sleep. Consider also the consumption method; a mix of fast-acting smoking or vaping or even a sublingual at certain times may be best, while the longer onset of an edible may be helpful at other times.

Gastroesophageal reflux disease (GERD)

Gastroesophageal Reflux Disease (GERD) is a digestive disorder in which stomach acid and/or food and fluids back up from the stomach into the esophagus. Symptoms include heartburn, chest pain, difficulty swallowing, chronic cough, disrupted sleep, and new or worsening asthma. According to some estimates, 10 to 20 percent of the U.S. population suffers from GERD to some degree.

Some of the current medications used to treat GERD may do more harm than good. Long-term use of proton pump inhibitors (PPIs), for example, weaken bones (due to poor absorption of calcium) and increase risk of pneumonia, kidney disease, and dementia.

Cannabis has several properties that may help to alleviate symptoms of GERD, including anti-inflammatory and pain relieving properties. In one study, THC reduced transient sphincter relaxations (TSLERs) and acid reflux in study participants. TSLERs, which occur after gastric stimuli and distention, have been identified as the primary cause of GERD. In addition, some studies show that cannabis and the attachment to CB1 and CB2 receptors associated with the endocannabinoid system can also help by modulating the responses between the gut and the brain.

REMEMBER

Because of GERD's association with asthma and because smoking (tobacco or cannabis) may worsen symptoms, consumption methods other than smoking may be best. Vape products, tinctures, and even edibles may be better options. With edibles, however, consider the other ingredients. Chocolate, caffeine, and spicy ingredients may exacerbate the condition. THC seems to play the biggest role in potential symptom relief, but consider starting with a product that has a more balanced CBD-to-THC ratio, such as 1:1.

Glaucoma

Glaucoma is a condition in which fluid builds up in the front part of the eye. The resulting pressure can damage the eye's optic nerve.

WARNING

The American Academy of Ophthalmology, American Glaucoma Society, and Canadian Ophthalmological Society caution against the use of cannabis in the treatment of glaucoma. While evidence shows that THC may reduce pressure in the eyes for people with glaucoma, up to 20mg of THC may be required to accomplish this goal, and effective treatments must control pressure 24/7.

In addition, cannabis is known to reduce blood pressure, which can interfere with blood flow to the optic nerve, worsening the condition. And because cannabis is not water-soluble, eye drop applications have not been well developed.

However, some research shows that cannabis may impact receptors that can offer neuro-protection for the optic nerve and possibly play a role in the prevention or treatment of glaucoma, but more research is needed before it can be recommended.

Hepatitis C

Hepatitis means inflammation of the liver. When the liver is inflamed or damaged, its function can be diminished. Viral infections (hepatitis A, B, or C), heavy alcohol use, toxins, some medications, and certain medical conditions can all cause or contribute to the onset or worsening of the condition. In the U.S., the most common hepatitis viruses are hepatitis A, B, and C. The condition may be acute (short-term) or chronic (lifelong) and may range in severity.

Cannabis alone isn't a treatment for Hepatitis C nor is it a treatment for any complications such as liver disease and cirrhosis. Where cannabis may be of value is in helping to relieve the nausea associated with certain medications used to treat Hepatitis C.

As with other symptom relief for nausea, choose a strain that works for you but consider starting with a product that has a 1:1 or higher CBD-to-THC ratio.

HIV/AIDS

Human immunodeficiency virus (HIV) is a virus that spreads through certain bodily fluids and attacks the CD4 (T cells) that play an important role in immune system function. Left untreated, the immune system's ability to fight infection is diminished, and if the condition is severe enough, opportunistic infections or cancers take advantage of the weakened immune system and signal that the person has *acquired immune deficiency syndrome (AIDS)* — the most severe phase of HIV infection.

No evidence shows that cannabis is effective in treating HIV or AIDS. It's primarily used to alleviate the adverse side effects of antiretroviral therapy and other medications used to treat HIV/AIDS and its symptoms, including pain, nausea, vomiting, loss of appetite, and corresponding weight loss and wasting (see "Cachexia"). Cannabis has been shown to be helpful in mitigating the effects of all these symptoms. In addition, some new studies suggesting that cannabis may interrupt the progression of the disease, which can help patients live longer with a higher quality of life.

If you are considering using cannabis to help with your symptoms consider the strain Blue Dream to combat nausea and stimulate your appetite. Girl Scout Cookies may also help in that area, and with its high THC content may help alleviate pain, as well. Blackberry Kush may be helpful for appetite and for pain.

Huntington's disease

Huntington's disease is a progressive brain disorder that causes uncontrolled movements, emotional problems, and diminished cognition (thinking ability). Two forms of Huntington's disease are distinguished by age of onset:

>> Adult-onset Huntington's disease typically strikes people in their 30s or 40s. Life expectancy is about 15 to 20 years after signs and symptoms appear. Early signs may include irritability, depression, small involuntary movements, poor coordination, and trouble learning new information or making decisions. As the disease progresses, patients develop involuntary jerking or twitching movements known as *chorea*. They may eventually experience trouble walking, talking, and swallowing; changes in personality; and diminished thinking and reasoning capabilities.

>> Juvenile Huntington's disease begins in childhood or adolescence. Symptoms include mental and emotional changes, slow movements, clumsiness, frequent falling, rigidity, slurred speech, drooling, and diminished performance in school. Seizures occur in 30 percent to 50 percent of children with this condition. The disease tends to progress more quickly than the adult-onset form; affected individuals usually live only 10 to 15 years after symptoms appear.

Research shows that those suffering from Huntington's disease have fewer CB1 receptors in a particular area of the brain and that by using cannabis to further stimulate those remaining CB1 receptors, specifically with THC, patients may see improved motor function, a slow-down in the symptom progression, and maybe even an improvement in that specific area of the brain.

Because evidence points to THC as the chemical compound in cannabis that has the greatest potential for helping patients with Huntington's disease, products with higher amounts of THC are likely to produce the best results. Of course, this also means "high" in general, so consider the psychotropic effects of different products when choosing them. Products with higher amounts of both THC and CBD may be most appropriate, so that the CBD may help mitigate the high, while the THC stimulates the CB1 receptors.

Inflammation

Inflammation plays a key role in a number of illnesses and diseases. In fact, every illness whose name ends in "-itis" is characterized by inflammation — appendicitis, arthritis, bronchitis, colitis, conjunctivitis, dermatitis, gastritis, sinusitis, and the list goes on.

Cannabis has proven anti-inflammatory properties. In particular, the CB2 receptor plays a starring role. When activated, the CB2 receptor signals the cell to release fewer pro-inflammatory messengers called *cytokines*. Both CBD and the terpene beta-caryophyllene, which comprises 12 to 35 percent of cannabis plant's oil concentration, activate CB2 receptors. THC also has anti-inflammatory properties.

Your choice of product varies depending on the illness and the symptoms you're experiencing. In general, whole plant products blend the benefits of all cannabinoids and certain terpenes, with some strains having a higher concentration of CBD. Strains you may want to consider, include ACDC with a 20:1 CBD-to-THC ratio and little psychotropic effect; Harlequin with a 5:2 CBD-to-THC ratio; and Charlotte's Web with 0.3 percent THC and a high CBD concentration.

REMEMBER

Your choice of product also depends on your preferred consumption method. Smoking and vaping deliver the fastest onset but also tend to wear off the fastest. Edibles have a slower onset but last longer. Tinctures and edibles are more discreet. Topical lotions or creams may be more effective for inflammation that affects the skin, such as various forms of dermatitis.

Insomnia

Insomnia is difficulty falling asleep or staying asleep, assuming the person wants to sleep and conditions are suitable for that to happen. As a result, those who suffer from insomnia typically suffer also from fatigue, low energy, mood irregularities, difficulty concentrating or thinking, and decreased performance at work or school.

THC, CBD, CBN, and certain terpenes may all help with sleep issues. THC has strong sedative effects and has been shown to reduce the amount of time required to fall asleep, but too much can worsen anxiety in some people. CBD has somewhat weaker sedative effects but its pain relieving anti-inflammatory properties may help people who have trouble sleeping due to pain and inflammation. CBD also has the ability to reduce daytime drowsiness. Myrcene is the terpene of choice for relaxation and sedation.

For a good night's sleep consider higher THC products that also include CBD and myrcene. Also consider edibles, which require more time to take effect but last longer than smoke or vapor. Specific strains that may be better for enhancing sleep include Tahoe OG Kush, Granddaddy Purple, God's Gift, and Afghan Kush.

Irritable bowel syndrome (IBS)

Irritable bowel syndrome (IBS) is a disorder that affects the large intestine resulting in cramping, abdominal pain, bloating, gas, nausea, and diarrhea, constipation, or both. It differs from irritable bowel disease (IBD), which includes Crohn's disease and ulcerative colitis, which are autoimmune disorders (see the later section "Ulcerative colitis and Crohn's disease.")

The main cause of IBS remains unknown, but research suggests that the problem may be traced to the gut-brain axis (GBA) — the communication network that between the central nervous system and the enteric nervous system, which helps to control peripheral intestinal functions. Some evidence suggests that an underlying deficiency of endocannabinoids may be partially responsible for diminished communication along the GBA that results in producing IBS symptoms. Supplementation with plant-based cannabinoids may help restore balance in the endocannabinoid system.

REMEMBER

If you have IBS, consult your doctor about treatment options, including medical marijuana. If your doctor recommends it, ask about specific cannabinoid and terpene profiles that may be of most value. You may want to start with a product that has a higher CBD-to-THC ratio and move on from there. The anxiolytic (anti-anxiety) properties of CBD may help to reduce the stress-like symptoms that many people with IBS suffer.

Lupus

Lupus is a systemic autoimmune disease that occurs when the body's immune system attacks its own tissues and organs. Inflammation caused by lupus can affect many different body systems including joints, skin, kidneys, blood cells, brain, heart, and lungs. Lupus can be difficult to diagnose because its signs and symptoms often mimic those of other ailments. The most distinctive sign of lupus — a facial rash that resembles the wings of a butterfly unfolding across both cheeks — occurs in many but not all cases of lupus. Some people are born with a tendency toward developing lupus, which may be triggered by infections, certain drugs or even sunlight. While lupus has no cure, treatments can help control symptoms.

Because the endocannabinoid system plays a role in regulating the immune system and controlling inflammation, there's some rationale for using cannabis for potential relief of symptoms related to lupus. Specifically, CB2 receptors modulate the body's inflammatory response. Clinical trials are ongoing in several countries to study how cannabinoids may help in the treatment of lupus.

Given the prevalence of inflammation in lupus high CBD strains would be a wise choice. The addition of some THC may help relieve the pain associated with this condition. A strain with a high CBD-to-THC ratio such as ACDC (20:1 CBD-to-THC) would be great option and one that will mitigate psychotropic effects of the THC.

Menopause

Menopause is a stage in a woman's life that begins 12 months after her last period. The seven to 14 years leading up to that point (perimenopause) are typically marked by changes in her monthly cycle and by hot flashes, mood swings, insomnia, pain, low libido, weight gain, fatigue, and osteoporosis. The onset of menopause or any of the symptoms may also trigger anxiety or depression, as well. Women may exhibit none, one, or a multitude of menopause symptoms at differing points during the years of transition.

Cannabis may help alleviate various symptoms associated with menopause. Product choice varies depending on the nature of the symptoms:

» **Emotion:** During menopause, estrogen levels drop. Some evidence points to a connection between estrogen and endocannabinoids in regulating mood and emotional response. Many cannabis strains are uplifting and energizing. Combinations of CBD and THC may be helpful to combat mood swings, anxiety, and depression. High CBD strains and products can be good support for social anxieties during this time.

» **Hot flashes:** Anandamide is an *endocannabinoid* (occurring naturally in the body) that's thought to play a role in regulating body temperature. Larger doses of THC have been associated with lowering body temperature, but some reports suggest that small amounts may do the opposite. Each individual is different and should explore dosing and strains for themselves. Perhaps high THC consumption at night can help both insomnia and night sweats.

» **Pain:** Some women experience pain during menopause, and THC has been well documented in its ability to relieve pain.

» **Low libido:** Evidence is mixed regarding cannabis' ability to improve sex drive. Because emotion and setting are a big part of determining the degree of pleasure obtained from sex or cannabis, combining the two experiences may enhance or diminish the experience of both depending on the emotions and mind-sets of the participants.

» **Vaginal dryness.** Although some women swear by their cannabis-infused vaginal lube, vaginal dryness, already a symptom of menopause, may be exacerbated by certain strains. Be sure to check the terpene profiles and ask your budtender if the strain you're considering causes dry mouth because, if it does, it'll probably affect other areas of the body as well. Vaginal lubes may counteract this effect in addition to improving vaginal and clitoral sensitivity.

>> **Bone density loss:** Some cannabinoids have been known to stimulate bone growth. Loss of bone density is a potential symptom of menopause, which increases the risk of breaks and bruises. Some studies suggest that CBD along with a multitude of cannabinoids including CBG, CBC, and THCv may offset or increase bone density. Considering your strain choices for combating other symptoms, this can be a nice side effect.

>> **Weight gain:** Weight gain during menopause is well-documented. Strains high in THCv have shown an ability to lower appetite and regulate blood sugar levels and reduce insulin resistance. The most noted high THCv strain is Doug's Varin at 24.3% THCv. However, if you're choosing a different strain, go for one with high CBD or a product with a high enough CBD-to-THC ratio to counteract any appetite stimulation from THC.

Migraines and headaches

Migraines are recurring headaches characterized by moderate to severe pain that's throbbing or pulsing. They're often accompanied by nausea, vomiting, and extreme sensitivity to light and sound.

Cannabis can be relaxing and help mitigate pain and anxiety from migraines and headaches as well as possibly stop an attack before it starts, although that may require more regular use. Nausea is also a common symptom in migraines that may benefit from cannabis.

For migraine sufferers, strain may be a very important decision because the wrong choice in cannabis can trigger anxiety or other symptoms that can actually cause a headache. OG Kush is a popular and prevalent strain that has enough THC to relax and mellow you out and relieve pain fast but enough CBD for more lasting relief. A high CBD, low THC strain such as ACDC and Remedy can do the trick as well.

Though very few studies suggest which consumption method is best, edibles are not usually recommended for migraine pain because sufferers need quick relief. Smoking, vaping, and possibly sublingual tinctures are typically preferred.

Multiple sclerosis (MS)

Multiple sclerosis (MS) is an autoimmune disorder in which the body's immune system attacks the myelin (which surrounds and insulates the nerve cells of the brain and spinal cord), the cells that make myelin, and the nerve cells themselves. Symptoms include numbness, speech impairment, loss of muscle coordination, blurred vision, and severe fatigue. Cannabis may mitigate some symptoms of MS, including pain, tremor, and spasticity.

If you're looking to add cannabis to your treatment regime for symptom relief, choose specific strains based on the symptoms you're trying to mitigate. For severe pain, inflammation, and fatigue, lean toward strains that are higher in THC such as Sour Diesel. Uplifting, sativa-dominant strains may help alleviate depression, and both Redwood Kush and Afghan Kush may help to calm muscle spasms.

Nausea and vomiting

Cannabis has an excellent track record for helping to combat nausea and vomiting. The brainstem's *dorsal vagal complex (DVC)* is the overall regulator of nausea and vomiting. Research shows that endocannabinoid receptors in the DVC and gastrointestinal tract become antiemetic (reduce vomiting) when activated by THC and that CBD activates a neurotransmitter that decreases the sensation of nausea.

As with other symptom relief for nausea, choose a strain that works for you, but consider starting with a 1:1 CBD-to-THC ratio to mitigate the "high," which may be uncomfortable when combatting nausea. Blue Dream, Durban Poison, Sour Diesel, and Northern Lights are all good choices. As for consumption method, consider smoking, vaping (oil or bud) for quick relief. You probably want to avoid edibles or even sublingual tinctures if you're feeling queasy.

REMEMBER

Cannabis typically relieves nausea and vomiting, but it can have the opposite effect when consumed regularly over a long period of time. See "Cannabinoid hyperemesis syndrome (CHS)" for details.

Pain

Cannabis' ability to relieve pain, especially chronic pain, has been one of the primary factors fueling medical marijuana advocacy and its growing acceptance in society. It's fast becoming a popular alternative to traditional pain medications such as opioids, which are highly addictive and far more dangerous than cannabis. Both THC and CBD appear to be helpful for alleviating pain. While THC binds to CB1 receptors in the brain that play a primary role in inhibiting neurotransmitter release, CBD seems to work in a different way, binding to a specific receptor called vanilloid TRPV1. One study showed that even low doses of CBD administered over seven days was effective in relieving both pain and anxiety.

Because both THC and CBD have some evidence to support their use in relieving pain, you have a wide variety of options based on the desired overall experience — whether and to what degree you want to experience the intoxicating effects of THC. A blend of THC and CBD is probably most effective, so consider starting with a 1:1 CBD-to-THC ratio. If you opt for a CBD-only product, be sure to give it seven to ten days to take effect. For faster relief, you may want to use a CBD-THC blend for seven to ten days and then wean yourself off the THC. Consumption method also affects the speed of onset, with smoking, vaping, or sublingual products taking effect more quickly and edibles requiring more time but providing longer-lasting relief. Topical lotions and creams are better for localized pain. Transdermal patches are also a good choice for both localized pain and long-term relief, but they do deliver the cannabinoids into the bloodstream and can make you high if they contain THC.

Popular strains used for pain relief include White Widow, Blue Dream, and Bubba Kush. Jack Herer and AK-47 are more uplifting but also effective pain relievers.

Parkinson's disease

Parkinson's disease (PD) is a long-term degenerative illness that affects the central nervous system and involves the loss of cells that produce *dopamine* — a neuro-transmitter (chemical messenger) that plays a key role in muscle coordination, reward, and memory. The reduction in dopamine causes motor system disorders with symptoms that include dyskinesia (involuntary muscle movement); rigidity (stiffness of the limbs and trunk); *bradykinesia* (slowness of movement); and postural instability (impaired balance and coordination). Symptoms may also include mood changes (particularly depression); sleep disruptions; difficulty speaking, chewing, or swallowing; constipation; and urinary problems.

REMEMBER

Any evidence to support the use of cannabis for Parkinson's disease is anecdotal. According to the Parkinson's Foundation, "despite several clinical studies, it has not been demonstrated that cannabis can directly benefit people with PD." In fact, researchers caution against the use of cannabis for PD patients, because both PD and cannabis can impair the brain's executive function, which is responsible for making plans and limiting risky behavior.

Post-traumatic stress disorder (PTSD)

Post-traumatic stress disorder (PTSD) is a serious mental health disorder triggered by a violent, disturbing, or life-threatening event. Symptoms include anxiety, depression, unwanted memories or dreams of the trauma, heightened reactions, and avoidance of situations that remind the person of the event.

Many returning veterans who've had battlefield experiences show signs of PTSD. Although the military prohibits the use of marijuana to treat symptoms of PTSD, many retired military personnel are finding relief in cannabis. Cannabis may help to relieve anxiety and depression, improve sleep, and reduce the frequency or intensity of nightmares. (Several studies show that cannabis reduces the rapid eye movement (REM) stage of the sleep cycle, during which the most vivid dreams occur.)

WARNING

Don't consume cannabis when you're in a heightened emotional state. Research suggests that it's most valuable when consumed in smaller doses before an emotional event to prevent the symptoms from occurring.

Consider strains higher in THCv, which may help to curb anxiety attacks without suppressing emotion. Blue Dream and OG Kush are favorites among those using cannabis for PTSD. These strains are higher in THC and lower in CBD. However, because high doses of THC may also cause anxiety, start lower and go slower with these strains until you know how they affect you.

Restless legs syndrome

According to the National Institute of Neurological Disorders and Stroke, "Restless legs syndrome (RLS), also called Willis-Ekbom Disease, causes unpleasant or uncomfortable sensations in the legs and an irresistible urge to move them. Symptoms commonly occur in the late afternoon or evening hours, and are often most severe at night when a person is resting, such as sitting or lying in bed. Since symptoms can increase in severity during the night, it can become difficult to fall asleep or return to sleep after waking up." Poor sleep often results in exhaustion, fatigue, and an inability to concentrate, which can negatively affect performance at work or school and relationships.

Much of the evidence to support the use of cannabis in relieving RLS symptoms is anecdotal. However, in one small study, five out of six subjects taking an inhaled form of medicinal cannabis (higher in CBD) experienced full remission and all participants reported having improved sleep after the study ended. Results from another study found that Sativex (a medication made from cannabis that contains both CBD and THC) improved sleep for about half the participants.

Because both CBD and THC may improve sleep in those with RLS, product selection is wide open and depends primarily on your personal preferences. If you have trouble falling asleep, products that contain some THC may be helpful, because it has stronger sedative effects. If you're looking for relief without the intoxicating effects of THC, consider products with higher CBD content or CBD-only products. However, if you go the CBD-only route, you may need to take the product for seven to ten days before you experience any relief. Products that contain the terpene myrcene may also be beneficial.

Also consider consumption methods. Smoke, vape, and sublingual tinctures provide the fastest relief. Many patients report that edibles are less effective in controlling RLS symptoms.

TIP

When discussing options with your doctor or budtender ask about the indicas Granddaddy Purple or Purple Kush for helping to relax and fall asleep. If you need a clearer head, consider high CBD options such as ACDC or Charlotte's Web that may help to alleviate pain and anxiety and help you relax but with lower THC content.

Schizophrenia/psychosis

Schizophrenia is a severe, chronic psychiatric illness that affects how a person thinks, feels, and behaves. It impairs a person's ability to think clearly, make decisions, manage their emotions, and establish and maintain relationships. They commonly experience anxiety, paranoia, delusions, and (mostly auditory) hallucinations.

WARNING

Don't consume cannabis, especially products high in THC, if you have schizophrenia or a family history of mental illness. Research shows that cannabis may trigger psychotic illness in youth, especially those with genetic predispositions, and it can worsen symptoms in those already diagnosed.

Researchers are exploring the potential of pure CBD for alleviating symptoms. CBD has properties that may help with anxiety and psychosis and is not psychoactive. However, no strong evidence supports the use of CBD for helping people with schizophrenia. If you're interested in exploring the potential of CBD, discuss the option with your doctor and stick to hemp-derived CBD-only products from companies that offer online batch information that matches your exact product purchase and batch with third-party lab testing and proof of 0 (zero) percent THC. Some companies, but not all, offer this type of guarantee. Definitely stay away from CBD products labeled "whole plant," even if they're hemp-derived.

Sexual dysfunction

Sexual dysfunction refers to any difficulty an individual or couple experiences during any phase of the sexual response cycle (excitement, plateau, orgasm, and resolution) that leaves one or both individuals feeling unsatisfied. It affects about a third of the population — women more than men.

Cannabis consumption may enhance or diminish sexual desire and satisfaction. It may help in the following ways:

>> Alleviate anxiety and depression

>> Improve focus, so participants are less distracted

>> Reduce inhibitions

>> Increase blood flow

>> Intensify physical sensations

Cannabis also carries some potential adverse sexual side effects, including the following:

>> **Dependence:** Frequent cannabis use in association with sexual activity may create a situation in which the individual requires the increased dopamine experienced during consumption and is even less open to sexual experience without the assistance of the substance.

>> **Orgasm issues:** Some studies suggest that daily consumption for men may create orgasm and premature ejaculation issues.

>> **Lower testosterone:** Daily consumption may lower testosterone levels in men.

>> **Mucosal dehydration:** Certain strains promote mucosal dehydration, most notably dry mouth. Some women may experience vaginal dryness that may further inhibit arousal and intercourse or result in painful intercourse.

As with any other medical application of cannabis for potential symptom relief, consult your physician and consider strains, consumption methods and frequency of consumption. A budtender at your dispensary may also provide some insight based on interactions with other customers. Consider starting with a balanced 1:1 CBD-to-THC product. THC is associated with a mental shift and increased physical sensitivity, but too much can increase your heart rate and cause anxiety. CBD holds the anxiety at bay. Steer clear of products with skunky, woody, earthy terpenes, which have a stronger sedative effect and lean toward products with limonene.

TIP Consider a cannabis-infused lube, which may increase blood flow to your nether regions, thus increasing sensitivity. These lubes are also great if you experience vaginal dryness from consuming cannabis via other methods. However, do your homework. Some lubes are not to be used with condoms and other rubber or latex products.

Skin conditions

Cannabis may help with certain skin conditions, such as eczema (atopic) dermatitis and psoriasis and some of the symptoms associated with these conditions, including itching, pain, poor sleep, and anxiety. Both eczema and psoriasis can cause itchy and painful, red, scaly spots or patches on the skin. In a human trial, 60 percent of participants experienced improvement in severity of itching and sleep loss when using a topical endocannabinoid cream, and a good number of those were able to stop their other medications, including topical immunomodulators (20 percent), oral antihistamines (38 percent), and topical steroids (33.6 percent).

Cannabis has several properties that may improve these conditions in the following ways:

» Reduces the severity of itching.

» Slowing uncontrolled cell growth (characteristic of psoriasis).

» Regulating the body's immune response. (Eczema)

» Reducing inflammation.

» Alleviating pain and anxiety.

» Killing bacteria to prevent or treat infections.

» Improving sleep.

If you have eczema or psoriasis, consult your dermatologist about the possibility of using cannabis-infused lotions, creams, or oil-based tinctures and ask for specific product recommendations. Some products may contain other ingredients that can irritate the skin. Other products and consumption methods, including smoking, vaping, and tinctures, may be useful for relieving symptoms associated with these skin conditions, such as pain, anxiety, and poor sleep.

Sports medicine

Cannabis use in competitive sports is still banned both by national and international sports bodies on the professional and collegiate levels. However, in some instances and for some sports such as marathons and mixed martial arts (MMA), many of the pros use both THC and CBD in their training, competitions, and recovery.

Many athletic individuals use cannabis to improve recovery and relieve sore muscles after workouts, taking advantage of cannabis' analgesic and anti-inflammatory properties. Some athletes also use specific strains that promote energy and focus to improve their competitive drive. Research is now showing that the famed "runners high" — that euphoric, energized feeling after extended exercise — originates in the same endocannabinoid system that's active in the "high" produced from cannabis. Even some famed long-distance runners are signing with cannabis companies, openly showcasing the value of cannabis for exercise and recovery.

Tourette syndrome

According to the National Institute for Neurological Disorders and Stroke (NINDS), "Tourette syndrome (TS) is a neurological disorder characterized by repetitive, stereotyped, involuntary movements and vocalizations called tics." The average onset of this condition is between the ages of three and nine years. The tics and outbursts associated with this syndrome cause serious quality of life issues for sufferers, as well as their families.

One study published in *Behavioral Neurology* entitled "Treatment of Tourette Syndrome with Cannabinoids," concludes that "THC is recommended for the treatment of TS in adult patients, when first line treatments failed to improve the tics. In treatment resistant adult patients, therefore, treatment with THC should be taken into consideration."

Strain choices should be based on the needs of the patient, though whole plant products that contain a 1:1 ratio of CBD-to-THC are considered the most therapeutic and offer the "entourage effect." Strains that offer relaxation, calming, and uplifting responses may work best but consider terpene profiles when making a choice of what is available in your dispensary.

When choosing a consumption method, consider speed of onset, duration of effect, and discretion. Smoking and vaping deliver the fastest relief but wear off sooner. Tinctures taken sublingually provide relatively quick relief and are more discreet. Edibles, which are the most discreet means of consuming cannabis, have a slower onset but the effects last longer.

Ulcerative colitis and Crohn's disease

Ulcerative colitis and *Crohn's disease* are two types of *inflammatory bowel disease (IBD)*. Ulcerative colitis is characterized by inflammation and the formation of ulcers in the lining of the colon (large intestine). Crohn's disease is a chronic inflammatory condition of the gastrointestinal tract that typically affects the end of the small bowel (the ileum) and the beginning of the colon, but it may affect any part of the digestive tract, from the mouth to the anus. Symptoms of either condition include abdominal pain and cramping, diarrhea, fatigue, weight loss, and malnutrition.

While neither condition has a known cure, certain therapies can greatly reduce symptoms and even bring about long-term remission. Diet and lifestyle changes along with treatments to restore a healthy balance of gut microbes seem to hold the most promise. Cannabis may also be beneficial in helping to restore healthy immune function, reduce inflammation, and alleviate pain and anxiety.

CB1 and CB2 receptors both seem to play a role in these conditions, so consider trying whole-plant products that contain a 1:1 CBD-to-THC ratio. Both cannabinoids also play a role in alleviating pain. Consider smoking, vaping, or sublingual tinctures for fast relief. Edibles may provide longer-lasting relief, but avoid products that contain any ingredients that may irritate your colon.

Accounting for Potential Adverse Side Effects

Although cannabis has numerous properties that may be useful in providing symptomatic relief for a wide range of symptoms, it also has the potential to negatively impact a person's health. Potential adverse side effects vary depending on the individual, frequency of consumption, types and potencies of products used, and other variables.

Possible adverse short-term side effects include the following:

WARNING

>> Impaired short-term memory, which may make learning and retaining new information difficult.

>> Impaired motor coordination, which may increase the risk of injury to self and others.

Don't drive high.

>> Altered judgment and lowered inhibitions, which can lead to unhealthy choices.

Possible adverse long-term side effects include the following:

>> Altered brain development, including lower IQ, among those who frequently consumed THC in adolescence.

>> Bronchitis, among those who smoke cannabis.

>> Increased risk of chronic psychiatric disorders, such as schizophrenia, in people who have a genetic susceptibility.

>> Nausea and vomiting, among long-term, frequent consumers. (See "Cannabinoid hyperemesis syndrome (CHS)" for details.)

>> Psychological dependence on cannabis, though there are no physical addictions to the cannabinoid due to the lack of receptors in the medulla oblongata.

WARNING

Medical cannabis use is not legal for those under the age of 21 unless directed by a physician.

Chapter **10**

Using Pot for Pets

C hapter 9 explores many of the possible health benefits of medical cannabis for people, but pets are members of the family too, and they suffer from many of the same maladies. Cannabis may also be of value to them, not only for symptom relief and palliative care but also for prolonging and improving their quality of life.

In this chapter, we explore the use of medical marijuana for providing symptomatic relief for pets — primarily dogs and cats, along with horses, because most of the published studies are related to the efficacy and dosing in these animals. (Few studies reveal the potential benefits of using cannabis in the treatment of other pets or animals.) We look at the potential health benefits of cannabis and provide guidance on consulting with your veterinarian and determining the proper dosing for your pets. We describe many of the conditions that cannabis is used to treat, introduce you to some of the commercial cannabis products currently on the market, and offer suggestions on preparing a few of your own cannabis home remedies.

Recognizing the Potential Benefits of Cannabis Treatment

Like humans, dogs, cats, and other animals have an endocannabinoid system (ECS) that acts as a communication network for helping to regulate other systems in the body related to healthy function. For example, the ECS is thought to play a role in regulating the immune system, possibly helping to alleviate symptoms of allergies and asthma. The body contains its own endocannabinoids, which serve as chemical messengers across the ECS. Cannabis contains cannabinoids that serve a similar function, mimicking the activity of the body's own endocannabinoids. As a result, cannabinoids, including cannabinol (CBD) and tetrahydrocannabinol acid (THCa — a precursor to THC that's non-psychoactive) may have a positive impact on a wide range of health conditions, including the following:

- Aging and mental function
- Allergies and asthma
- Anxiety
- Arthritis
- Autoimmune disorders
- Bone and joint health
- Cancer
- Cardiovascular health
- Colitis
- Diabetes
- Epilepsy/seizures
- Glaucoma
- Inflammation
- Loss of appetite/weight loss
- Nausea and vomiting
- Obesity
- Obsessive-compulsive disorder
- Pain
- Skin conditions
- Spinal injury

More importantly, cannabis is being used increasingly in pets to maintain health and improve the quality of life over the course of the natural aging process. Cannabinoids, especially CBD, may make pets feel better overall as they age by reducing pain and discomfort, boosting their mood, and keeping them more active, making them feel and appear more youthful. If you're like most pet owners, you want your pet to live a long, healthy, and happy life, and certain cannabis products place additional tools at your disposal that may help you toward achieving that goal.

REMEMBER

While you can find plenty of anecdotal evidence online for the effectiveness of cannabis in treating a variety of maladies in dogs, cats, horses, and other animals, research into the effectiveness of cannabis in treating specific health conditions in pets is very limited and further restricted almost entirely to CBD. While THCa may also offer health benefits, especially when combined with CBD, federal restrictions on products that contain THC limit its availability for research. However, several studies have been conducted to evaluate the safety of CBD in treating cats, dogs, and horses, and the evidence indicates that CBD is indeed safe. In short, CBD may help alleviate symptoms of certain health conditions your pet is struggling with, and it is very unlikely to harm your pet.

TIP

With your pet's health and wellness in mind, the best direction to go when contemplating cannabis for your pet may be the hemp-derived CBD route. Because hemp-derived CBD contains little to no THC, your pet can reap the many potential health benefits of cannabis without getting high. In addition, products made from hemp-derived CBD are federally legal, so you can find a vast array of products online and at most stores that carry a variety of pet supplies. You don't have to be over the age of 21 or buy these products from a dispensary.

Consulting Your Veterinarian First

Before giving CBD or any other supplement to your pet, discuss it with your veterinarian, if he or she is willing to do so. Although hemp-derived CBD is safe and federally legal, some veterinarians may be reluctant to engage in any discussion of cannabis products due to fear of possible legal repercussions and the lack of guidance from their state veterinary medical associations and state boards. However, if you're thinking about giving your pet any CBD supplement, asking your vet about it is certainly worth a try.

REMEMBER

As laws change and as more research becomes available related to the safety and potential health benefits of cannabis for pets, veterinarians will begin to feel more comfortable having these discussions with pet owners. If your veterinarian is reluctant to discuss CBD now, don't hesitate to bring up the topic during your next visit. Many veterinarians would like to recommend CBD or at least discuss it with pet owners and simply feel that they don't yet have the information and freedom to do so.

WARNING

Cases of THC toxicity have been reported in pets (especially young pets) overconsuming cannabis. Don't let your pet chow down on your bud, don't blow your smoke or vapor toward your pet's face, and be especially cautious with edibles, because other ingredients such as chocolate and raisins can also be toxic to pets. Proceed with caution if you decide to give your pet any cannabis product, even CBD. Start low and go slow until you see how well your pet tolerates it.

TIP

Look for a holistic veterinarian who has experience using a variety of cannabis products for treating pets. One of the most famous is Gary Richter, MS DVM, author of *The Ultimate Pet Health Guide: Breakthrough Nutrition and Integrative Care for Dogs and Cats* (Hay House, Inc., 2017).

Treating Specific Conditions in Pets

Cannabis has many components in addition to CBD that may provide health benefits to pets, so different cannabis products may be more suitable for some conditions than others. In this section, we provide general guidance on using cannabis to treat some specific conditions in pets. As we encourage in the previous section, consult your veterinarian for more specific guidance.

REMEMBER

For some types of symptom relief such as pain or inflammation, you may need to treat your pet for several days before seeing any improvement.

Anxiety

Hemp-derived CBD products are on the market that specifically target pet anxiety. THCa products for pets may also be available for helping with anxiety. THCa is a form of THC that doesn't have the same psychoactive properties as THC, so it doesn't get you (or your pet) high. THC starts out as THCa and is decarboxylated when heated to form THC.

Sweet Mary Jane offers two tincture products that include THCa — Re-Leaf and Creature Comfort. They're both great for dogs with anxiety without getting them high. You can put it under their tongue or put the drops on a piece of bread.

WARNING

Too much THC can actually trigger and worsen anxiety in both humans and animals, so proceed with caution. If you decide to use a product that contains THC, make sure the CBD-to-THC ratio is a minimum of 1:1 and that the THC the product contains is the non-psychoactive form — THCa.

Appetite loss

Age, illness, and certain medical treatments may cause appetite loss in both people and pets. If loss of appetite leads to excessive weight loss or malnutrition, the problem can be very serious. Fortunately, cannabis has a strong reputation as an appetite stimulant. If the rotisserie chicken trick doesn't get Fido or Felix to start eating again, consider trying an appetite stimulant made from cannabis.

While THC is the cannabis component most responsible for stimulating appetite, cannabinol (CBN) products may be of more value for stimulating your pet's appetite. CBN stimulates appetite without the strong psychotropic effects characteristic of THC.

Cancer

Evidence supporting the effectiveness of cannabis in treating cancer in pets is still mostly constrained to stories from pet owners and some treatment providers. Some preliminary studies show that cannabis may help to prevent the spread of cancer in people, so a reasonable conclusion would be that it can help prevent the spread of cancer in certain pets, as well. However, cannabis is mostly used for relieving the symptoms associated with cancer and with certain cancer treatments such as chemotherapy. If your pet has cancer, cannabis may be able to help alleviate the following symptoms:

» Pain

» Inflammation

» Discomfort

» Nausea, vomiting, and loss of appetite

While cannabis used to treat cancer in pets is typically administered orally, topical applications to tumors may also be beneficial.

A LAST RESORT

If you read personal accounts of pet owners who've used marijuana as medicine for their pets, you start to notice a familiar thread running through many of these stories. Many of the pet owners are medical marijuana consumers themselves. They've taken their pets to the vet and tried every available remedy recommended. Some feel so sorry for their pets that they're almost to the point of deciding to "put them down."

Finally, it crosses their mind that medical marijuana has helped them, so why not try it on their pet? They give their pet a small dose of whatever it is they're taking and see remarkable results. Pets that can barely move a muscle are up walking again. Those that had stopped eating have their appetite restored. Pets who whined and cringed when being touched or held no longer have these reactions.

Digestion issues

Cannabis has anti-inflammatory and analgesic (pain relieving) properties that make it potentially useful in treating gastrointestinal issues in both humans and pets. Research has also revealed that the ECS helps to regulate the digestive system. Stimulation of the CB1 and CB2 receptors (see Chapter 2) helps to regulate gastric secretion, gastric emptying, and intestinal *motility* (the contraction of the muscles used to mix and propel contents in the gastrointestinal tract).

WARNING

High doses of CBD in pets has been associated with diarrhea, so start with a low dose and slowly increase it while observing your pet's stools. If your pet experiences diarrhea, reduce the dose.

Epilepsy/seizures

The most (and most promising) research on the health benefits of cannabis for pets is in the area of treating epilepsy and preventing seizures. Several studies have explored the effectiveness of cannabis — CBD oil in particular — in treating dogs with epilepsy. Epilepsy and seizures are actually quite frequent in pets, especially in certain dog breeds. Initial findings suggest dramatic improvements in reducing the number of seizures these dogs experienced.

AKC TO THE RESCUE!

The American Kennel Club Canine Health Foundation (AKCCHF) is funding a major clinical trial to study the use of CBD to treat drug-resistant epilepsy in dogs. According to the AKC:

Canine epilepsy is the most common cause of recurrent seizures in dogs. Unfortunately, the medications used to treat epilepsy, such as phenobarbital, potassium bromide, diazepam, and other anticonvulsant drugs, can cause serious side effects in some dogs. Even with medication, up to 30 percent of dogs with epilepsy continue to experience seizures.

Hopefully, the results from the study will provide clear evidence, beyond the anecdotal evidence available online, that CBD is a safe, effective treatment for reducing epileptic seizures in dogs. Such results would be likely to give veterinarians the green light to start talking about the potential health benefits of CBD and other cannabinoids with pet owners.

Nausea/vomiting

While cannabis may not be effective in preventing your cat from hacking up hair balls on your pillow, the antiemetic (anti-nausea) properties of cannabis may be valuable in helping reduce nausea and vomiting in pets. CBD may also be safer than other antiemetic medications, such as Metoclopramide or Maropitant. Cannabis also has anti-anxiety properties that may be helpful if anxiety (such as separation anxiety) is the root cause of your pet's nausea and vomiting.

TIP

Prior to trying cannabis to treat a pet's nausea and vomiting, try to identify the root cause of the problem. You may need to address other issues first, such as your pet's food, possible infection with worms or parasites, pregnancy, overeating or eating too quickly, sources of anxiety, and so on.

Pain

Cannabis has anti-inflammatory and analgesic (pain reducing) properties that may be helpful for some pets suffering from pain or inflammation. The most common use is for arthritis or hip and joint pain affecting older pets. A number of cannabis products on the market specifically address these issues and are often combined with glucosamine to increase mobility in older pets.

As pet owners, we use Up and Moving (www.therabis.com/shop/up-and-moving) on our pets' food. We've also used treats called HemPup (hempupinc.com). Both products are CBD only and are great for reducing pain and improving mobility.

Palliative care

Palliative care involves relieving pain and discomfort without addressing underlying (usually untreatable) conditions. Such care is usually provided to patients as they struggle with debilitating or terminal illnesses. Palliative care may prolong and improve the quality of your pet's final months, weeks, or days. Cannabis products containing a variety of cannabinoids and other ingredients can be useful for this purpose.

Tumors

A *tumor* is any abnormal growth of tissue. It can be *benign* (not spreading) or *malignant*, which means it can spread to other parts of the body. Like humans, pets are susceptible to developing tumors, and certain cannabinoids may help in their treatment. However, most of the evidence that supports the use of cannabis in treating tumors is anecdotal — few, if any, scientific studies support its effectiveness. Some pet owners have reported success eliminating or reducing the size of tumors (or stopping their growth) through oral or topical application of various cannabis products.

Noting the Potential Adverse Effects of Cannabis on Pets

Cannabis, especially products with higher concentrations of THC, can have adverse side effects on both people and pets. Hemp-derived CBD products are safest, but they can still cause some undesirable side effects, such as the following:

>> Drowsiness

>> Itching

>> Nausea or vomiting

>> Diarrhea

If you're giving your pet CBD and notice any of these symptoms, stop the CBD or decrease the dosage.

The adverse side effects of too much THC can be more serious and even quite severe:

>> Lethargy

>> Dilated pupils

>> Drooling

>> Poor balance (staggering)

>> Muscle twitching

>> Vomiting

>> Involuntary urination

>> Unconsciousness (coma)

If your pet accidently ingests a product containing THC, or you notice any of these symptoms, contact your veterinarian immediately.

Administering Cannabis to Pets

If you decide to use cannabis to support your pet's health and wellness, you now have to figure out how to administer it. You have to choose a consumption method and figure out the right amount to give your pet.

The easiest approach is to find a product that's suitable for your pet and for the desired purpose and follow the instructions on the packaging or those provided by your veterinarian. A suitable product has the right concentrations of cannabinoids and terpenes to meet your pet's needs, is something your pet likes or at least tolerates well, and is made by a reputable manufacturer. (See the later section "Obtaining Commercial Cannabinoid Products" for details on how to find suitable cannabis products for pets.)

If you decide to use a product that's not designed specifically for pets, continue reading for guidance on how to administer the product and figure out the right dose.

Deciding on a way to administer it

While many people consume cannabis by smoking it or vaping, those modes of consumption aren't suitable for pets. However, you have several other options for getting your pet to take her "medicine," including the following:

» **Sublingual:** If you're giving your pet CBD oil or a similar product, place the recommended number of drops under your pet's tongue. The benefit of sublingual administration is that the product is absorbed and takes effect almost immediately. Unfortunately, convincing your pet not to swallow for a few seconds is a challenge.

» **Edibles:** You may be able to purchase treats that contain CBD or other cannabinoids and medicinal ingredients. Assuming your pet likes the treats, this option is easiest. You can also find cannabis oils and powders to add to your pet's food or on a piece of bread or other human food your pet likes. The drawback of edibles is that they require more time to be absorbed and take effect. Your pet may not start to experience the benefits for 30 minutes or longer but with daily doses, you should begin to see the symptom relief you're looking for.

» **Topicals:** You can apply creams, lotions, or oils to your pet's skin for localized treatment or apply it to the less furry side of your pet's ears where it can be absorbed into the bloodstream.

Choosing an initial dose

Without your veterinarian's guidance, figuring out how much CBD to give your pet can be a major challenge. You have two options:

» Buy a hemp-derived CBD product developed especially for pets and follow the instructions included with it.

>> Search the web for "CBD dose for pets" or "CBD dosing chart for pets" and follow the dosing guidance provided on a trustworthy site. (Many companies that develop CBD products for pets post their dosing charts online.)

WARNING

CBD concentrations vary, so three drops of one product may contain significantly more or less CBD than three drops of another product. One 30 ml bottle may contain 500 mg, whereas another bottle of the same size contains 250 or 125 or 75 mg CBD. After you figure out how much CBD to give your pet, in milligrams (mg), you need to figure out how many milligrams of CBD are in each drop of oil:

1. **Multiply the number of milliliters in the bottle by 20.** A standard eyedropper dispenses 0.05 ml per drop, meaning each milliliter consists of about 20 drops. A 30 ml bottle contains 30 ml x 20 drops or about 600 drops.

2. **Divide the total number of milligrams of CBD (or other substance) in the bottle by the total number of drops calculated in Step 1.** For example, if the 30 ml bottle contains 250 mg CBD, 250 mg ÷ 600 drops = 0.42 mg/drop.

Now, the math becomes pretty easy. If your dog is 30 pounds and you want to start her on a low dose of CBD of about 0.75 mg daily, then 0.75 mg ÷ 0.42 mg/drop = approximately two drops.

You also have the option of spreading out the dose over the course of the day; for example, if you calculate that your dog should be getting two drops a day, you may want to give her one drop in the morning and one in the evening.

WARNING

For products that contain THCa, the recommended dosage is significantly less than the amount of CBD. However, don't use any products that contain THC or THCa on your pet unless your veterinarian expressly recommends it and prescribes a specific dosage, which isn't likely for reasons given earlier in this chapter.

Monitoring your pet's reaction

Whenever you start your pet on any medication or supplement, observe her closely and note any changes, positive or negative. If you applied a topical, look for any changes to the skin in the area where you applied it. Look for any changes in behavior or activity level. Does your pet seem happier? Is she more or less lethargic? Does she seem more or less aggressive? Have you noticed any improvement in symptoms? Any changes you notice provide valuable information and guidance for adjusting the dose, as explained next.

Adjusting the dose

Arriving at the right dose for your pet is, to some degree, a process of trial and error. Start with a dose at the low end of the scale. If you observe no improvements in symptoms within five days increase the dosage slightly. Continue to increase the dose over several weeks being careful not to exceed the upper limit, unless instructed to do otherwise by your veterinarian.

If you notice any adverse side effects, such as excessive sedation, disorientation, excitement, vomiting, and so on, stop administering the cannabis until the symptoms subside and then restart the cannabis at a prior dose that didn't produce those adverse side effects.

REMEMBER

Your goal is to arrive at the lowest effective dose possible.

Preventing and responding to overconsumption

Overconsumption of cannabis in pets typically occurs when a pet chows down on her owner's flower or edibles and consumes an excess amount of THC. Wherever cannabis becomes legal, veterinarians see a huge increase in cases of pets accidentally ingesting cannabis, and the experience is not pleasant for these animals. Pets don't understand the way cannabis makes them feel; being high can make them fearful and anxious. They may feel disoriented, may be unable to walk normally, and may even end up in a coma.

WARNING

To prevent overconsumption in pets, keep all cannabis products, especially those that contain THC, away from your pets when not in use. Never get your pet high intentionally, which constitutes cruelty to animals and is a felony in certain jurisdictions. If your pet accidentally ingests some of your cannabis, take your pet to the vet and be open about what happened, so your vet can provide the necessary treatment.

You also need to be careful about overconsumption if you're administering cannabis to your pets for medicinal purposes. Follow the standard industry advice of starting low and going slow with your pets. Start at the low range and increase the dose slowly over the course of several days or weeks.

Obtaining Commercial Cannabinoid Products

A wide selection of cannabis products for pets is now readily available, including doggie biscuits, soft-chews, and hemp oil. Hemp-derived CBD products are most readily available, because these products are federally legal. You can buy hemp-derived CBD products for pets online and have them shipped across state lines, and you don't even need to be 21 years old to place the order.

REMEMBER

Hemp-derived CBD oil is treated as a supplement, and if you follow the news at all, you know that the quality of supplements can vary considerably. At the very least, read the labels closely to find out how much CBD the manufacturer claims the product contains. Even better, do your homework — research manufacturers and specific products to find a reputable supplier.

A few companies are also manufacturing medical marijuana products that contain THCa for pets, but these are available only in states in which medical marijuana is legal, and you must obtain them from a marijuana dispensary. CBD products that contain even relatively small amounts of THCa may be more effective for pets due to the *entourage effect* — the synergy among the various cannabinoids, terpenes, and other components of the cannabis plant, especially in products that are identified as *whole plant*.

Preparing Your Own Concoctions

While the industry has begun to develop more cannabis products for pets, many cannabis consumers are simply sharing their own cannabis with their pets. After all, CBD oil is CBD oil, whether it's labeled for pets or people. You just need to adjust the dose accordingly. However, dosing becomes more complicated if you're creating your own cannabis dog or cat treats and especially if those treats contain THC.

You can find plenty of recipes online for creating your own pet treats, so just follow the recipe and add cannabis or CBD oil as an ingredient. You may even find recipes that include cannabis in the list of ingredients. Another option is to simply add the cannabis to your pet's favorite food or cook your pet a special meal that includes cannabis. If you're baking treats, just be sure to mix the ingredients thoroughly, so the cannabis is spread equally throughout the batter; otherwise, dosing will be inconsistent.

WARNING

Don't forget about the potential danger of other ingredients. For example, chocolate, coffee, and caffeine all contain methylxanthines, which can cause vomiting, diarrhea, panting, excessive thirst and urination, hyperactivity, abnormal heart rhythm, seizures, and even death. Grapes, raisins, nuts, coconut, onions, milk, dairy, and the sweetener xylitol should also be avoided.

4

Grasping the Basics of Cannabis Cultivation, Post-Harvest, and Production

Grow your own cannabis indoors or outside, assuming that growing cannabis is legal where you live.

Build your own grow room, for indoor cultivation.

Ensure that your plants have all the nutrients they need and nothing that threatens their health or the quality of your product.

Know when and how to harvest your plants to ensure a bountiful crop of the highest quality.

Properly cure and manicure your plants post-harvest.

Transform cannabis plants into concentrates, edibles, lotions, tinctures, and other awesome products.

Chapter **11**

Growing Cannabis

Some people get pretty excited about growing certain plants, such as orchids, roses, and even tomatoes. They take great pride in growing a bumper crop of succulent vegetables or having the fullest most colorful blooms in the neighborhood. However, nobody gets more excited about their plants than cannabis growers, and you can't really blame them — after all, they're growing their own medicine or their own recreational drug of choice, saving tons of money, and perhaps even sharing their harvest with friends and earning bragging rights for the smoothest, most potent product.

Another factor that makes growing cannabis such a great hobby is that it's pretty easy to grow. Or maybe we should say that it's pretty difficult *not to grow*. It is a weed after all. Left to its own devices, it would thrive in just about any fairly sunny location with decent soil and a sufficient precipitation. But if you're going to grow it, you probably want to do it right, so you can maximize the quality and the quantity of your harvest without investing too much effort. In this chapter, we provide the guidance you need to do just that.

TIP

Although we provide the general guidance you need to grow quality cannabis and maximize your harvest, we encourage you to find a nearby nursery or (in legalized states) a cannabis grow outlet where you can consult with a knowledgeable salesperson about equipment and supplies, have your questions answered, and obtain assistance when your plants aren't as green and perky or your buds aren't as big and beautiful as you expect.

Wrapping Your Brain Around the Cannabis Growth Cycle

Before you get into the nitty-gritty of actually growing cannabis, you should grasp the basics of the cannabis growth cycle. With a clear understanding of the growth cycle, you're better able to meet the needs of your plants, which vary with the different stages of growth:

» **Germination:** All cannabis plants begin their lives as hard, dry seeds. Within one to seven days of being placed in a warm, dark, moist environment, the seeds sprout (germinate); they split open, and the tap root appears. The tap root grows down into the soil or substrate while the stem grows upward.

» **Seedling:** When the first fan leaves appear, the plant is considered a *seedling*. This stage lasts for about two to three weeks, during which time the seedlings require 18 to 24 hours of light. Initially, fan leaves may have a limited number of fingers (one or three). As plants mature, the fan leaves have more fingers (typically five or seven). Seedlings require plenty of light to avoid becoming spindly. At this stage they're very susceptible to overwatering, so water sparingly.

» **Vegetative:** When plants begin to develop leaves with the full complement of five or seven fingers, they've entered the vegetative stage, which lasts for two to eight weeks. During this time, plants need 18 to 24 hours of light and sufficient water and nutrients, especially nitrogen, to support growth. You'll also want to stake and trellis your plants to support them. As the plants near the flowering stage, you can distinguish between male and female plants (see Chapter 2), at which point you should separate the two to prevent fertilization (unless you're breeding plants or need seeds).

» **Flowering:** When you're ready to flower (when plants are about half their adult size), switch the plants to a light cycle of 12 hours on, 12 hours off. Without 12 hours of darkness, plants may not flower. About four weeks into the flowering stage, switch to a fertilizer that's higher in potassium and phosphorous and lower in nitrogen. (See the later section "Prepping Plants for Harvest" for details of what to do a few weeks prior to harvest.)

You can tell when a plant is ready to harvest by looking at its buds. If half the buds have red and orange hairs and about 70 percent of the trichomes are milky white and the other 30 percent are amber, the plant is ready to harvest. (See Chapter 12 for more about harvest and post-harvest.)

REMEMBER

Plants can be auto-flowering or photoperiod. Auto-flowering plants enter the flowering stage after a certain number of weeks regardless of whether they get 12 hours of darkness. Photoperiod plants may not flower unless they get the full 12 hours of darkness.

Choosing a Cultivation Method

One of your first choices as a grower is where and how you intend to grow your plants — the cultivation method. Do you want to grow plants indoors or outdoors, in the ground or in containers, in soil or hydroponically (in water)? In this section, we weigh the pros and cons of the various options to enable you to make well-informed decisions.

Indoor

Before you decide to turn your walk-in closet into a grow room, weigh the pros and cons of growing indoors:

>> **Pros:** Privacy, security, easy access, and the ability to grow in any climate during any season of the year.

>> **Cons:** High-costs of equipment and electricity to run that equipment, loss of available living/storage space, work involved in setting up a grow room, the mess (and potential water issues) in your living quarters, odors inside (and outside) your home, noise from fans.

If you decide to grow indoors, consider the following factors when choosing one or more rooms to use for your grow operation:

>> **Electrical capacity:** Grow lights, fans, timers, and other electrical equipment can consume a significant amount of electricity. If your home has a 100 amp system that's already having trouble meeting your electrical needs, a grow room can put it over the top, potentially increasing safety risks and the risk of damage to expensive equipment. Consult an electrician to ensure that your home has sufficient capacity and that the room is wired properly.

>> **Light leakage:** The room should have no light leaking in from outside or from neighboring rooms. The smallest light leaks can cause plants to produce seeds, which isn't desirable for your bud. (As explained later, you can purchase a grow tent to overcome this challenge.)

>> **Ventilation:** You must be able to ventilate the room — to ensure airflow into and out of the room without making your entire home smell like your grow (unless, of course, that's your goal), while ensuring the outgoing air doesn't contain odors that irritate the neighbors.

>> **Drainage:** Some spills are unavoidable, but if you don't have a way to drain away excess water from plants, you can end up ruining the floor in a grow room and creating an environment in which excessive humidity provides the perfect environment for molds and fungi, which are unhealthy for both you and your plants.

>> **Different areas:** You may want or need to segment the room (or use separate rooms) for different stages of plant growth — germination, seedling, vegetative (veg) state, and flowering. Light and nutrient requirements vary during the different stages.

See the later section "Creating a Grow Room for Indoor Cultivation" for more about setting up a grow room.

Outdoor

If you have an area outside that's private, secure, and gets at least five hours of direct sun and five hours of indirect sun, you have the option of growing cannabis outdoors. Before you decide to grow outdoors, consider the following pros and cons:

>> **Pros:** Larger yields, significantly lower costs, less mess, a more organic and flavorful product. Growing outdoors is also generally easier because nature does a lot of the work.

>> **Cons:** Less privacy and security (in general) and increased exposure to disease, pests, and weather events (wind, hail, floods, extreme heat or cold), which can damage the plants or even wipe out your entire crop.

REMEMBER

You can grow cannabis outdoors in a wide variety of climates, but in colder regions, your growing season may be relatively short. The good news is that you need only six to ten weeks (usually eight) to produce a crop.

See the later section "Preparing for Outdoor Cultivation" for details about choosing a proper grow site and preparing it for cultivation.

Hydroponics

Hydroponics is a method of growing plants without soil. Instead, plants are grown in a nutrient solution with the use of a substrate such as coco coir, clay pebbles, or vermiculite to support the plant. The benefits of hydroponics are the following:

>> Bigger yields

>> Higher potencies

>> Faster growth

>> Reduced risks of pests and disease

>> Less water required

>> More plants in less space

The main drawback of hydroponics is that it isn't as forgiving as soil. If you make a mistake with the nutrients, you can easily and quickly kill all the plants in your hydroponics system. Another drawback is the cost and complexity of setting up and maintaining a hydroponics system. (See the later section "Using a hydroponics system" for more details.)

WARNING

If you're a novice, steer clear of hydroponics. Soil is much easier and more forgiving.

Soil

Soil is a tried and true method for growing cannabis. It offers the following benefits over hydroponics:

>> Easier

>> Lower cost (dirt cheap)

>> Lower maintenance

>> More forgiving

See the later section "Prepping Your Soil or Other Grow Medium" for details.

Creating a Grow Room for Indoor Cultivation

Growing cannabis isn't like growing a house plant. For optimal quality and maximum yield, you should set up a grow room, so you have more control over the lighting, ventilation, air circulation, temperature, and humidity. If you're growing photoperiod plants (which require 12 hours of darkness during the flowering stage), a grow room is essential.

In this section, we cover the basics of creating your very own grow room.

Tackling the initial setup

The first thing you need is a room — an unused bedroom or closet does the trick. If you don't have a suitable room, consider putting up a grow tent (or grow box) in an open space in your home, basement, or garage. You can buy a grow tent or build your own. Your grow room or tent must have the following features:

>> Sufficient space for the number of plants and size of plants you want to grow. The space also must be tall enough to accommodate the plant height and hang a grow light far enough above the plant to prevent it from burning the plant. A three-feet square, six-feet tall area is sufficient for growing one or two plants.

>> Light sealed. No outside light should penetrate the walls. If you close yourself into the room during the daytime or when lights are on in surrounding areas, the room should be pitch black inside. (This isn't as important for auto-flowering strains.)

>> White or reflective interior walls, floor, and ceiling. If the interior isn't reflecting light, it's absorbing it, which is a waste of light. You want all light to be reflected back into the room, so that your plants can absorb it.

>> Floor drain or waterproof tray. You need something in place to catch anything that drains off from the plants.

>> Openings for ventilation fans. The room needs at least two openings, typically one near the bottom at one end of the room and another near the top at the opposite end of the room.

>> Outlets for plugging in lights or fans or an opening for power cords and other wiring.

>> Some type of framework near the top for hanging the grow lights and other equipment.

Simulating the desired climate

When you're growing outdoors, Mother Nature dictates the climate. When you're growing indoors, you play that role. Controlling the climate involves regulating the temperature, humidity, and airflow. Ideal conditions vary according to the growth stage:

>> **Germination:** During germination, seeds need to be kept warm and moist in the dark. You can start seeds in dampened soil plugs in a mini greenhouse (available at most hardware stores). Just make sure the seeds don't dry out; otherwise, they'll be ruined.

>> **Seedling/vegetative:** During the vegetative stage, maintain a temperature between 75 and 80 degrees Fahrenheit and relative humidity between 60 and 70 percent. Proper ventilation is necessary to pull in outside air that helps cool your room and deliver a steady supply of carbon dioxide (CO_2). The CO_2 concentration should be between 700 and 900 parts per million (ppm). (See the later section "Supplying carbon dioxide" for details.) Proper circulation is also necessary to keep the plants healthy. See the next section for more about ventilation and circulation.

>> **Flowering:** During the flowering stage, maintain a temperature between 72 and 78 degrees Fahrenheit and relative humidity between 50 and 55 percent. Lowering the humidity discourages fungal growth on the buds. The CO_2 concentration should be between 1,200 and 1,500 parts per million (ppm). (See the later section "Supplying carbon dioxide" for details.)

REMEMBER

In terms of temperature, remember this rule: No colder than 60, no hotter than 85, and never above 90.

Focusing on air flow

When you grow plants outdoors, air naturally circulates around the plants. When you grow plants indoors, you need to ensure proper ventilation and circulation. *Ventilation* carries outside air into the room and stale air out of the room, whereas *circulation* moves air around inside the room. Ventilation and circulation keep plants healthy and support growth in the following ways:

>> **Help to regulate heat and humidity:** Grow lights kick out a lot of heat, which also increases the humidity in the grow room. An exhaust fan pulls hot and humid air out of the grow room, creating a vacuum that pulls in cooler, drier air (assuming the room has intake holes or vents).

>> **Deliver CO_2 to plants:** Plants breathe in carbon dioxide (CO_2) and breathe out oxygen (O_2). Without proper ventilation, the CO_2 supply in the room is depleted, and the plants "suffocate."

>> **Prevent pests and diseases:** Warm, humid, stagnant air provides an ideal environment for mold, mildew, fungi, and certain pests. Pulling in cooler, drier air eliminates this problem, and having a breeze in the room helps to discourage infestations of small flying insects such as gnats.

>> **Strengthen plant stalks and stems:** Plants sense the breeze in the room and grow hardier as a result, which provides more support for buds during the flower stage.

REMEMBER

Improper air flow in grow rooms is the number one reason for reduced yields and complete crop failure.

In this section, we explain how to properly ventilate a grow room and circulate air within the room.

Ensuring proper ventilation

The first order of business is to install one or two fans to ventilate the room — an exhaust fan, an intake fan, or both. With an active system, you have an exhaust fan on one end of the room and an intake fan of the same size on the opposite end. In a passive system, you use only one fan. As the exhaust fan pulls air out of the room or the intake fan pushes air into the room, air flows in or out through one or more holes on the opposite end of the room. In passive systems, the hole (or holes) without the fan must be larger than the hole with the fan.

Most grow rooms use in-line duct fans, which are very easy to install. Installation is similar to connecting a flexible duct pipe to a clothes dryer. You can buy 4-, 6-, or 8-inch diameter in-line duct fans depending on the size of the room and the size of any existing holes. Six-inch fans are common. If you have a grow tent, check the size of the exhaust and intake holes and buy fans to match.

Also check the cubic feet per minute (CFM) rating of the fan(s) and buy a fan with a CFM rating that's higher than the volume of the room in cubic feet. The general idea is that you want sufficient ventilation to completely replace the air in the grow room once every minute. Simply measure the room's length, width, and height in feet and multiply the three numbers. For example, if the room is 3-by-3-by-6 feet, $3 \times 3 \times 6 = 54$ cubic feet, so a fan with a rating of 100 CFM would be sufficient. However, you may need a fan with a higher CFM rating if you're pumping the air over a long distance or have one or more bends in the duct pipe.

REMEMBER

Your intake hole should be near the bottom at one end of the room with the exhaust hole at the top of the opposite end of the room. The exhaust hole is higher, because heat naturally rises to the top.

Whether you use one or two fans, install a filter on the intake and exhaust ducts. The intake filter keeps out bugs, mold spores, dust, and other contaminants. The exhaust filter is usually a carbon filter that helps to reduce the odors from the cannabis exiting the room. You attach the filters directly to the fans or use a piece of flexible duct pipe between the fan and filter.

TIP

Use as little duct pipe as necessary and run it as straight as possible. The longer the distance the air has to travel and the more bends in the pipe, the less efficient the air flow. If you must run pipe a long distance or add a bend, consider buying fans with higher CFM ratings.

Circulating the air

Air circulation is also important. Plants don't "exhale" with any type of force during respiration. Fans used to circulate the air move the O_2 surrounding the plants and replace it with CO_2 that the plants can "breathe in." You need one or more fans inside your grow room to maintain proper circulation. Deciding on the number of fans and positioning them in the room is mostly a process of trial and error. The goal is to have all parts of all plants "dancing" — all the leaves should be shaking gently. If you notice any part of any plant that's not dancing, you may need to reposition the fan(s) or add a fan.

TIP

Start with two small fans in opposite corners of the room or one slightly larger oscillating fan in one corner of the room and make adjustments from there.

Supplying carbon dioxide

Plants require CO_2 to survive. This is the symbiotic relationship plants have with animals. Animals breath in O_2 and exhale CO_2; plants "inhale" CO_2 and "exhale" O_2. If your grow room has adequate air flow, CO_2 sublimation isn't necessary, but it increases overall yields if you're using higher intensity lighting.

Several methods are available for adding CO_2 to a grow room. You can buy a tank of CO_2 and simply pump it into the room, allow dry ice to melt inside the room, or buy CO_2 canisters or bags that release the gas slowly into the room over a period of time. If you're adding CO_2 to your grow room, keep the following important points in mind:

>> Add CO_2 only when the lights are on. When the lights are off, plants slow down their use of CO_2 considerably, so any CO_2 added is CO_2 wasted.

>> Turn off the intake and exhaust fans for a few minutes when releasing CO_2; otherwise, you're pumping out the gas, and wasting it.

>> Add CO_2 from the top of the room and in front of one of your circulating fans. It's denser than air, so it tends to drop toward the floor. For example, if you're using a CO_2 tank, run a hose to near the top of the grow room and lower it so it's in front of one of the fans.

> » Maintain a level of 900 parts per million (ppm) of CO_2 during the vegetative stage and 1,150 ppm during the flower stage. You'll need a CO_2 meter to monitor CO_2 levels.

REMEMBER

Additional CO_2 is necessary with higher light intensity, enabling the plant to take advantage of the added light with greater photosynthesis.

Setting up grow lights

Lighting is a key factor in a successful indoor grow operation. The types of lights, the way you set them up, and other pieces that control and direct them are the keys to your yield and the flavor of your end product. In this section, we guide you through the process of choosing and installing your grow lights.

Calculating your lighting needs

Before you head out to your local nursery or hardware store to shop for grow lights figure out how much light you need. In general, a standard 1,000 watt grow light will cover four plants that have a fully grown diameter of about 3 feet, depending on strain. If you set up your grow lights and plants and notice that some parts of one or more plants aren't receiving light, you'll need to add one or more lights.

Choosing light fixtures and bulbs

Most standard household light fixtures and bulbs are insufficient for growing cannabis. They don't provide the intensity and quality of light the plants need for optimal growth. The exception is fluorescent lights (typically T5s) or compact fluorescent lights (CFLs), which are okay, but result in smaller, lower-quality buds. We don't recommend fluorescent lighting.

After ruling out fluorescent lighting, your choice of grow lights depends on your goal and the stage of growth:

> » If your goal is high yields, choose a high intensity discharge (HID) bulb — metal-halide (MH) for the vegetative stage and high pressure sodium (HPS) during the flower stage. These bulbs emit a lot of light and a lot of heat, so you need to position them at a greater distance from the plants.

> » If you're looking for better terpene yields for extraction, use light-emitting diode (LED) or ceramic metal halide (CMH) bulbs, because these preserve the terpenes without bulking up the flower weight and density the way high-intensity discharge (HID) lighting does.

Your choice of light fixture depends on the bulbs you want to use. After choosing a bulb type, shop for grow light system that includes all the lighting components you need, including the bulbs. Components/features of a grow room lighting system include the following:

>> **Fixture with reflector hood:** The fixture holds the bulbs, and the reflector hood directs the light down to the plants. Reflector hoods come in different types:

- **Closed hood:** Shaped like a box, a closed hood reflector creates a more focused beam of light (and heat).

- **Vented hood:** Similar to a closed hood reflector but with openings on the ends for connecting the hood to in-line duct fans for cooling.

- **Wing:** Typically a curved and textured aluminum sheet that provides a less focused beam of light than a closed hood reflector. The light covers a greater area but is less intense (so is the heat).

- **Parabolic:** Shaped like an umbrella, a parabolic hood distributes light like a wing but in a more circular pattern.

Your choice of hoods is a personal preference. Go with a closed hood if you're concerned about heat or with an wing or parabolic if you're not.

>> **Ballast:** The ballast provides control over the current that the lightbulb draws from the power source. The following two types of ballasts are most common:

- **Magnetic:** Less expensive, heavy, hot, potentially noisy, susceptible to flicker, and supports only bulbs of a certain wattage. If you want to change from a 400W bulb to a 600W bulb, for example, you need to replace the ballast.

- **Digital:** More expensive, smaller, lighter, cooler, quieter, less susceptible to flicker, more efficient, may be equipped with a dimmable option, may cause radio frequency interference.

>> **Hooks and pulleys:** Grow light systems often include hooks and pulleys for hanging the light fixtures in your grow room. Pulleys enable you to more easily raise and lower the light fixtures to place them at the right distance from the tops of the plants.

>> **Timer:** Grow light systems typically come with a timer, or you can purchase a timer separately, which automates the process of cycling the lights on and off on schedule.

Mounting your light fixtures

Mount the light fixtures to the ceiling of the grow room above the plants, positioning the fixtures to ensure equal distribution of light over the entire canopy. How you mount the light fixtures depends on the fixture and how your grow room ceiling is configured. Using hooks, ropes, or chains and possibly pulleys, you can hang your fixtures in a way that you can easily raise and lower them to the proper distance from the tops of your plants.

Position the lights above the plants, so all parts of all plants are receiving light. The light should be as close to the top of the tallest plant as possible without burning it. Keep a close eye on the plants whenever adjusting the lights, and if the top of any plant is getting burned, raise the light.

WARNING

Don't place anything flammable close enough to the light that there's any possibility the light will ignite it.

Setting and resetting timers

During the vegetative stage, plants require 18 to 24 hours of light. During the bloom/flower stage, they need 10 to 12 hours of light and at least 12 hours of total darkness (for photoperiod strains); auto-flowering strains will flower without 12 hours of darkness. Putting your grow lights on timers greatly simplifies the process of managing the required light/dark cycles, but you still need to manage the changes in lighting over the growth cycle.

REMEMBER

If you plan to have a continuous garden with some plants in veg and some in bloom, set up your lighting differently in those two areas. For photoperiod strains, use a separate grow tent or grow room for plants that are in the vegetative stage and those that are in the flower stage.

To monitor your plants through the growth cycle and adjust the lighting, take the following steps:

1. **Position the lights at the proper distance above the canopy for the vegetative stage.**

2. **Adjust your light timer(s) to provide 18 to 24 hours of light.**

   Experiment with different settings in that range over several grows to find the optimum amount of light for each strain you grow.

3. **Keep an eye on your plants, adjusting the lighting as necessary to keep the lights the proper distance from the tops of the plants as they grow taller.**

   When your plants are about half the size of full-grown plants, they're ready to switch from the vegetative to the flower stage. (At this point, you either adjust the lighting, as explained in the remaining steps or move the plants to the flower tent or room.)

The size of a full-grown plant is strain dependent and impacted by light, container size, and other environmental influencers such as CO_2. You may have to go through several rounds of growing a particular strain to develop a clear idea what the size of a full-grown plant is and when the plant is ready to switch from the vegetative to the flower stage.

4. **If you were using MH bulbs during the vegetative stage, change to HPS bulbs for the flower stage.**

   You don't need to change out fluorescent, CFL, or LED bulbs.

   When changing to the brighter HPS bulbs, shade the plants for a couple days to prevent them from getting blasted by the more intense light. You can place a piece of cardboard between the light and the plants to serve this purpose, but make sure it's as far as possible from the light to prevent a fire.

5. **Adjust the height of your lights to position them the proper distance from the tops of the plants for the flower stage.**

6. **Adjust the timers, so that the plants receive at least 12 hours of total darkness and 10–12 hours of light.**

   Auto-flowering strains don't need 12 hours of darkness; experiment with the lighting between grows to determine what's best.

7. **Continue to monitor your plants during the flower stage, adjusting the height of the lights as needed to keep them the proper distance from the tops of the plants as the plants grow taller.**

   When the stigma (the hair-like strands that cover the bud) on half the buds turn orange and red, your plant is ready for harvest.

Measuring the light

Light intensity has a big impact on yield. All parts of all plants should have exposure to the light, and the lights should be as close to the plants as possible without burning them. If the top of any plants are wilting or burnt from the light, raise the lights.

For more sophisticated grows, obtain a photosynthetic active radiation (PAR) meter and take measurements at several different locations above the canopy to measure the PAR output of the lights. The PAR measure should never rise above 1,200 PAR.

Deciding on a watering/fertilizing system

Whether you're growing indoors or outdoors, you need to decide on a system for watering and fertilizing your plants. You basically have two options: manual and automatic. During your first grows, we recommend the manual method as you develop a sense of how much water and fertilizer your plants generally need. (See the later section "Watering and fertilizing your plants.")

After developing an understanding of your plants' water and nutrient needs (which may vary depending on the strain), consider installing an automated irrigation system. These systems are equipped with timers that water and feed plants automatically on a pre-set schedule. They provide the same benefits of lighting systems — the convenience and reliability of automation. However, you still need to monitor your plants to be sure they're getting enough and not too much water and nutrients.

Using a hydroponics system

In all hydroponics systems, plants are placed in trays or containers that contain a grow medium other than soil, such as pea gravel, expanded clay aggregate, coco coir, or vermiculite. Various systems are then used to deliver water and nutrients to the roots (see Figure 11-1 for illustrations of these systems):

>> **Aeroponic:** Plants sit in a tray above a water/nutrient reservoir with their roots dangling down. Solution from the reservoir is sprayed up onto the roots at regular intervals, and excess solution drips down into the reservoir.

>> **Drip:** Nutrient-rich water is dripped slowly at regular intervals into the grow medium where the roots can absorb it. Unused water drains back to the reservoir to be reused or to a waste reservoir and then discarded.

>> **Deep water culture (DWC):** Plants sit in baskets above an aerated (and typically chilled) water/nutrient reservoir with their roots submerged in the solution, which allows for continuous feeding.

>> **Ebb and flow:** Plants sit in pots in a grow tray. Nutrient-rich water is pumped into the grow tray at regular intervals and flows into holes at the bottom and sides of the pots. The pumping stops and water is allowed to drain back into the reservoir from which it was pumped.

>> **Nutrient film technique (NFT):** NFT is like a cross between DWC and ebb and flow. Plants sit in baskets above a grow tray. Nutrient-rich water is continuously pumped from a reservoir into the grow tray and then drains from the opposite end of the grow tray back into the reservoir. This arrangement delivers a continuous flow of nutrient-rich water to the roots.

>> **Wick:** A plant sits in a container above an aerated, nutrient-rich water reservoir, and a rope or other absorbent material (such as felt) is placed through the middle of the growth medium and into the reservoir. Through capillary action, the solution from the reservoir "climbs" the rope, providing the plant with as much or as little water and nutrients as it demands.

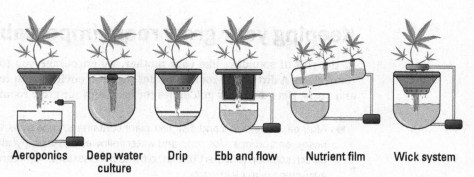

FIGURE 11-1:
Various
hydroponic
systems.

Aeroponics   Deep water culture   Drip   Ebb and flow   Nutrient film   Wick system

© John Wiley & Sons, Inc.

Here are a few suggestions for increasing your odds of a successful hydroponics grow:

>> Disinfect all your hydroponics equipment with isopropyl alcohol or bleach between grows to kill off any bacteria or other infectious agents. Anaerobic bacteria can build up in dirty systems and kill your plants from the roots up.

>> Use clean, pH neutral water. Water from a reverse osmosis (RO) system or distilled water is suitable.

>> Aerate the nutrient-rich water solution. You can place an aeration stone in the bottom of the reservoir attached to a small air pump like those carried by local pet stores. Without aeration, your plants may not receive the oxygen they need.

>> Replace the water/nutrient solution every couple weeks. Don't merely add nutrients, because nutrient concentrations may become too high as a result. (Remember to use a fertilizer with a higher nitrogen concentration during the vegetative stage and higher potassium and phosphorous during the flower stage.)

>> After dumping the old nutrient solution, run a dilute water and hydrogen peroxide solution through the system to clear out any infectious agents and then rinse with plain water.

>> Consider flushing the grow medium with plain water whenever you change the nutrient solution.

TIP

When choosing and setting up a hydroponics system, research to find out the type of system that's best for your grow space and skill level. Simpler is usually better. Use high quality food grade plastics in your system and make sure it's leak free before starting your grow.

Keeping your grow room impeccably clean

At the risk of sounding like your mother, we encourage you to keep your grow room clean. A dirty grow room provides the ideal environment for bacteria, fungi, and pests. Here are a few guidelines for keeping your grow room clean:

>> After each use, wash and disinfect plant containers, grow trays, irrigation hoses, and pumps. Use soap and water followed by isopropyl alcohol or a bleach solution (one part bleach to three parts water). Then, carefully rinse everything with plain water.

>> Keep your grow room free of any dead plant mater and debris. This is where many pests and pathogens can get a foothold in a garden of healthy plants.

>> Watch for common pests such as aphids, fungus gnats, spider mites, and thrips. If you see even one of these nasty critters, identify it and find an effective pesticide. This is where your friendly garden store or grow store staff comes in handy.

Preparing for Outdoor Cultivation

Growing plants outdoors is generally easier than growing them indoors because Mother Nature chips in to do some of the work. Even so, you have to lay the groundwork for a successful grow to ensure that your plants receive the nutrients they need. In this section, we lead you through the process of preparing a site for outdoor cultivation.

REMEMBER

As long as you have a sunny location in an area where you get at least eight to ten weeks of relatively sunny weather and temperatures between 60 and 90 degrees Fahrenheit, you can grow cannabis outdoors. If your growing season is short, you can get a jump on things by starting your plants indoors and then transplanting your seedlings (after a brief hardening period). If you live in a warmer climate, you can simply plant your seeds outside after the threat of frost passes.

Choosing a site

If you decide to grow outdoors, choose your grow site carefully. Consider the following factors:

>> **Compliance:** Your grow site must comply with all local rules and regulations. It must be private property owned by you. In most locations, your garden must be secure with a privacy fence and plants no taller than the fence. Any

gates must be locked to prevent kids from getting to the plants and to discourage theft.

REMEMBER

» **Space:** The amount of space you need depends on the number and types of plants you want to and are legally permitted to grow. Your plants will need to be spaced at least three to five feet apart, so they all get plenty of sun and breeze.

Think ahead. Will each plant have enough space when fully grown? Will plants shade other plants from the sun?

» **Soil:** Cannabis can grow in a wide variety of soil types, as long as the soil has sufficient drainage. If it doesn't, you can amend the soil or plant in containers. (See the later section "Evaluating the soil" for details.)

» **Sunlight and darkness:** Cannabis plants need at least five hours of direct sunlight plus at least five hours of indirect sun daily. They'll reward you for more sun with a bountiful harvest. Also, don't plant a photoperiod strain under or near a bright street lamp; otherwise, it may not flower properly.

REMEMBER

Consider surrounding objects such as buildings and trees and how the angle of the sun changes over the course of the growing season. As a result, an area that gets full sun all day long during one part of the growing season may be shaded part or all of the day during another part of the growing season. Ideally, your grow site will get sun all day long throughout the growing season.

» **Convenient access:** You'll be tending to your plants regularly and be eager to watch them grow, so pick a location with easy access. A backyard garden may be ideal.

» **Access to water:** Unless it rains every few days, you'll need to water your plants regularly, so pick a site that has easy access to water.

REMEMBER

Cannabis must be grown on private property, so you must own the land. Growing on public land, such as a national park or forest, is illegal.

Evaluating the soil

Prior to planting in an outdoor grow site, check the soil. Quality soil has the following characteristics:

» **Loamy:** Loam soil is a combination of approximately equal parts of sand and silt along with relatively little clay. It retains moisture, but it also drains well, so plants aren't sitting in saturated soil in which they're susceptible to root rot and other diseases. Loam soil crumbles easily in your hands. If the soil is rock hard when dry, it contains too much clay. If it doesn't hold together at all when you squeeze it into a ball, it may be too sandy.

>> **Fertile:** Healthy soil also contains organic matter, such as decomposing wood and other plant matter. You can mix mulch and other amendments into the soil to increase its fertility, if necessary.

>> **Slightly acidic:** You can use a pH meter to test the soil's pH, which should be in a range of 5.5 to 6.5. Anything lower is too acidic, and anything higher is too alkaline.

>> **Alive:** Good soil is home to many critters, including earthworms and beneficial bacteria and other microorganisms. If you don't see anything crawling around in your soil, it's probably lacking in organic matter.

TIP

Take a soup can of soil from several areas around your grow site to your local nursery or university extension office to have your soil tested. Test results show pH levels; levels of key nutrients, including potassium, phosphorous, and nitrogen; concentrations of organic matter; and so on. You may also receive specific recommendations on amendments needed to improve soil quality.

TIP

For a more thorough guide to evaluating outdoor soil, check out the free Willamette Valley Soil Quality Card Guide at `catalog.extension.oregonstate.edu/sites/catalog/files/project/pdf/em8710.pdf` published by Oregon State University.

Deciding whether to grow in-ground or in containers

When growing outside, you have the option of growing your plants in containers or in the ground. Sometimes, the choice is easy; for example, if the only place with enough sun is a concrete or wood deck, you have no choice but to grow in containers. If you do have a choice, consider the pros and cons of each option:

>> Planting in-ground is generally easier and more forgiving. With quality soil, you don't have to worry so much about plants becoming root bound or developing root rot, and you may not have to water as frequently.

>> Containers add height which may make your plants taller than allowed by law or taller than the privacy fence you built.

>> If containers are too small, plants can get root bound, preventing them from absorbing the water and nutrients they need. In containers, plants may also be more susceptible to root rot if the plants don't drain properly.

>> You can move containers around if the sunny locations in your space change over the course of the growing season.

>> If you have poor quality soil, you need to amend the soil prior to planting, which adds to the cost and work involved.

>> In a container, you can easily customize your soil mix to create the perfect grow medium for your plants.

For more about preparing your soil for planting, see the later section "Prepping Your Soil or Other Grow Medium."

Hardening off your plants

If you start your plants inside (in a grow room or on a windowsill), harden them off before transplanting them to an outdoor location. *Hardening off* is a process in which plants gradually become acclimated to the outside environment over a period of seven to ten days.

Take your plants outside for 30 minutes or so on the first day and place them in a sheltered area where they receive indirect sunlight and perhaps a gentle breeze. Continue to increase this time by 30 minutes or so each day, gradually increasing their exposure to more direct sun. Watch your plants carefully for signs of heavy stress such as burning or wilting. Light stress is good, and it will accelerate the hardening off process, but heavy stress can kill a plant or severely impact its ability to flourish.

You should also harden off your plants against the cold. If frost is possible, keep the plants inside at night. Otherwise, gradually expose them to the cold nights. You may want to place them in a cold frame or under a box or bucket at first to provide some shelter from the cold without having to bring them inside, just be sure to uncover them the next day or they may overheat. Over the course of seven to ten days, they should be able to make it through a cool and frost-free night.

Supporting and protecting your plants

When growing plants outside, you may need to provide them with support and protection from the elements, especially cold and frost as the summer growing season ends.

First, focus on providing your plant with structural support throughout its growth cycle especially in the flower stage. The idea is to provide your plant's branches the support they need to grow big fat buds without becoming too heavy and breaking off from the main stalk. Bamboo stakes, along with twine or Velcro plant straps, are great and provide a variety of ways to stake your plants, such as the following:

>> Place a stake alongside the stalk, and tie the stalk to the stake.

>> Place three or four stakes around the periphery of the plant, and tie branches that need support to the stakes. You can also wrap twine around the stakes to create your own "cage."

>> Place a row of stakes in front of or behind several plants, and then tie stakes horizontally to the vertical stakes (or weave them together) to create a trellis. You can then tie branches to the trellis.

Tomato cages are also great and readily available at any garden or hardware store. Place them over your young cannabis plants, and the plants will grow up through the cage and be well supported. Even better are Screen of Green (ScroG) kits (see Figure 11-2), which provide support along with a means for scrogging (see the later section "Training your plants for maximum yield" for details).

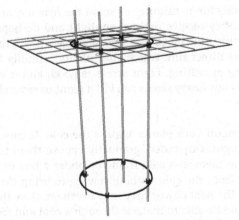

FIGURE 11-2:
A ScroG kit.

© John Wiley & Sons, Inc.

Prepping Your Soil or Other Grow Medium

The process for prepping your soil or other grow medium prior to planting depends on whether you're planting indoors or out, in-ground or in containers, or in a hydroponics system:

>> **Outdoor, in-ground:** Evaluate your soil or have it professionally tested (see the earlier section "Evaluating the soil") and work in any amendments necessary to make the soil suitable for growing cannabis.

>> **In containers:** Ask the horticulturalist at your nursery to recommend a soil mixture suitable for cannabis. If you don't feel comfortable asking about soil for cannabis, ask about a soil mix for tomatoes, which will be fine for your cannabis plants, as well.

Be sure your containers have good drainage. If you're growing indoors, also be sure to place the containers on trays to catch excess water.

REMEMBER

>> **In hydroponic grow medium:** Rinse the grow medium with plain water before using it in your hydroponics system. Hydroponic media typically have before-use instructions. Follow those, and you'll be golden.

Planting Seeds or Cuttings

You can grow plants from seeds or create a clone of a plant from a cutting. To decide, consider the pros and cons of seeds versus cuttings:

>> Growing from a cutting of an existing plant essentially clones the plant, so you know what you're getting. If you clone a female plant, you get a female plant.

>> Although technically you can clone an auto-flowering strain, it's usually not worth the trouble because the clone doesn't produce nearly the same yield. If you want to grow auto-flowering strains, buy seeds.

>> Unless you buy feminized seeds, which have a very high likelihood of growing into feminine plants, you can't tell just by looking at a seed whether it's a seed for a male or female plant. You have to plant a bunch of seeds, wait until you can determine whether the plant is male or female (see Chapter 2), and then dispose of the male plants.

>> You also can't tell the strain of a plant by looking at a seed, so unless you know which strain of plant the seed came from, you have no idea what strain the seed will produce.

>> Plants from seeds generally are more vigorous. In fact, sometimes growers grow cuttings and allow them to go to seed to revitalize the plant's genetics.

WARNING

If you're in a location where cannabis is illegal, growing it is probably illegal too. Bringing in seeds or cuttings to your location can very well be a felony, and reputable sellers won't ship to you. You can probably purchase and grow hemp seeds and plants, which have a negligible amount of THC, but these plants won't produce the psychoactive effects of plants that contain higher levels of THC. Check with your seller to be certain you're getting what you think you're purchasing. If you buy seeds for CBD-only hemp plants by mistake, you can end up being very disappointed post-harvest.

Acquiring seeds or cuttings

You can usually find cannabis seeds for sale at most dispensaries in areas where growing cannabis for personal use is legal. You may also find growers who sell cuttings/clones. You can expect to pay $50 to $100 for a pack of ten seeds. When shopping for seeds or cuttings, read the labels and any other information the manufacturer provides on their website or in their catalog to make sure you're getting the right seeds or cuttings (the strain) for the plants you want to grow.

TIP

One way to get your mitts on some seeds is to collect seeds when you find them in flower you purchased or get some from friends if they're collecting.

When buying seeds or cuttings, here are some key characteristics to consider:

>> **Feminized seeds:** Nearly all seeds sold by reputable companies are feminized, but make sure they are. These seeds are specially treated to grow into female plants.

>> **Auto-flowering or photoperiod:** Auto-flowering plants are easier, because they enter the flower stage after a certain number of weeks regardless of the light/dark cycle. If you're a beginner, seriously consider going with auto-flowering plants.

>> **Genetic background:** If seeds are from a well-established strain, such as O.G. Kush or Bubble Gum or a cross-breed, the genetic background should be stated.

>> **Blend:** The blend represents the percentage of the three species — sativa, indica, and ruderalis. All auto-flower strains contain some percentage of ruderalis, which is responsible for the auto-flowering nature of the plant.

>> **Yield indoors:** The number of grams of bud per square meter of plant when grown indoors.

>> **Yield outdoors:** The number of grams of bud per plant (after drying) when grown outdoors.

>> **Plant height indoors:** Shorter than when grown outdoors.

>> **Plant height outdoors:** Taller than when grown indoors.

>> **Time to harvest:** Approximate number of weeks after germination the flower should be ready to harvest.

>> **Potency:** Percentages of CBD and THC.

>> **Effect:** The type of experience you can expect when consuming product from the plant.

WARNING

KNOW THE LAWS

Before buying cannabis seeds or cuttings, research the country, state, province, and local laws regarding buying, selling, possessing, and transporting seeds or cuttings across borders. Rules and regulations vary considerably:

- In some European countries laws prohibit growing cannabis but seed is legal, which is quite confusing. You're allowed to buy and eat cannabis seeds because they're non-psychotropic, but you can't buy them to grow cannabis. Other countries in Europe, such as Germany, have their own seed laws.

- In Canada, where cannabis is federally legal, seeds can be shipped across provincial lines.

- In the U.S., in some states in which cannabis is legal, you can purchase seeds from some dispensaries or other locations to grow plants as long as you keep them in the state. Other states may bar selling to non-licensed growers. Shipping or transporting seeds across state or international borders is illegal, although a few reputable online seed stores ship to individuals with success.

If you choose to buy seeds online and have them shipped to you, research the store carefully and check reviews to make certain they have a solid track record.

Cuttings are typically treated in a similar manner as seeds in legalized locations. They may be available from some dispensaries or outlets for pick up or delivery with a fee. They're prohibited from crossing U.S. state lines or international borders. You can buy individual plants and mix and match strains. Prices vary and are often determined by plant size. Buy cuttings (clones) only from a reputable source who understands proper backcrossing of strains for stability. *Back-crossing* involves pollinating a plant with one of its parent plants to promote sexual stability, so that when you have a female it won't hermaphrodite into a male during flowering.

Both seeds and clones are often able to be purchased from commercial locations already in your state.

REMEMBER

In the U.S. transporting any part of the cannabis plant over state lines is illegal. This applies to seeds and clones and technically even to tissue samples.

Germinating seeds

Germinating seeds requires a dark environment that is around 70 degrees. There are many ways to germinate seeds (in soil, in a wet paper towel, in starter plugs) You can also sow them directly into the soil in a garden or container, as long as the soil is light and fluffy, so the roots can easily grow down and the stalk can break through the soil. Plant seeds about 1/4 to 1/2 inch deep and cover them loosely with soil.

REMEMBER

Most importantly, seeds need a moist environment; they won't germinate if they get too dry. You can use a heat mat to increase the success of germination in colder climates.

Planting seedlings

WARNING

When planting seedlings, handle them very gently, being careful not to damage the roots. Plant the seedling firmly in the soil but not so deep that it rots in the soil. When planting from a starter plug (such as a rooting cube) tease the roots a little if the cube is root bound to allow the roots to spread through the new medium.

Start with a small pot and transplant to bigger pots as the plant grows to avoid root bound plants. A plant is usually ready to transplant when the top of the plant is nearly the same circumference as the top of the pot. By starting your seeds in small cups, you may be able to get away with transplanting your seedlings only once — into a gallon or larger container that the plant can grow in over the course of the rest of its grow cycle.

WARNING

Don't wait too long to transplant plants and don't use containers that are too small. Otherwise, you increase the risk that the plants will get root bound, which can stunt their growth, and the plant may not fully recover.

Cloning plants

To clone a plant, you cut a branch from the plant and soak the base of the cut branch in water until roots form. Follow these more detailed steps:

1. **Wait until near the end of the vegetative stage, just before the flower stage.**

2. **Examine lower, sturdy branches and find a healthy segment about seven inches long with at least two nodes above the location where you'll make your cut (see Figure 11-3).**

3. **Using a sharp pair of scissors or a razor blade, cut the branch at a 45 degree angle below the lowermost node.**

4. **Dip the base of the cutting in a rooting solution and then insert it 3/4 of the way into a root cube or rockwool cube.**

   Roots will grow directly from the stem of your cutting through the opening in the bottom of the cube.

5. **Place each cutting with the root cube at its base into a clone dome or mini-greenhouse like the one shown in Figure 11-4.**

6. **Keep your plants in the clone dome with the vents closed for at least the first week. Water the cubes regularly without completely saturating them, and allow them to dry out slightly between waterings.**

7. **During the first week, wipe the condensation off the inside of the domes daily to prevent rot.**

8. **After your cuts have started to root, transplant them into a container and start hardening them off by exposing them to increasing amounts of time with the dome off to acclimate them to their un-domed environment.**

   See the later section "Transplanting" and the earlier section, "Hardening off your plants."

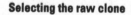

Selecting the raw clone

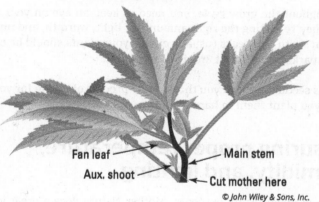

FIGURE 11-3:
Cut a branch on a
45-degree angle
below at least
two nodes.

Fan leaf — Main stem
Aux. shoot — Cut mother here
© John Wiley & Sons, Inc.

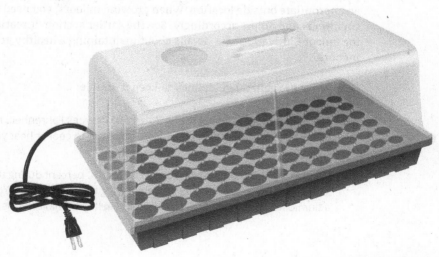

FIGURE 11-4:
A typical clone
dome.

© John Wiley & Sons, Inc.

Transplanting

When transplanting any plant, whether it started from seed or a clone, handle it gently being very careful not to damage the roots. Center the plant in the pot, and plant it deep enough to cover the root ball completely in soil. If the plant is root bound, you can gently tease the roots apart to encourage outward growth. Pack your soil or other grow medium down around the roots well enough to support the plant while new roots grow, but not so tight that the soil restricts outward root growth. Water the soil around the roots.

Keeping Your Plants Healthy

Throughout the grow cycle, you need to keep an eye on your plants and ensure that they're getting the right amounts of light, warmth, and nutrients to flourish. Within six to ten weeks (usually eight), your plants should be covered with beautiful sparkling buds that are ripe for harvest.

In this section, we lead you through the process of caring for your plants from the time you plant them to harvest time.

Ensuring proper temperature, humidity, and lighting

When growing plants outdoors, Mother Nature does a great job of ensuring the proper temperature, humidity, and lighting, assuming your plants are located in an appropriate outside location. When growing indoors, you need to monitor these conditions and adjust accordingly. See the earlier section "Creating a Grow Room for Indoor Cultivation" for details about maintaining a healthy grow environment indoors.

Here are some general guidelines to keep it simple:

>> Maintain temperatures between 70 and 80 degrees Fahrenheit, never below 60 degrees or above 90 degrees. You may need to cool or heat your grow room to maintain the proper temperature.

>> Relative humidity should be between 60 and 70 percent during the vegetative stage and between 50 and 55 percent during the flower stage. You may need a humidifier or dehumidifier to maintain healthy humidity levels.

>> For photoperiod plants, ensure that they get 18–24 hours of light during the vegetative stage. When you're ready for the flower stage (when plants are about half their adult size, switch to a 12 hours on, 12 hours off schedule. Auto-flowering strains don't need 12 hours of darkness to flower.

Watering and fertilizing your plants

Whether your plants are in the ground or in containers, water and feed them regularly but only when necessary. Here are some guidelines to get you started on the right foot:

>> When growing in containers, make sure the containers have holes in the bottom or sides for drainage, and place a tray below each pot to catch any excess water. To prevent root rot, discard any excess water from the trays, so your plant isn't sitting in it.

>> When plants are young, water near the stalk, so the roots can access the water and any nutrients (fertilizer) it contains. As plants mature, water farther from the stalk to encourage roots to grow out from the stalk.

>> Before watering, stick your finger in the pot about a quarter to half inch. The soil should be moist, neither dry nor sopping wet. If it's wet, skip the watering and let it dry. If it's dry, go ahead and water. This applies to the total life cycle of the plant from veg to bloom. (You're generally better off erring on the side of too little water than too much.)

TIP

If you observe wilting and the soil feels moist, hold off on watering and check the container (if the plant is in a container) to make sure it's draining properly. Sometimes, the drainage holes can get clogged.

>> If you use a soil mix that contains fertilizer, ask your supplier when you should start adding fertilizer. You usually need to wait four to six weeks for the plant to use up most of the fertilizer in the soil before adding more fertilizer without burning the roots.

>> Consider using organic fertilizers, which release nutrients into the soil more gradually and are more forgiving than chemical fertilizers. Organic fertilizers include bat guano, bone meal, kelp, and earthworm casings.

>> When using chemical fertilizers, use half the recommended amount to prevent harming the plants accidentally. As you gain experience, you can gradually try using more fertilizer while watching for any signs of stress or toxicity. Different strains may have slightly different nutritional needs.

>> During the growth stage, use a fertilizer that's higher in nitrogen, such as one that has a nitrogen-to-phosphorous-to potassium (NPK) ratio of 3-1-1. From the early to the middle of the flower stage, switch to a fertilizer with an NPK ratio of about 1-3-2 followed by 0-3-3 for late bloom. (These are general guidelines. You can change things up as you gain experience.)

TIP

If your plant suddenly wilts or you notice yellow or brown leaves near the bottom of the plant or exposed roots near the top of the soil or growing out of the drainage holes in the container, the roots may have outgrown the container. Remove the plant from the container, gently tease the roots to separate them, and then transplant to a larger pot with fresh soil.

Checking and adjusting the pH

Throughout the growth cycle, keep the soil slightly acidic — the pH level should be between 5.5 and 6.5. If the pH is outside that range, add pH up or pH down (available at nurseries and hardware stores) to the water/feed mixture when watering your plants to adjust the pH of the grow medium. Also, use a digital pH meter or pH test drops to test the pH of your nutrients solution before feeding it to the plants; this will help maintain the proper pH of the soil.

Battling common pests

The best defense against pests is a good offense. Keep your room and garden clean. Properly compost all discarded plant material. Quarantine any plants from outside sources until you're sure they're healthy and pest-free before bringing them into your grow room or garden. Shower and wear clean clothes before stepping into your grow room or garden. While these precautions may seem excessive, they keep out the pests and diseases and save you time, money, and effort in the long run.

TIP

If you're growing indoors, be sure to add a filter to your intake fan or vent to keep incoming air free of pests and pathogens.

If you find pests in your garden, take a picture of them and search the internet to identify them. Google's image search feature can come in handy with this. After you've identified the critter, look up effective pesticides for eradicating it. If you're unable to identify the pest or find the appropriate information to fight the infestation, take your picture to your local garden or grow store or university extension office and ask for advice from the staff.

Preventing and treating common diseases

As with pest control, the best defense is a good offense. Cannabis is most susceptible to common diseases when plants are stressed or when the environment promotes the growth and spread of infectious fungi, bacteria, and viruses. To prevent the most common and serious infections, take the following precautions:

» Provide sufficient space between plants. All parts of all plants should be exposed to light and fresh air.

» Prune plants, as discussed in the next section, to further increase the plants exposure to sun and fresh air.

» Water only during the day and avoid getting water on foliage and flower, if possible. Damp leaves are more susceptible to fungal infections.

» Maintain healthy levels of light, heat, and humidity when possible. Heat plus humidity is an ideal combination for fungal growth.

» Make sure soil/containers have proper drainage, and don't overwater.

» If you're growing in conditions with high humidity that can't be avoided, consider spraying plants with an organic anti-fungal solution as a preventive measure.

The following three diseases are most common in cannabis:

» **Root rot:** Overwatering or poor drainage can lead to root rot. The roots turn brown and soft and struggle to absorb water and nutrients, making the entire plant sick. If the plant has some healthy (white) roots, you can cut away the rotting roots and replant the plant in fresh, well-drained soil. Be sure to sanitize the pot and all tools used during the repotting process with a solution of one part bleach to three parts water. If the entire root system is brown, discard the plant.

» **Powdery mildew:** Mildew is a fungus that's closely related to mold. It typically appears first on the lower part of the plant and quickly spreads. If you see white spots on leaves that have the consistency of flower, remove the infected leaves, being very careful not to stir up the mildew or touch leaves that aren't infected, and dispose of them properly, not in the compost pile, even if it's legal to compost cannabis in your state or country (it may not be). Spray the foliage with an organic fungicide, being careful not to spray any buds. For serious infections, you may need to remove infected leaves and quarantine any infected plants. Mildew can spread quickly through airborne spores.

WARNING

Mildew can be hazardous to your health, especially if it gets on your buds and you ingest it. It makes cannabis unfit for commercial sale.

>> **Leaf septoria:** This disease typically appears first on the lower part of the leaves causing them to develop brown scabs and turn yellow and then brown. It's another fungal infection typically caused by a combination of heat and humidity. Nitrogen deficiency can increase susceptibility. Leaf septoria probably won't kill your plant, but it will reduce yields. If you notice signs of infection, remove and dispose of infected leaves (not in the compost pile). You may be able to control the infection simply by reducing the heat and humidity and improving air circulation. If that doesn't work, spray the foliage with an organic fungicide, being careful not to spray the buds.

Pruning your plants

Pruning is a way to keep plants healthy while redirecting the plant's energy to growing flower. You start pruning in the vegetative stage when plants begin to get bushy and stop two or three weeks into the flower stage. Here are some pruning guidelines to get you started:

>> Use sharp scissors to make smooth, clean cuts, which are less prone to making the plant susceptible to infection. You may want two pairs of scissors — small for removing leaves and larger/sturdier for removing branches.

>> Wash your hands and disinfect scissors in a solution of one part bleach and three parts water before moving from one plant to the next to avoid spreading disease.

>> Start by removing branches from the bottom of the plant where the light doesn't reach. (This process is called *skirting*.)

>> Remove dead and yellowing leaves whenever they appear. (Do this over the entire course of the growth cycle.)

>> Remove branches that are growing up through the middle of the plant. They won't receive enough sunlight to become very productive.

>> During the bloom stage de-fan your plants. *De-fanning* involves removing the large leaves so they don't sit on each other and block light from penetrating the canopy to reach all the plant and each of the plants. De-fanning also allows air to flow through the canopy and is important for growing heathy, disease-free plants.

Training your plants to maximize yield

You can train your plants to create more branches and grow more horizontally to increase the area of the canopy. The result — more buds. Here are a few ways to encourage a plant to spread out and produce more buds:

>> **Trellising:** When plants get bushy, parts of the plant may not receive enough light to fuel their growth. By trellising the plant, you can spread out the branches while providing them with additional support. You can build a basic trellis by weaving together bamboo stakes or thin strips of wood, or using a piece of fencing. Tie branches to the trellis to train them in the direction you want them to grow (see Figure 11-5).

TIP

Position the trellis as perpendicular to the light source as possible to maximize exposure.

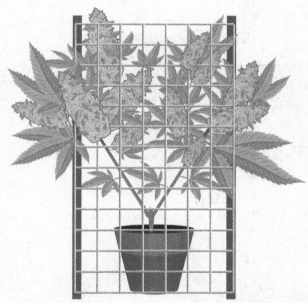

FIGURE 11-5:
Use a trellis to support the plant and increase exposure to light.

© John Wiley & Sons, Inc.

>> **Topping:** Wait until the plant has two or more nodes, then cut the stem between the topmost growth and the two nodes just below it (see Figure 11-6). By topping the plant, the *growth tips* (where the bases of the fan leaves attach to the stem) grow into separate stems that extend out from the main stem. You may top each secondary stem sometime later to encourage the growth of two new branches from each stem.

>> **Low-stress training (LST):** As secondary stems grow (stretch), gently pull down on them and anchor them in place, so they grow horizontally (see Figure 11-7). You can use wires pushed into the soil or strings tied to the rim of the container to hold down the stems, but be sure to use thicker wires or strings, so they don't cut into the plant.

>> **Scrogging:** Place a grid called a Screen of Green, or ScroG (typically made of wire or string to produce three- to four-inch square openings), about four to eight inches above the plant, and train the branches to spread in different directions. When buds begin to form, gently tuck them up through the nearest square. This spreads out the buds, so they're all about the same distance from the light source (see Figure 11-8).

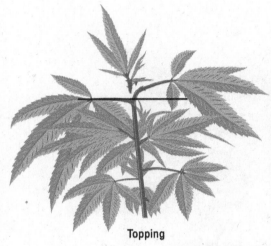

FIGURE 11-6:
Top a plant
to encourage
the growth of
secondary stems.

Topping

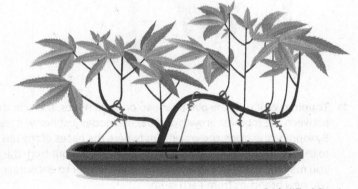

FIGURE 11-7:
Low-stress
training
encourages
branches to grow
horizontally.

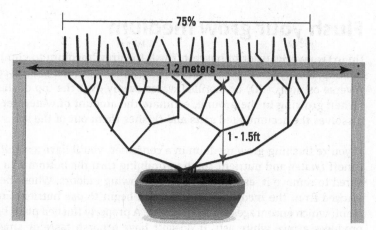

This is the sort of thing you are aiming for when doing a SCROG.
Try to fill 75% of the width of your screen before you begin flowering.

© John Wiley & Sons, Inc.

FIGURE 11-8:
Scrogging spreads out the buds to give them equal light.

WARNING

Although you can use these techniques with auto-flowering plants, their stems may not bend easily, making them susceptible to damage.

Prepping Plants for Harvest

A few weeks prior to harvest, start to prepare your plants for their final days. Preparation consists of restricting water to the roots (not spraying the foliage) and flushing the grow medium, as explained in the following sections.

Stop spraying the foliage

As buds start to form, limit spraying the foliage, and end spraying three weeks prior to harvest to mitigate trichome damage.

WARNING

Alter any integrated pest management (IPM) spraying regiments to preserve the integrity of trichomes. Excessive spraying or high pressure spraying with phyto-toxic products (some pesticides and nutrients can be toxic to the plant if misused) can damage trichome heads and negatively affect potency and taste. Never spray oil-based foliage sprays or pesticides (such as Neem oil) on flowers, because they have the potential to adversely affect the taste of the flower and are difficult to wash off entirely.

Flush your grow medium

Up to two weeks prior to harvest, flush the grow medium to eliminate excess salt buildup. Slowly pour up to three times the volume of the plant's container of pure reverse osmosis (RO) or distilled water evenly over the top of the grow medium. (When growing in the ground, estimate the amount of water needed.) The water dissolves the accumulated salts and flushes them out of the soil.

If you're flushing grow medium in a container, you'll have a significant amount of runoff (water and nutrient solution draining thru the bottom of a pot), so be prepared to remove it, especially if you're growing indoors. When the salts have been leached from the medium, the plant will begin to use nutrients remaining in the plant, which encourages leaf senescence. A properly flushed plant burns cleanly and produces a nice white ash. It doesn't have a harsh taste or smell from residual nutrients.

Cultivating Cannabis in an Industrial Setting: Special Considerations

Size matters in commercial cannabis cultivation and the number of plants, the size and configuration as well as the expense will be determined by the local laws.

Considering space locations and rules

Each state or province will have its own rules about the number of plants that can be grown per your license. In some states, there are plant count limits and different levels of licenses. You may need to prove sale of a certain percentage of plants grown and harvested through legally connected or wholesale sales of plants before you are permitted to move up to the next level and grow more plants.

Grow facilities will be closely monitored and rules will be strictly reviewed. Compliance is as important in the Grow as in any other stage of the industry. Most rules are designed to combat diversion, which is when legally grown cannabis moves out of the legal stream from seed to sale and winds up on the black market.

Considering the use of pesticides and nutrients

As with any commercial agricultural operation, regulations exist regarding pesticides and nutrients. Even if you are not growing "organic" cannabis, there will be rules, oversight and testing required of all cannabis plants and products.

In some large operations, it will be cost effective to create electronically monitored and timed watering with nutrients. You may also find it cost effective to mix your own nutrients though special expertise will be required and base chemicals will still need to be purchased.

Handling green waste

While there is much less oversight regarding green waste in home grows, commercial endeavors will find strict rules involved with the disposal of green waste. This is classified as any part of the plant that does not end up in a product sold to customers. Laws will vary but in general, any unused plant matter such as stems, leaves, and stalks, if not legal to be sold in your state will require treatment.

In some cases, this will mean waste must be ground and mixed with dirt or other products to render it unusable and unrecognizable. In some locations it must be placed in special locked containers to await pick up by a waste management company. You should check with your regulators to see what is legal in your area.

Arranging third party testing

In a commercial cannabis operation, products must be tested by a third-party lab for pesticides, pests, mold and mildew as well as other contaminants. As with everything else about cannabis, local rules govern everything from the amount to be tested for each harvest to the specific protocols involved in the testing by the grow as well as the lab. You can reach out to your local regulatory body for a list of approved labs in your area. Don't forget to do your due diligence and learn all you can about the requirements and the reputation of the labs you intend to use. If the lab doesn't meet and comply with all state or province rules and regulations, then neither will your product.

Tracking plants from seed to sale

With the development of each legalized state or provincial regulatory body, a tracking system will be put in place by the government. This is meant to keep track of all the product moving around the location and prevent diversion into the black market.

The systems will be electronic and may be online. They will include product tagging as well as codes to be batched and follow the product from "seed to sale." For example, in Colorado we start each plant receives an RFID tag at 8 inches tall. The physical plant has the tag attached and that number will follow every part of the plant by being entered into the system, whether it is the stalk and leaves being disposed of as green waste; the buds being trimmed and sold; the trim being used in pre-rolled joints; or the ground bud, trim or shake going to the MIP to be extracted and then turned into concentrates, edibles, lotions or tinctures.

Nothing escapes the tracking for the compliant company and this will take technology, protocols and staff to maintain.

Chapter **12**

Harvesting and Post-Harvest

You just invested eight to ten weeks of diligent effort and expertise to grow the perfect cannabis bud/flower. Now what? As harvest time approaches, you need to start thinking about when and how to harvest your plants and then dry and cure them to create the highest quality product available. After all, your harvest and post-harvest activities can make or break the final product. They can be the difference between smooth, tasty bud and a mushy or a dry and brittle mess. The time and effort invested in doing it right (and figuring out how to do it right) will be well worth it!

REMEMBER

Biological and chemical activities continue long after the plant is cut down. Properly drying and curing your plants is essential for ensuring the quality of the final product. You don't want your bud too wet or too dry coming out of the drying and curing process. Too wet, and mold becomes an issue; too dry, and you lose terpenes. Strike the right balance, and you preserve the health and flavor of your bud and maximize its potency.

In this chapter, we walk you through the process of harvest and post-harvest, beginning with deciding when to harvest and ending with storing and packaging your end product.

Deciding When to Harvest: Timing Is Everything!

As soon as buds begin to form on your carefully cultivated plants, your eagerness to harvest begins to build, and you become more susceptible to making the common mistake of harvesting too early. The other, less common, mistake is to wait too long, at which point the cannabinoids and terpenes begin to break down. So, how do you know when to harvest your plants?

In this section, we answer that question by presenting several methods for figuring out when to harvest your plants at their peak.

Keeping an eye on the trichomes

The best way to tell when your plants are ready for harvest is to keep an eye on the *trichomes*, which comprise the glistening, sticky substance that covers the cannabis buds. Upon closer examination (which usually requires a microscope), you can see that these trichomes actually look somewhat like tiny mushrooms, with a head and a stalk. (See Chapter 2 for more about cannabis plant anatomy.) The trichomes contain a large majority of the cannabinoids and terpenes in the plant.

When your plant is covered in buds, and you can see the glistening masses of trichomes, use a small, hand-held magnifier (30–100x magnification) or a jeweler's loupe to examine the trichomes closely. Depending on the plant strain (and your eyesight), you may be able to distinguish changes in trichome opacity and color without magnification; trichomes may be considerably larger on some plant strains than on others. Changes in color indicate ripeness:

>> **Clear/translucent:** When the plant is in its early flowering stage, trichomes appear clear or translucent.

>> **Opaque:** Trichomes gradually become more opaque (white or cloudy) as the buds mature.

THE LIFECYCLE OF A TRICHOME

As a plant matures, trichomes change both in color and size. A trichome starts small and swells up like a balloon as it ages. Cannabinoids and terpenes accumulate in the trichome. The trichome gland head grows heavier and more bulbous as its secretory vesicles synthesize oil. The gland head eventually degrades and falls off as the plant nears the end of its life. When the heads fall off the trichomes, the bud's potency declines dramatically.

>> **Amber:** When buds are fully mature (ripe for harvest), the trichomes turn amber. At this point, the buds may start to degrade.

>> **Brown:** When buds are past their peak, the trichomes turn a darker and darker brown.

TIP

You can now purchase microscopes that attach to smart phones and display magnified images on the smart phone's screen, which can really come in handy for this task.

Depending on personal preference, most growers begin their harvest when a quarter of the trichomes have turned amber. Others prefer to not let any trichomes begin to degrade and start harvesting as soon as they see a majority of cloudy trichomes.

Observing the pistils and stigmas

The *pistil* is the reproductive organ of a female cannabis flower. *Stigmas* are the vivid, hair-like strands of the pistil designed to collect pollen from male plants. (As explained in Chapter 11, you don't want your female plants pollinated because they then spend more energy on producing seeds than on producing quality buds. In addition, unless you're breeding plants, you don't want seeds in your bud.)

Over the course of a plant's life, the stigmas start out white and gradually change to yellow, orange, red, purple, and then brown depending on the strain. A good rule of thumb is to harvest your plants when about half the buds are covered with orange and red stigmas. When they begin to turn purple and then brown, bud quality is on the decline.

REMEMBER

Pistils and stigmas have an important role in reproduction and are useful for determining when to harvest, but, unlike trichomes, they generally don't affect a flower's potency or flavor.

Tracking leaf senescence

Leaf senescence is a term that describes the process of deterioration of a plant's leaves as it ages. Chlorophyll degradation during leaf senescence results in an increase in *carotenoids* (mainly yellow, orange, or red fat-soluble pigments) and *anthocyanins* (mainly blue, violet, or red flavonoid pigments), which cause fall colors. These same colors appear late in a cannabis plant's flowering cycle. When most of a plant's leaves turn yellow, it's a good sign that the plant is ready for harvest.

REMEMBER

If a plant is properly flushed, waiting until it's mostly or entirely senesced ensures that very little to no residual nutrients remain in the plant. These residual nutrients can contribute to a harsh or unpalatable smoke. See the later section "Flushing Your Plants Prior to Harvest."

WARNING

Don't mistake plant stress for ripeness. Leaf senescence in the earlier stages of a plant's growth cycle indicate stress, possibly from too much or too little water, a disease, or a pest. By knowing the average time-to-harvest for the plant your growing (as explained in the next section), you'll have a better idea of whether the senescence is due to stress or is a sign that the plant is ready for harvest.

Find out the strain's expected time-to-harvest

If you buy seeds or clones from a legal and reputable seller or they show up in bud you or someone you know purchased, and you know the strain, you can usually find out the approximate number of weeks required for the plants to mature. This information is included in seed catalogues (such as Royal Queen Seeds at www.royalqueenseeds.com) and printed on the label of seed packets. It may also be included when you purchase clones.

WARNING

Using time-to-harvest estimates is the worst way to determine when plants are ready to harvest. These estimates are great for planning your grow schedule and knowing when to start checking the pistils, stigmas, and trichomes more closely, but harvest times vary considerably based not only on plant strain but also on growing conditions.

Harvesting Your Plants

Harvesting is easy — you simply cut down the entire plant just below the lowest branch using large, sharp pruning shears or harvesting loppers. The other option is to cut off branches individually. However, if you're growing commercially, you must cut down the entire plant, so you can determine and record its wet weight (see the next section for details).

WARNING

Mitigate cross contamination of any plants that aren't being harvested by limiting movement of harvested plants thru the grow space and covering or culling any plants that may be infested or infected.

After harvesting your mature plants, you can either weigh and calculate your yield, as explained in the next section, or skip to the drying process as explained in the later section "Drying, Curing, and Trimming Flower Post-Harvest." If you're harvesting commercially, you have no choice but to weigh and calculate your yield first. If you're a home grower, the choice is yours. Some home growers like to weigh and calculate their yields and keep detailed records, so they can tell the impact of changing variables, such as light exposure and nutrients used for each crop.

Weighing and Calculating Your Yield (Dry/Wet Weights)

In a commercial setting, regulations require that all plant matter be weighed and tracked through different stages of harvest and post-harvest to prevent *diversion* — having any of the plant matter transferred outside the system used to regulate it. Commercial growers may be required to report weights of product as it's harvested, dried, and cured along with the weight of all green waste. By weighing product as it proceeds through the various stages of harvest and post-harvest, you can also identify points at which weights change, especially from wet to dry and pre- to post-trim weights.

If you have a home grow you may have less need to weigh your plants, but you may be interested in tracking for yourself and comparing or predicting yields.

REMEMBER

Calibrate your scale(s) prior to weighing anything to ensure accuracy; check the scale's manual for instructions. If you're a commercial grower, use a certified scale with buckets or tubs into which you will load the plant matter. Sterilize the buckets or tubs between batches. If your weights are off at any weigh-in, you may have some explaining to do to the regulators and can be at risk of losing your license.

Determining the plant's wet weight

Wet weight is the weight of the total plant including fan leaves and stems. Much of this is green waste not included in the final weight of the yield after the plant has been manicured (trimmed).

ESTIMATING DRY WEIGHTS

Regulations don't allow companies to report ballpark figures, but if you're a home grower, you can make a rough estimate of the dry weight of a yield based on the wet weight.

In general 50 percent of a plant's wet weight is stem weight. If it's a long-stalked sativa, up to 80 percent can end up as green waste including stems, leaves, and final trimming. However, bud density and whether you trim the buds wet (as opposed to dry trim) can also impact the accuracy of that estimate.

In essence, depending on the strain, you can estimate between 20 and 50 percent to be viable bud weight after drying.

Weighing after bucking or shucking and maybe rough trimming

After determining a plant's wet weight, you buck or shuck and perhaps rough-trim the buds and then weigh the buds without all the plant matter you removed. *Bucking* and *shucking* is the act of removing buds from stem. In your home grow you do this with a knife or scissors. Commercial operations may use a "munch" or "twister" machine:

>> A *munch machine* is comprised of rollers and blades. You stick the end of the stem between rollers that draw it into the machine and kick it out the other side into a collection bag leaving mostly bud behind. The machines are becoming standard for the larger grow operations, but most smaller operations still hand shuck. (A person can hand-shuck about 10 pounds per hour depending on the cannabis strain, the weight of the buds, and the length of the node space. In contrast, a munch machine can shuck up to about 150 pounds per hour.)

>> A *twister machine* rotates buds down a large, slowly spinning tube equipped with tumblers or blades to not only separate buds from stems but also to perform a *rough trim* — removing some excess sugar leaves from the buds. However, they're accused of damaging the buds and knocking off trichomes. Organizations that hand trim their buds without these machines usually make a big deal of the effort (and it takes a lot) that provides a higher quality bud. As an end user you pay for the quality upgrade.

WARNING

Whether you're hand-shucking or using a machine, wear gloves and safety goggles. When using machinery, read and follow all safety precautions, including wearing earplugs or headphones to protect your hearing. Sterilize all equipment with isopropyl alcohol before and after use, between working with different strains to prevent contamination, and at the end of the day.

TIP

Although many commercial and home growers dry and cure their cannabis before trimming it, we recommend wet trimming for a higher quality product. The trichomes on fresh plants are more pliable and malleable; they won't break off as easily during the process. The loss of trichomes (kief) lowers the potency of the bud. The benefit of trimming dry bud (over wet trimming) is that you can make it look the way you want it to. It won't change shape or size after trimming as a wet bud typically does as it dries. See the later section "Trimming bud" for instructions on how to hand-trim bud (wet or dry).

Weighing green waste and wet bud

After bucking or shucking and perhaps trimming your bud, you now have two piles — a pile of bud, and a pile of everything else (green waste). You may have a third pile of trim, because trim has some value, as well, but keep it separate from your bud. Now you're ready to weigh your green waste and wet bud and perhaps your trim. Simply take turns loading each onto your scale and taking and recording your readings.

In addition to being required by law for commercial operations, weighing wet buds helps you determine how much moisture you're losing during the drying and curing phases. In general, you can anticipate a 90 percent loss from wet to dry due to loss of water and other volatile compounds such as terpenes. However, weight loss from wet to dry varies depending on the plant strain and other variables.

REMEMBER

Green waste rules vary among jurisdictions. Some allow you to use green waste for products, and some may even let you sell it to a third party to create hemp products such as rope (which is still used by the U.S. Navy). Others bar you from using it at all. Rules may also vary regarding disposal; for example, whether you're permitted to compost it. As always, check your regulations.

REMEMBER

Don't forget to record dry trim and green waste weights. Refer to your jurisdiction to find out which weights you need to report, but a good rule of thumb is to weigh everything before and after each stage of the harvest and post-harvest process.

Drying, Curing, and Trimming Flower Post-Harvest

After harvesting your plant (and bucking, shucking, and weighing it, if grown commercially), you're ready to dry, cure, and trim — the final steps before selling or consuming your product (or gifting some of it to someone you really like). In this section, we lead you through the process.

Drying your plant or buds

Plants and buds must be dried to remove most of the moisture in preparation for curing. The drying process differs a little depending on whether you're a home or commercial grower:

>> **Home grower:** Home growers and small commercial operations generally hang entire branches or stems that hold the buds. You can use clothes hangers or string a clothes line across a room to hold the branches or stems. Whatever rig you use make sure it's sturdy enough to hold your plants and not in a highly trafficked area. Space the branches and stems far enough apart so they're not touching each other. The benefit of this method is that you don't need to handle the buds (to flip them over, for example), so buds retain their trichomes, and you have more symmetrical buds that are more potent. The drawback is that more space is required.

>> **Commercial grower:** Use a tray rack like those used in cafeterias, with removable food-grade drying trays (trays with fine mesh screens at the bottom that allow the air to circulate). Place buds evenly on the trays with sufficient space between them to allow the air to circulate freely. Place the trays on every other level of the racks, so you have six to ten inches of space between trays.

WARNING

Before you hang your buds or place them on trays, clean and sterilize your equipment with isopropyl alcohol and let it dry to mitigate mold, bacteria, and pests.

Regardless of whether you're a home or commercial grower, the key to drying your bud is consistency and evenness throughout the process. Proper drying relies on the right temperature and humidity, as explained later in this section.

REMEMBER

Go low and slow! Dry your cannabis in a cool, dry, dark, and well-ventilated place. Time will do the rest. The goal isn't to completely dry out the bud but to remove most of the moisture and distribute the remaining moisture evenly through the bud. The outside surface naturally dries faster. Time allows the moisture trapped inside the bud and stem to migrate outward, resulting in a more uniform distribution of moisture.

THE CHEMICAL PROCESSES YOU DON'T SEE

During the time in the drying room, buds undergo certain chemical changes that increase the potency and quality of the product:

- Certain compounds break down and combine with other compounds to create THCa and other cannabinoids. Proper drying and curing increases THCa content, which increases the potency of the final product.

- Chlorophyll — the pigment that gives plants their green color — is broken down, which results in a smoother smoke (not harsh).

- Nitrogen is also broken down during the process.

- Sugars remaining in buds are broken down by beneficial microbes, so the buds burn more evenly. Sugars don't evaporate when you smoke, leaving behind black, clumpy ash.

The moral of this story is to be sure to give your bud the time necessary to allow it to dry and cure properly. The time invested will pay handsome dividends in the final product.

Plan for two weeks at the designated temperature and humidity with daily fluffing activities and rack rotation as we cover later in this section.

Choosing a suitable room or space

Your drying room environment is critical to success. Your dry room should meet the following criteria:

REMEMBER

» A closed space that's light-tight, has adequate ventilation, and is constructed of a material that doesn't hold moisture. For example, cinder block is a poor choice, because it soaks up moisture, unless it's sealed.

During the dry cycle, allow as little light as possible into the room. Some people use a green headlight so they can work in relative darkness inside the room but still see what they're doing.

» Temperature controlled — heat or air conditioning along with a thermostat to maintain a consistent temperature.

» Be equipped with thermometers and hygrometers distributed around the room to check for hot spots, cold spots, and areas that are too damp or dry.

>> Be equipped with small fans to circulate the air in the room. Think gentle breeze, not gale force wind. Fans serve three purposes: 1) they ensure equilibrium across the room, so all flower dries at the same rate, 2) along with temperature and humidity control, they help to prevent mold and mildew, and 3) they expedite the drying process.

REMEMBER

In a square room, place a fan in each corner and face each fan at an angle to the wall that's slightly less than 45 degrees, so all the fans are blowing clockwise or counterclockwise. This creates a vortex that ensures circulation throughout the entire room.

WARNING

Clean and sterilize all equipment before bringing it into the room. Wiping everything down with a solution of one part bleach and three parts water does the trick.

Some companies including Autocure (autocure.us) in San Diego can fabricate a dry room to your specifications. They can build in airflow like that used in wind chambers for testing airplanes and cars but with a gentler breeze.

Sterilizing the room

After setting up your room and before bringing any bud into it, run an ozone or hydroxyl generator in the closed room:

>> **Ozone generator:** An ozone generator is more effective and requires only two hours to sterilize all surfaces in a room. However, it's more dangerous. Also, ozone has a strange smell that may be unpleasant.

WARNING

Evacuate the building (all people and pets) before running the ozone generator. Ozone damages mucosal tissue, including tissue in nasal passages and lungs. People aren't safe simply being in another room. They need to be out of the building and wait for the ozone to dissipate before re-entering the building.

>> **Hydroxyl generator:** A hydroxyl generator requires at least 48 hours to sterilize a room, but it's safe, even if people are in different rooms in the building.

Don't run the generator in the room when your plants are in it. The gasses may degrade the various chemical compounds in plants. Plants may be left in the building, but in a different room.

After turning off the generator and waiting a couple hours for the room to air out, you can bring in your plants and start to fine-tune the temperature and humidity.

Setting the temperature

Set and maintain a temperature in the room of 65 degrees Fahrenheit, and never let it get any higher than 68 degrees. Check the thermometers throughout the room and make sure all areas are a uniform temperature. If you have warm spots or cold spots, you may need to adjust your fans or add one or more fans.

If the temperature is any higher than 65, terpenes start to evaporate at a faster rate, and once you lose them, they're gone. Myrcene, the fruity mango terpene, is the most volatile and is lost at 68 degrees with Limonene following at 70 degrees.

TIP

Too cold isn't ideal either. Certain molds thrive in cool, damp environments. Also, everything takes longer to dry in a cooler room. A setting of 65 degrees is low enough to prevent terpene evaporation and high enough for faster production drying.

Controlling the humidity

Relative humidity dictates the quality, consistency, and pliability of final product. Maintain humidity in a range of 50–65 percent and check humidity regularly with your hygrometer.

REMEMBER

Controlling your room for humidity can be a constant battle, especially if you're in a high humidity location. Use a humidifier and/or dehumidifier if necessary.

High humidity is bad because it results in longer than necessary dry time and, more importantly, promotes mold and mildew. The last thing you want on that bud you spent so much time and effort growing is fungus!

Lower than 50 percent humidity isn't favorable either. While it allows for quicker drying, you end up with buds that are crusty on the outside but mushy inside. Remember, you want moisture distributed evenly throughout the bud.

Fluffing your buds. . . or not

If you're a home grower, hanging whole branches and stems, *fluffing* your buds (turning them over) isn't necessary, because they're not sitting on trays. If you're a commercial grower, drying your buds on trays, fluffing is necessary to ensure that the buds dry evenly and don't get flat spots.

REMEMBER

Fluff every bud every day. You can flip them over individually using your hand or tongs or place an empty tray upside-down over a full tray, flip both trays over, and remove the top tray — like flipping a cake from a cake pan onto a plate. After fluffing the buds, make sure they're evenly spaced on the tray; you don't want them overlapping or touching. Also, rotate the racks, moving those from the periphery of the room toward the middle of the room and vice versa.

Deciding when your buds are dry enough

The best way to tell whether your buds are dry enough for curing is by performing the old-school *stem test*. Take an average size bud and bend the stem. If the stem snaps on several buds on different tray racks, the buds are sufficiently dry. If the stems bend over without breaking, more drying time is needed.

REMEMBER

Not every stem on every bud in the room needs to snap, but if several average sized buds from all over the room snap, then you have an indicator that the total room drying is done. Now you're ready to cure.

Curing dried cannabis

Curing is any process used to preserve and sometimes add flavor to consumable products. It's generally done by adding a preservative, such as salt, nitrates, nitrites, vinegar, or sugar; removing water; or cooking or smoking (as in the case of smoked fish). Regardless of the process, the goal is to make the product inhospitable to microbes that would otherwise cause it to spoil. The same is true for cannabis — proper curing results in a consistent, shelf-stable bud with a flavorful terpene profile.

The curing process requires minimal moisture. You don't necessarily want to remove more moisture from your bud; some moisture is required to enable healthy chemical and biological processes to continue during the cure cycle. Sugars and chlorophyll are still being broken down over the course of the cure process, thus improving the quality of your bud. Air circulation is also important. Although you cure buds in airtight containers, the containers need to be burped regularly to allow gases that are harmful to the curing process (such as ethylene) to escape and allow oxygen in — to prevent anaerobic (non-oxygen-breathing) microbes from ruining the bud. For the same reason, buds need to be fluffed as they cure.

Start by loading your buds loosely into a hermetically sealed (airtight) container, such as a mason jar, Tupperware container, or a five-gallon bucket with an airtight lid. Leave enough room to fluff the buds. Seal the container with the lid. Now, the buds are ready to be cured.

The cure process takes anywhere from three to eight weeks depending on the mass and density of the bud and the amount of moisture remaining in the buds after drying. Over the course of the cure, your involvement varies, as explained in the following sections.

During the first week

The first week of the cure is the most critical, because the risk of mold is highest. During this time, take the following steps every day:

1. **Burp the container and fluff the buds.**

   Burping consists of opening the lid of the container for a few minutes to allow bad gases out and fresh air in. Fluffing consists of gently hand mixing the buds, so they shift places.

2. **As you burp and fluff the bud, check whether they're all sticking together, which may be a sign they're too wet.**

   Condensation on the inside surfaces of the container may also indicate that the buds are too wet. If no buds are sticking together or they sound like gravel rolling around in the container, they may be too dry.

3. **Gently squeeze and release several buds.**

   If the buds bounce back like a dry sponge, they're doing great. If they feel squishy, they're probably too wet. If the buds are crunchy, they're probably too dry.

4. **Take a whiff inside the container.**

   If it smells like bread, which means that yeast is growing, or smells like a damp basement, indicating mold or mildew, the buds are too moist.

5. **Proceed as follows, based on conclusions drawn from your observations:**

   - **Acceptable moisture:** Seal the container and repeat these steps daily for the first week.

   - **Too moist:** Depending on how excessive the moisture is, burping and fluffing more often and/or leaving the lid off the container for 20 minutes if just a little too moist to 20 hours for a bit more may be sufficient. If the moisture is more excessive, you may have to go back to the previous section and continue drying the bud.

   - **Too dry:** Depending on how dry the buds are, burping less often (every second or third day) may be sufficient, but continue to fluff the buds daily. You can also add a moisture pack, such as Boveda, to the container. However, moisture packs add to the cost and may add too much moisture.

TIP

Stick a note on the outside of the container that includes the time and day of the last burp and fluff and the condition of the product. You may also want to include instructions on how to proceed, such as "Burp & fluff on Friday." Also keep a log of when you started the cure, so you know how long the product has been curing.

WARNING

Don't leave your buckets unattended. Daily fluffing and inspection is essential for at least one week.

After the first week

After the first week, burp, fluff, and inspect once a week for four to six weeks. Your buds still require oxygen to fend off the anaerobic microbes and fuel essential chemical processes, and you still need to release any harmful gasses. Continue to keep notes recording your inspection observations, the activities you performed, and instructions on how to proceed.

After these five or six weeks, assuming your buds are sufficiently dry, they're ready for trimming. If you already trimmed your buds wet, you may want to do a second, finishing trimming to prepare them for storage.

Trimming bud

Trimming bud consists of snipping off all or most of the sugar leaves that stick out from the bud and shaping the bud to make it look more uniform and compact (see Figure 12-1). You want a nice, tight bud, not something that looks scraggly, but you also don't want to remove too many trichomes.

Grab a small pair of sharp scissors and follow these steps:

1. **Snip off any stem that extends from the base of the bud.**

2. **Snip off the crow's feet of small leaves at the base of the bud.**

3. **Snip off the less resinous portions of sugar leaves that stick out from the bud.**

   Some trimmers prefer to remove the entire portion of the sugar leaf that protrudes from the bud, while others prefer to remove only the less resinous portions of the leaves.

WARNING

Wear safety goggles, a long-sleeve shirt, and rubber gloves when trimming, especially if you're sensitive to trichomes. Sterilize all equipment with isopropyl alcohol before and after use, between working with different strains to prevent contamination, and at the end of the day.

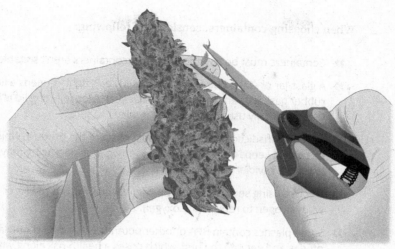

FIGURE 12-1:
Trim your buds.

Storing your buds

To store buds, you may keep them in the storage containers you used to cure them or transfer them to other clean, sanitized airtight storage containers. Airtight is key. You also want to store your buds in a cool, dark place.

TIP

For long-term storage (more than a couple months) or commercial storage or packaging, vacuum seal your buds or pack them with an inert gas, such as nitrogen. If you're a home grower, you can use a device for vacuum-sealing mason jars or for vacuum-sealing food items in plastic bags. You can use plastic bags for packing and storing clothing that allow you to use a standard vacuum cleaner to suck air from the bags prior to sealing them. Strongly consider using glass or stainless steel containers—plastic, may contain BPA or other harmful chemicals that can leach into your bud. If you're a commercial grower, more sophisticated vacuum packaging equipment and supplies are available and necessary.

Packaging for commercial use

The variety of packaging options for selling bud commercially is mind blowing. All packaging needs to be opaque and child-resistant and hermetically sealed, but beyond that, a package can be a jar, a vial, or a pouch; glass, plastic, foil, or metal; vacuum packed or packed with an inert gas such as nitrogen. You can find plenty of vendors that specialize in cannabis packaging and packing equipment, such as vacuum chambers.

When choosing containers, consider the following:

» Containers must be airtight. Plastic pill containers aren't suitable.

» A glass jar or vial is fine as long as the lid seals tight. It needs a lid with a rubber gasket or an O-ring or a similar seal. A loose-fitting lid is insufficient. Glass is usually used for the finest quality products.

» In many jurisdictions, packaging must obscure the product, which is fine because it keeps the light out, too. Even opaque packaging may benefit from having ultraviolet (UV) protection.

» If you're using sealable bags, consider vacuuming out the air or filling the bags with nitrogen to replace the oxygen.

» Some plastics contain BPA or other potentially harmful chemicals that can off-gas and get into the bud, which poses a health risk along with degrading the aroma or flavor of the flower.

WARNING

Follow all weighing, packaging, and labeling rules in the jurisdiction in which you operate to remain in compliance. For example, in some locations, dispensaries are permitted to sell only pre-packaged cannabis; they're prohibited from weighing and packaging it themselves. Clear packaging, which enables you to see the bud inside, may also be prohibited.

When packaging, follow these precautions:

» Be sure the bud has been properly cured prior to packaging. Otherwise, your product is at a higher risk of developing mold. See the earlier section "Curing your bud" for details.

» Make sure the package is clean, sterilized, and dry before you weigh and insert your cannabis product.

Chapter **13**

Making Concentrates and Marijuana Infused Products (MIPs)

Marijuana consumption methods have expanded dramatically over the years. While consumers of the past mostly smoked it in joints or with a pipe or bong and occasionally baked it into a batch of brownies, today's consumers smoke, vape, eat, drink, and dab it; take it sublingually (under the tongue); apply it topically (to the skin); and even bathe with it (for example, soaps and bath bombs).

Many of the commercial products available today are referred to as *marijuana infused products (MIPs)*, and they're made in facilities referred to in the industry as MIPs. All these commercial products are either concentrates or are made with *concentrates* — extracts from cannabis plants such as hash, oil, resin, and crystals. Concentrates can be consumed as is (via dabbing, for example) or infused into other products such as edibles, capsules, or creams, thus creating MIPs. (See Chapter 2 for descriptions of concentrates and extracts.)

In this chapter, we bring you up to speed on concentrate basics, explain various extraction methods, and lead you through the process of creating your own concentrates and MIPs.

Grasping Concentrate Basics

Concentrates are products from cannabis plants that contain higher potencies of desirable substances (mostly cannabinoids and terpenes) without most of the plant matter. They're created through a variety of extraction methods that involve subjecting the harvested and usually cured plant matter to temperature (heat or cold), pressure, solvents, or a combination of the three. The result is an oil or semi-solid product (such as resin), which is much more potent than the flower from which it was extracted.

REMEMBER

Technically, a *concentrate* is any product made by removing the desirable substances from a plant; for example, orange juice concentrate is made by removing the skin and seeds and most of the pulp and water from oranges. An *extract* is a concentrate made with the use of a solvent to draw the desired substances from the plant; for example, you can make vanilla extract by soaking vanilla beans in consumable alcohol, such as vodka. In this chapter, we use the terms "concentrate" and "extract" interchangeably to some degree.

The quality and potency of the concentrate is a factor of the flower from which it's made along with the efficiency and effectiveness of the extraction process. Most extraction processes start with flower, frozen flower, kief, and/or trim. The goal is to extract as much of the cannabinoid and terpene content as possible and remove most of the inert parts of the plant, although some plant waxes and fats may also have commercial value.

Exploring Different Extraction Methods

Concentrates and extracts can be made through a variety of extraction methods, some more complex and dangerous than others. The extraction method of choice is based on the desired end product, as presented in Table 13-1.

TABLE 13-1   Choosing an Extraction Method

Desired End Product	Concentrate/Extract	Extraction Method	Starting Material
Various concentrates and MIPs	Kief	Dry sift	Flower
Smoke product or edible	Hash	Ice water and agitation	
Hand rolling	Flower		

Desired End Product	Concentrate/Extract	Extraction Method	Starting Material
Dab and other products	Rosin or whipped rosin	Pressure and heat	Bubble hash, kief, flower
Dab and other products	Shatter, wax, live resin, THC crystalline, or terpene juice	Butane or propane	Flower for shatter and wax
			Frozen flower for live resin, THC crystalline, and terpene juice
Vape oil and other products	Oil	CO_2	Flower and trim
Edibles	Butter	Heat	Flower and trim
Tinctures	Tincture	Alcohol or glycerin	Flower and trim

Non-solvent extraction methods

The most common non-solvent extraction methods use water or a combination of heat and pressure. These methods are much easier than solvent methods to perform safely and typically are less strictly regulated. In this section, we cover the basics of these extraction methods. See the later section "Creating Your Own Concentrates" for instructions.

Dry sift

Dry sift consists of physically knocking the trichomes off the flower and collecting them to produce kief. Many herb grinders have three chambers; as you grind your flower, it falls into the second chamber that has a screen on the bottom through which the kief passes, collecting in the third chamber. To produce larger volumes of kief, you can use silk screening equipment to separate the kief from the plant matter. See the later section "Making kief" for detailed instructions.

Hand rolling

One of the oldest methods for making hash is hand rolling. You start with fresh cannabis (not dried or cured) and gently roll it between the palms of your hands. The sticky trichomes come off the plant and stick to your hands. You can then scrape the substance off or continue to rub your hands together to create a sticky ball or stick of hash — commonly referred to as "charas." See the later section "Making your own charas" for details.

Ice water or dry ice

If you're interested in creating your own concentrates, the ice water and dry ice methods are safest and easiest. The process consists of placing flower in ice water to freeze the trichomes and then agitating the mixture to knock the trichomes off the flower. You then filter the mixture through progressively smaller screens to remove the plant matter. You place the wet hash in a cool, dark place to dry it, and then you press it into cakes to create hashish — technically referred to as *bubble hash*. See the later section "Making bubble hash" for complete instructions.

REMEMBER

You can smoke bubble hash or use it as an ingredient in edible products.

Pressure and heat

To create rosin, you apply pressure and heat to flower, kief, or bubble hash. You can purchase a rosin press that's built specifically for the job or use a hair straightener or T-shirt press. You place your starting flower, kief, or bubble hash between two pieces of parchment paper or in a small-micron bag and squeeze it between two heated metal plates. See the later section "Making rosin" for details.

TIP

You can whip rosin by stirring it to create a consistency that's more like peanut butter, which may make it easier to handle and to mix with other edible ingredients, but whipping may reduce its potency.

Heat and butter

By baking cannabis and then simmering it in butter and water, you can create your own cannabis-infused butter. When it cools, the butter separates out from the water, and you can discard the water. You can then use the butter to create your own edibles. See the later section "Making cannabis butter."

Alcohol

By baking cannabis and then simmering it in alcohol, you can create your own tinctures, which you can take sublingually or add to beverages. See the later section "Make your own tinctures."

Solvent extraction methods

In solvent extraction processes, a solvent is added to the plant material. Pressure and temperature are then altered to enable the solvent to dissolve the desired components of the plant. Any remaining solvent is removed, leaving behind the oils, cannabinoids, and terpenes extracted from the plant. Think of solvent extraction methods like brewing a pot of coffee. You pour hot water over coffee grounds contained in a filter. The hot water acts as a solvent, extracting the caffeine and the substances that give coffee its aroma and flavor. The filter removes all the plant matter — the ground coffee beans. Although hot water isn't the greatest solvent for cannabis, the concept is the same.

In this section, we describe several different solvent extraction methods, so you have a general idea of what's involved in each process.

WARNING

Don't try any solvent extraction method at home. Combinations of solvents, heat, pressure, and even static electricity can result in deadly explosions.

If you work in an extraction facility, safety is your top priority. Many regulatory bodies require closed loop systems, which allow only minute amounts of solvents into the surrounding air; the result is that volatile fumes can easily build up in the contained spaces of a facility.

Facilities employing this type of extraction should include filters, fire resistant building materials, sensors, alarms, and safety protocols. Personnel should be required to wear fireproof coverings and anti-static footwear (to prevent sparks). Any plastic materials, including plastic bags, which are susceptible to creating static electricity, should be banned. Even the smallest spark can ignite the volatile gasses and cause an explosion. Personnel must be trained properly on all processes and procedures and should perform their duties with the utmost care and diligence.

Butane, propane, or both

Butane and propane are commonly used as solvents to create extracts referred to as *butane hash oil (BHO)* or *propane hash oil (PHO)*. Depending on the raw materials and the process, the extracts produced vary in consistency and include shatter, wax, budder, live resin, THC crystalline, and terpene juice, most of which you can purchase at a dispensary.

Regardless of whether the solvent used is butane, propane, or a combination of the two, the process is generally the same. Plant matter is placed in a column with a screen at one end, and butane passes through the column, extracting the cannabinoids and terpenes from the plant matter. The solution is then placed in a vacuum oven to *purge* (evaporate) the solvent, leaving behind the BHO or PHO, which should contain very little to no solvent.

In commercial facilities, butane and propane extractions also involve manipulating pressure and temperature. Pressurizing and chilling the gas converts it to a liquid, which can then be mixed with the plant matter to create a "soup." A vacuum oven uses heat and depressurization to convert the solvent back into its gas form, and the gas is reclaimed.

The process is most safely performed using a *closed loop system* — an automated or semi-automated system that regulates the parameters of the process. Due to the hazards associated with these solvents, many regulatory bodies require special licensing and permits to perform butane and propane extractions. A closed loop system uses heat to reclaim the gas from the "soup" prior to placing it in the oven.

CO_2

CO_2 extraction is similar to that of butane and propane extraction (see the previous section) in that it manipulates the temperature and the pressure of a gas to extract substances from cannabis plants. However, CO_2 extraction has some notable benefits:

>> The CO_2 extraction process kills any mold or bacteria in the processed plant matter, as it does in the butane and propane extractions.

>> Pressure and temperature can be manipulated to extract selected compounds from the plant instead of just a combination of all compounds blended together.

>> The process doesn't involve the use of volatile gasses. However, due to high pressures, the process isn't completely safe. CO_2 tanks and other equipment have been known to explode.

The one potential drawback of CO_2 extraction is that the extracts may lack the flavor profile (due to a loss of terpene content) present in BHO and PHO.

Oil produced by CO_2 extraction is used in almost every vaporizer (vape) device on the market. It's also used for dabbing and to manufacture a wide variety of MIPs, including edibles and lotions. Terpenes are sometimes added back into the CO_2 oil to add desired flavors and aroma.

WARNING

You may have heard about Rick Simpson Oil (RSO), named after its creator, who claims it cured his cancer. He maintains a website at phoenixtears.ca where he provides instructions for making it. While we respect Mr. Simpson's work and especially his dedication to helping others, we caution you not to try it yourself. His method involves the use of toxic, volatile solvents along with boiling off the solvents. The fumes can be very harmful and, when combined with the heat needed for the boiling-off process, susceptible to explosion. While he provides guidance on how to reduce the risks, the process is still dangerous, especially if done indoors, which would be a big no-no.

Creating Your Own Concentrates

You can create your own respectable concentrates safely and without the use of dangerous processes, expensive machinery, and toxic solvents. In this section, you discover how to make your own kief, dry hash, bubble hash, rosin, charas, tinctures, and butter.

Making kief (dry sift)

Kief consists of the trichomes that cover cannabis buds. Trichomes contain most of the cannabinoids and terpenes a plant contains. Making kief is simply a matter of knocking the trichomes off the bud and collecting them. You can use one of the following methods to make kief:

>> Store your flower in a kief box or pollen sifter box. These boxes have two chambers, and the bottom of the top chamber is made of a fine mesh. You place your flower in the top chamber, and as kief naturally falls off the flower, it collects in the bottom chamber.

>> Use a three-chamber grinder to grind your flower. The top chamber grinds the flower, which falls into the second chamber. The kief that falls off the flower passes through a screen at the bottom of the second chamber and collects in the bottom chamber.

>> To collect larger quantities of kief, buy or make a large pollen sifter (shown in Figure 13-1) and obtain a slightly smaller box or tray to collect the kief. (You can make your own pollen sifter by stapling or gluing a fine screen or mesh to a wood frame.) With the sifter positioned above the tray, gently press down on and roll dried, cured flower against the mesh or screen causing the trichomes to fall off the flower, through the mesh, and onto the tray.

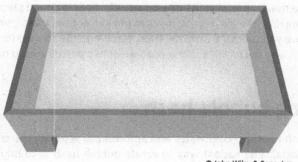

FIGURE 13-1:
A homemade pollen sifter.

© John Wiley & Sons, Inc.

TIP

The finer the mesh, the lower the yield and the higher the quality of your sift because less plant matter falls through the mesh. For the mesh material, consider using silk screens used for screen printing. Also consider cranking down the temperature in your work area or breaking up and freezing your flower before you start — the cold makes the trichomes less sticky, enabling them to more easily separate from the plant matter.

You can consume kief by rolling a joint in it or sprinkling it over flower after packing your pipe or bong bowl. You can also use kief to create other products, such as hash, as described in the next section.

Making dry sift hash

When you have some kief, you're ready to make your own dry sift hash. All you do is add a little heat and pressure to form it into a ball or patty. You have several options:

TIP

>> Load the kief into a pollen press or similar device and tighten the plunger.

Place a small piece of parchment paper under and over the kief to keep it from sticking to the press.

>> Ball up the kief and roll it between the palms of your hands, sort of like making meatballs but with more pressure.

>> Wrap it tightly in cellophane or parchment paper, tape it securely, and place it in a shoe below your heal. Walk around with it for a while, doing whatever you need to do.

>> Wrap your kief tightly in cellophane. Fill a glass jar or bottle with hot water, seal it tightly, and place the bottle on top of the wrapped kief and leave it for 30 to 60 seconds. Roll the bottle over the wrapped kief to press it into a patty.

>> Preheat your oven to 350 degrees. Wrap the kief tightly in cellophane and then a newspaper. Wet the newspaper with hot water and place it on a baking pan and into the oven for 10 minutes (no longer than that). Using a spatula, remove your package from the oven, place it on the counter (or on a cutting board), and roll it with a rolling pin (one or two passes should do the trick).

Making bubble hash

Bubble hash uses ice-cold water and agitation to separate the trichomes from the plant material. The easiest way to create bubble hash is to buy and use a bubble bag extraction kit, which you can find online or order from most hardware stores. The kit typically comes with a bucket and multiple bags with increasingly finer mesh screens at the bottom. See Figure 13-2.

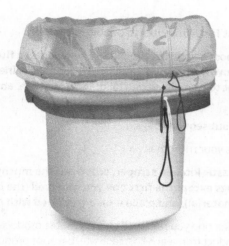

FIGURE 13-2:
A bubble-bag extraction kit.

Here's how you use a bubble bag extraction kit to make bubble hash:

1. Break up your plant matter and freeze it.

Your plant matter may be any combination of leaves, buds, trim, or shake, but the more trichomes it has, the better the yield and the quality of the end product. Cold is mandatory because it hardens the product and allows the trichomes to snap off the plant matter.

You can use a combination of indica and sativa or a single strain. The indica trichomes have fat heads that get caught in larger screens whereas the sativa trichomes require a smaller screen to catch.

REMEMBER

2. Place your bags in the bucket with the finest mesh screen on the bottom followed by bags with progressively wider mesh screens, as though you're double-bagging your groceries.

For example, you might have a 25 micron bag at the bottom that collects the trichomes followed by a 73-, 160-, and finally a 220-micron bag at the top. After placing each bag, fold its top over the bucket to secure it in place.

3. Fill the bucket about one-third full of ice.

4. Add your frozen plant matter until the bucket is about half full.

5. Add cold water, as cold as possible, until the bucket is about three-fourths full.

6. Mix the ice, water, plant solution thoroughly and vigorously.

You can use a paint mixer attached to an electric drill to ensure a thorough mixing. Mix until all flower is broken into tiny pieces and the solution appears frothy at the top.

7. Let the solution rest for 30 minutes to enable extraction.

8. Slowly lift the topmost bag out of the bucket, allowing the fluid to drain into the next bag down. When nearly all the water has drained from the bag, squeeze it tight to remove as much liquid as possible, and then set the bag aside.

9. Repeat Step 8 with subsequent bags.

   The last bag contains your trichomes.

10. Using a spoon or plastic kitchen scraper, scoop out the mushy trichome product from all bags except the first one you removed (the bag with most of the plant material), and place it on a tray lined with paper towel.

    All bags except the first one you removed contain usable product, but you may want to keep the product from each bag separate, because product quality from the different bags varies — product from the smallest mesh bag is highest.

11. (Optional) Repeat Steps 2–10 if you want to extract additional trichomes from the plant matter.

12. Place the tray with the mushy trichome product in a cool, dry, dark place to dry.

    The dried material can be pressed into cakes with your hands or used loose.

To avoid the added expense of a bubble bag extraction kit, you can use two clean buckets and rig your progression of finer mesh screens. You can even use a coffee filter as your smallest "screen," although it may drain very slowly. If you go this route, you still need to fill your bucket with ice, plant matter, and cold water and agitate it vigorously. Then, you pour from one bucket, into the other, through progressively finer mesh screens.

Making dry ice hash

Dry ice provides a quick and easy way to collect kief. Here's what you need:

>> Cannabis plant matter (fresh frozen or dried flower and trim) — amount can vary, but you don't want much more than will fill a five-gallon bucket more than a third of the way.

>> Dry ice (about three pounds for up to six ounces of plant matter). You may be able to purchase dry ice at your local supermarket or use your smart phone to search for "dry ice near me."

>> An ice pick, hammer, or screw driver to break up the ice.

>> A five-gallon bucket.

>> Three bubble hash bags (73-, 160-, and 220-microns) or similar devices for sifting the kief. Use bags made for a five-gallon bucket. (You can use one 220-micron bag, if you don't mind having different grades of kief all mixed together.)

>> Thick rubber or leather gloves, an oven mitt, or tongs (for handling the dry ice).

>> A clean, dry, flat surface.

>> Paper and tape to cover the work surface (newspaper, wax paper, or parchment paper will do).

>> A spatula, scraper, or plastic card (such as a credit card) to remove the kief from the work surface.

>> Three one quart storage containers for the kief.

WARNING

Use thick rubber or leather gloves, an oven mitt, or tongs when handling the dry ice. Never allow it to touch your bare skin — it can cause injury similar to a severe burn.

After gathering your supplies and plant matter, take the following steps:

1. **Cover your work surface in paper and tape down the paper so it won't move.**

2. **Break up your flower and/or trim into small pieces and place it in the bucket.**

3. **With your gloves on, break up the dry ice into ice-cube size pieces or somewhat larger and add it to the bucket.**

4. **Shake the bucket for about five minutes to distribute the cold and start knocking the trichomes off the plant matter.**

5. **Place a bubble hash bag or screen over the top of the bucket. Start with the smallest mesh bag.**

6. **Turn the bucket over your work surface, allowing the contents to drop into the bag and then remove the bag from the bucket, hold the top of the bag closed, and shake the bag over the work surface.**

7. **Continue shaking the bag until trichomes stop falling through the screen.**

TIP

For best results, shake the bag for 10 seconds, wait 5 seconds, shake again for 10 seconds, and repeat. This gives the ice a chance to cool the surrounding plant matter between shakes.

8. **Use your spatula, scraper, or plastic card to scrape the kief into a pile, remove it from the work surface, and place it into one of your storage containers.**

9. **Over the work surface, transfer the contents of the bag into the next smaller mesh bag and repeat Steps 7–8, and then repeat this step for the final, smallest mesh bag.**

You can use the kief you collected to make your own dry sift hash. See the earlier section "Making dry sift hash."

Making rosin

You can make your own rosin for dabbing without the use of harmful and dangerous solvents. All you need is a hair straightener (with a setting of about 300 degrees Fahrenheit), parchment paper, plant matter (cannabis flower, kief, or hash), heat-resistant gloves (for safety), and something to scrap the rosin off the parchment paper when you're done. After gathering your equipment and materials, take the following steps:

1. **Turn on your hair straightener and set it to between 280 and 300 degrees Fahrenheit.**

   If you don't have a degree setting on your straightener, start low and gradually increase the temperature.

2. **Cut a square piece of parchment paper that's slightly larger than twice the width of your straightener and fold it in half.**

3. **Place your plant matter near the middle of one half of the folded paper, fold the other half on top of it, and hold the two halves together to keep the plant matter from shifting.**

4. **Being careful not to burn your fingers, place the folded package between the metal plates of the hair straightener.**

5. **Close the straighter and squeeze as hard as possible but not so hard that you break your straightener. Squeeze for three to five seconds and release.**

   You may hear a sizzle indicating that the resin has been extracted.

6. **(Optional) Repeat steps 2–5 using the same plant matter to extract any remaining rosin.**

7. **Scrape the rosin off the paper and use it immediately to dab (see Chapter 6), or place it in an air-tight storage container for later use.**

Making charas

Charas is similar to hash and is thought to have originated in certain parts of Asia. The difference between charas and hash is that hash is typically made from dry, cured flower, whereas charas is made from fresh cannabis typically harvested two to three weeks prior to fully mature flower.

All you need to make charas are fresh cannabis and clean hands. To make charas, follow these steps:

1. **Wash your hands thoroughly with an organic, unscented soap, and dry them.**

2. **Slowly and gently rub flower between the palms of your hands.**

   The heat and friction loosen the trichomes and make them stickier, so they come off the flower and stick to your hands.

3. **When your hands are good and sticky and you've removed most of the trichomes, rub your hands together to create a stick or ball of trichomes.**

   This is charas.

4. **Repeat steps 2-3 until you run out of flower or have all the charas you want.**

You can vape charas with a dab rig, add it to a joint or bowl, mix it with tobacco and smoke it in a hookah, or use it to create rosin, as explained in the previous section. The traditional way to smoke it is with a *chillum*, which is like a one-hitter (see Chapter 6) but requires two people. You make a loose fist with one hand and place the chillum between your pinky and ring finger with your other hand cupped below the hand holding the chillum. You're essentially using your hands and the chillum to create a pipe. Then, someone lights the charas for you as you inhale. (See Figure 13-3.)

Make your own cannabis butter

Cannabis butter is a great MIP for using in various recipes to create your own edibles. To make your own cannabis butter, first gather the following ingredients and supplies:

» 1/2 pound of salted butter (it has a higher melting point than unsalted butter).

» 1/4–1/3 ounce flower. (You can adjust the amount to increase or decrease the potency, and you can add trim, if desired.)

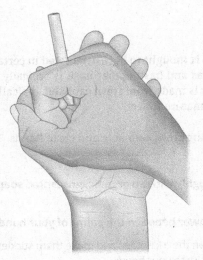

FIGURE 13-3:
Smoking charas
with a chillum.

© John Wiley & Sons, Inc.

>> 16–48 ounces of filtered or distilled water (amount depends on how long you choose to simmer).

>> Cookie sheet.

>> Parchment paper.

>> 2–3 quart sauce pan.

>> Sharp knife, coffee grinder, or blender.

>> Oven and stove (or crock pot).

>> Funnel.

>> Cheese cloth.

>> Storage containers (glass is best).

When you have everything you need, take the following steps to make your butter:

1. **Preheat your oven to 245 degrees Fahrenheit.**

2. **Line a cookie sheet with parchment paper and spread your cannabis out on the paper.**

3. **Bake your cannabis for 40 minutes to decarboxylate it and then remove it from the oven and allow it to cool.**

   See the nearby sidebar for more about decarboxylation.

4. Chop the cannabis with a knife, grinder, or blender.

5. Add the butter and one cup water to the saucepan and simmer on low until the butter is melted. (Don't let it boil.)

6. Add the chopped cannabis.

7. Continue to simmer uncovered for at least three hours, stirring occasionally and adding small amounts of water, if necessary. (Don't let it boil.)

8. Set a funnel lined with cheese cloth on top of a jar or other suitable container that's large enough to hold all the liquid.

9. Slowly pour the contents of the saucepan through the funnel to strain the cannabis butter.

10. Remove the funnel and place the jar in the refrigerator to cool. The butter will rise to the top, leaving water at the bottom.

11. Scoop your butter out of the jar and place it in your storage container.

THE IMPORTANCE OF DECARBOXYLATION

Raw cannabis contains tetrahydrocannabinolic acid (THCa), a precursor to tetrahydrocannabinol (THC) — the psychoactive substance that produces the "high." THCa has a number of properties that may help relieve symptoms of various medical illnesses. For example, it has anti-inflammatory and neuroprotective properties. However, it is non-intoxicating.

THCa has an extra carboxy ring (a group of chemicals) attached to its chemical chain. This ring must be removed to create THC. Various methods, referred to as *decarboxylation*, are used to remove this ring. The most common method is to apply heat. When cannabis is smoked or vaped, for example, the heat causes immediate decarboxylation. If you make cannabis brownies using chopped flower and trim, decarboxylation occurs during the baking process.

For decarboxylation, cannabis must be heated to 220 degrees Fahrenheit for 30–45 minutes. Unless you're smoking it, you should keep the temperature below 300 degrees to preserve the integrity of the cannabinoids and terpenes.

Make your own tincture

A *tincture* is a concentrated herbal extract. You can find THC+CBD tinctures at dispensaries and hemp-derived, CBD-only tinctures online and at many stores across the country. Various commercial processes are used to create tinctures, but you can create your own home-brewed version. Here's what you need:

WARNING

>> An 8 ounce or 16 ounce jar with a lid.

>> Enough dried cannabis to fill the jar.

>> Enough consumable alcohol to fill the jar — use Everclear or vodka.

Use only consumable alcohol — alcohol you buy at a liquor store, *not* rubbing (isopropyl) alcohol, which is toxic.

>> A sharp knife or blender.

>> A saucepan.

>> Water.

>> An oven and stove.

WARNING

Keep the alcohol away from the stovetop. High-proof, consumable alcohol is flammable. Use low heat and preferably an electric stove or hot plate instead of a gas stove. You can even use the heating plate on your electric coffee maker.

To create a tincture, take the following steps:

1. **Preheat your oven to 245 degrees Fahrenheit.**

2. **Line a cookie sheet with parchment paper and spread your cannabis out on the paper.**

   Use enough cannabis to fill your jar. You may use less for a less potent tincture.

3. **Bake your cannabis for 40 minutes to decarboxylate it and then remove it from the oven and allow it to cool.**

4. **Chop the cannabis with a knife, grinder, or blender.**

5. **Place the chopped cannabis in a jar and fill it with consumable alcohol.**

6. **Place the jar (uncovered) in a saucepan about half full of water and simmer on low for about 20 minutes.**

7. **Let the mixture cure and then strain it through a coffee filter.**

You consume tinctures typically by placing a few drops under your tongue and waiting a few seconds before swallowing. Start low and go slow. When you brew your own tinctures, you may have no idea how potent it is.

Cooking Up Edibles

You can use ground cannabis (flower and/or trim), cannabis butter, and other extracts to create your own edibles. In most recipes you use either cannabis butter or CO_2 extracted oil (or rosin), because you need a concentrate that blends in completely with the other ingredients. Otherwise the potency of different servings can vary considerably.

You can follow a recipe (see the Appendix) or simply add the cannabis or concentrate to your own favorite recipes. Here's a list of food items you may want to make yourself and enhance with cannabis:

>> Baked goods (cookies, cakes, brownies)

>> Candies (chocolates, gummies, lollipops, hard candies)

>> Beverages (tea, hot cocoa)

REMEMBER

The big challenge with making edibles is figuring out the concentration of cannabis in the entire batch and in each serving. It's much easier if you're using commercial products, because the label includes the information you need. If you're cooking with flower or homemade butter or rosin, it gets more difficult. We recommend trying any homemade concentrates to figure out the dosing before adding them to any recipe, so you have a better idea of how much to add.

WARNING

Clearly label all edibles as containing cannabis and store them in a secure place where children and pets can't get to them.

If you decide to sell your edible products commercially, you need a license and to follow a long list of rules and regulations, including having your products lab tested and labeled with potency information for both the entire contents of the package and for each serving, if selling for adult recreational use. In addition, packaging needs to be childproof, and the label must be designed in a way that's not appealing to children.

Preparing Tinctures, Lotions, and More

Using concentrates (those you buy or make), you can create your own cannabis tinctures, lotions, creams, soaps, and salves. Here are a few ideas to get you started:

>> Mix cannabis oil or rosin into an existing product; for example, your favorite skin lotion or body butter.

>> If you make your own soaps or lotions, you can add cannabis oil or rosin to your soap recipe.

>> Add cannabis oil or rosin to consumable alcohol or liquid sugar such as agave to make your own sublingual tinctures. This consumption method is second only to inhalation methods in terms of the speed at which the cannabis takes effect. Most people feel the effects within ten minutes.

When adding cannabis oil to a homemade recipe, the difficulty is in consistency of dosing, which requires calculating how much to add and then mixing the oil in thoroughly with the other ingredients. (See the Appendix for more on these calculations.) If you're adding cannabis oil to an existing lotion or cream for topical application, consider adding the oil separately for each application. If you mix it in and let it sit around for some time, the oil can separate out, and you'll get inconsistent doses.

5

Getting Down to Business

Explore the various types of businesses that comprise the cannabis industry and choose a business that's right for you.

Recognize the challenges that cannabis businesses commonly face, so you'll know whether you really want to do this and will be prepared to overcome the obstacles.

Lay a solid foundation for your cannabis business to improve your odds of success.

Explore various jobs in the cannabis industry and improve your odds of getting hired to fill the position you want.

Get up to speed on investment opportunities in the cannabis industry and recognize the potential upside and downside.

IN THIS CHAPTER

» **Recognizing the complexities of working with a Schedule I drug**

» **Exploring different cannabis business opportunities**

» **Understanding the business challenges you face**

» **Getting your business up and running — staffing and setup**

» **Making public relations a priority**

Chapter **14**

Starting Your Own Cannabis Business

Starting a business is a challenging and potentially risky endeavor in any industry, but toss in the complexities of working with a Schedule I drug that's still illegal in the vast majority of the world, and it can be close to insurmountable. As a cannabis entrepreneur, you'll find yourself having to navigate a labyrinth of rules and regulations, suffer through never-ending inspections, unravel the intricacies of the tax system, overcome restrictions on banking, and deal with community members who may not be overjoyed at having a cannabis business in their neighborhood. And you need to deal with all that in addition to all the other challenges of opening and running a successful business.

In this chapter, we bring you up to speed on the basics of starting and running a cannabis business. We introduce you to the complexities of working with a Schedule I drug, take you on a tour of common cannabis business opportunities, present the common challenges you're likely to face, explain the ins and outs of staffing and setting up your business, and provide guidance on how to keep peace with your neighbors and maintain a positive image in the communities in which you do business.

TIP

To avoid wasting time, money, and effort on a futile attempt to start a cannabis business and to give yourself a little bit of a head start, tackle the following preliminary tasks first:

>> Consult your city's business license department to find out whether the municipality allows the type of business you're thinking of starting.

>> Be sure that nothing on your record would cause a state or country to deny you a license, such as any criminal convictions.

>> Decide whether to focus on medical cannabis or adult recreational products. Your choice will narrow the opportunities and the complexities you'll have to address to ease your burden moving forward.

Working with a Federal Schedule I Drug

Marijuana is a Schedule I drug, which places it in the same class as heroin, lysergic acid diethylamide (LSD), ecstasy, methaqualone (Quaaludes), and peyote. These are drugs that have been determined by authorities of the U.S. government to have "no currently accepted medical use and a high potential for abuse." While we know that marijuana does, in fact, have medicinal properties and no biological potential for creating a physical dependency (but some potential for emotional and psychological dependency), it remains on the list of Schedule I drugs. This status poses several additional challenges for cannabis businesses:

>> The cannabis industry is highly regulated, and compliance is a huge and costly challenge. Business owners face an uphill battle to acquire and maintain licensing and to comply with continual tracking and reporting requirements. Owners and staff must be authorized to work in the industry and pass background checks to earn their badges.

REMEMBER

Each state has its own regulatory body. In Colorado, the Marijuana Enforcement Division conducts interviews and fingerprinting for all badge applicants. Key personnel in decision making roles can expect to pay approximately $250 for their badges, while all other staff pay $75. Badges must be renewed every two years for an additional fee.

>> You'll have to finance the business on your own or with the help of private investment. You can't get a loan from a federally insured bank, because they're prohibited by law from profiting from cannabis.

>> If your business will be buying or selling products containing THC (as opposed to hemp-derived CBD only), you won't be able to transport product across state lines. For example, you're prohibited from taking orders from and shipping product to out-of-state customers. If you want to do business in another state, you need to set up a separate operation in that state or establish partnerships with out-of-state operators.

>> Due to federal 280E legislation that disallows traditional income tax deductions for cannabis businesses, your business income will be taxed at an effective rate of 75–95 percent. When and if marijuana becomes federally legal in the United States, this will no longer apply.

Choosing a Business Type

The cannabis industry is open to a variety of business types that range from growing cannabis to selling and delivering it to consumers. The industry also supports a wide range of ancillary businesses that never come into contact with cannabis, such as companies that produce fertilizers, ventilation, and lighting equipment for growing cannabis and those that produce packaging and labels for cannabis products.

In this section, we describe some of the common types of businesses to assist you in choosing a business type that's most appealing and best suited to your interests and abilities.

VERTICALLY INTEGRATED OR NOT

A *vertically integrated* company is one in which the supply chain is owned by the company. In the cannabis industry, the term is used to describe companies that grow, manufacture, and sell cannabis products. Some jurisdictions encourage or require companies to be vertically integrated whereas others discourage or prohibit vertical integration.

Depending on the type of cannabis business you pursue, one of your early decisions is likely to be whether your business will be vertically integrated. Be sure to check the state and local laws to determine whether vertical integration is permitted or required in your area.

Grower

Growers represent the agriculture side of the business. In addition to structuring the business and procuring space to grow plants indoors or outdoors, growers have the following responsibilities:

>> Starting plants from seeds or cuttings and perhaps breeding plants to create new strains.

>> Growing and harvesting plants.

>> Separating the useable buds and properly disposing of the *green waste* — any organic waste that can be composted.

>> Drying, curing, and trimming the harvested bud.

>> Arranging for third-party lab testing for mold, contaminants, pests, and potency.

>> Packaging and perhaps transporting products to manufacturers or retail locations.

>> Tracking and reporting all processes as required by law to government regulatory agencies.

A grow business may be the perfect opportunity for you if you have a passion for the plant and the specialized knowledge to grow, harvest, and cure plants properly. If you don't have a green thumb, you may want to consider other opportunities in the industry.

Unfortunately, grow operations comprise the lowest profit margin segment of the industry. However, a grower can make up in volume for the low margins by selling product wholesale to multiple companies downstream, assuming the grower isn't part of a vertically integrated business. Another drawback is the high cost of entry into this segment due to the expenses of setting up for initial crops and meeting extensive regulatory thresholds.

Retailer

Cannabis retailers run the dispensaries and other retail outlets that sell products directly to consumers. Depending on the rules and regulations in your area, you may be permitted to run a medical dispensary, an adult recreational dispensary, or a dispensary that serves both medical and adult recreational clients.

A retail operation may be part of an integrated company that sells its own products, or it may be a standalone operation that purchases its products (flower, concentrates, lotions, tinctures, edibles, and so on) from third-party wholesale vendors. Retailers have a number of moving parts, must be fully compliant with all rules and regulations, and are responsible for any materials or individuals entering the premises.

Owners and operators of retail operations must enjoy working with people and be very diplomatic. Building and maintaining a thriving cannabis retail business requires the ability to make various stakeholders happy or at least keep them from becoming unhappy. As a retailer, you'll be dealing not only with a wide range of customers but also with regulators/inspectors and people in the neighborhood.

Here are a few of the specific challenges you're likely to face if you decide to start your own cannabis retail operation:

>> Locations must comply with set-back rules from other dispensaries as well as from schools and certain other establishments, so selecting a site can sometimes be challenging.

>> Although advertising is very restricted, retailers are highly visible, so they need to build strong relationships with their neighbors and their community. Not everyone will want you to open your cannabis store in "their backyard." Expect strong resistance and be pleasantly surprised if you're welcomed with open arms.

>> Retailers serve a wide variety of consumers, ranging from rank beginners to long-time users to medical patient seeking symptom relief. To thrive as a cannabis retailer, you and your staff must be able to appeal to and engage with consumers of various backgrounds and levels of experience and knowledge.

Retailing cannabis requires all the skills and talents of any retail operation plus the ability to comply with the highest levels of regulation of any industry. Think of starting a retail cannabis business as if you were starting a bank or a hospital. While other retailers may have to worry about secret shoppers and the competition, you'll have the added concerns of undercover stings — inspectors showing up unannounced to check whether you're allowing underage access, selling too much to individual customers, or selling even a second past your closing time.

Manufacturer of infused products (MIP)

MIP is an industry term used in reference to a company that makes marijuana infused products, including concentrates such as wax and shatter, oils and tinctures, lotions, and edibles. This segment of the industry acts as a laboratory as well as processing plant. It may be even more tightly regulated than other segments of the industry with additional rules and regulations that extend to manufacturing and commercial kitchens.

If you have a background in science and enjoy spending time in a laboratory or kitchen developing and manufacturing consumer products, then an MIP may be the right business opportunity for you. You'll be selling your products wholesale to retailers or, if your part of a vertically integrated company, you'll be in the middle of the supply chain, receiving flower from the grow operations and transforming it into end products to be sold through the company's dispensaries.

Under the umbrella of MIP are extraction and kitchen, discussed in the following sections. A business can do one or both. An extraction business can simply create the concentrates and sell them downstream to a dispensary or kitchen. Or a business can (and many do) purchase the oil and simply run a kitchen creating its own edibles or lotions. (These options are also available for hemp-derived CBD businesses.)

Extraction

Extraction involves various processes that pull the active ingredients from the plant to create concentrates, such as hash, wax, shatter, and live resin. (See Chapter 13 for more about extraction processes and the concentrates these processes produce.) Concentrates may be sold or used as ingredients in other products, such as edibles and topicals.

If you're into chemistry and think you would find job satisfaction in becoming highly efficient at extracting chemical compounds from raw plants, an extraction operation may be the right fit for you. However, extraction has two big drawbacks:

>> **Danger:** Some extraction processes involve heat, compression, and/or volatile and potentially toxic chemicals. Everyone on staff needs to know what they're doing and follow strict safety precautions to avoid blowing up themselves, each other, and the building and to avoid over-exposure to potentially toxic chemicals.

>> **Cost:** In addition to the high costs of machines and materials used in various extraction processes are the costs of safety sensors and equipment. Some MIPs use various extraction methods, which increases product selection but also increases costs. A single piece of equipment used for some extraction processes may cost several thousands of dollars.

Kitchen

Kitchen operations involve using the oil extracted from cannabis as an ingredient in a wide range of products, including vape oil, edibles, lotions, tinctures, and soaps. Running an industrial cannabis kitchen can be loads of fun. Although you may be required to follow recipes provided by your company or others to prepare products, you may also have the opportunity of developing your own recipes!

The main drawback of running an industrial cannabis kitchen is the burdensome rules, regulations, and inspections. You must meet the high standards already in place for traditional restaurants and industrial kitchens, but you have the added regulations that apply to cannabis. Keeping your kitchen impeccably clean and dealing with constant inspections and detailed tracking and reporting can be cumbersome in itself.

Processed product brand

A processed product brand can be a MIP or a combined Grow-MIP business that makes products and sells them to numerous retail outlets. For example, you can set up your own grow-MIP business to produce a line of infused chocolates that you sell to a variety of medical and recreational dispensaries in Oregon.

Another option is to set up all the business arrangements with a MIP and dispensaries, never producing the product on your own. You develop a strong brand presence and gain wide distribution of your product, essentially outsourcing the grow, MIP, and retail operations. In some cases, the processed product brand uses all wholesale products and outsources production of its product recipes right from the start, acting as a sales and marketing business without the production aspect.

The big challenge arises when you decided to expand distribution to other states. Because federal law currently prohibits shipping product across state or international borders, if you want to expand, you need to find a way to work around that restriction. Here are a couple ways processed product brands expand beyond state lines:

>> Set up a vertically integrated company in the other state. For example, if you begin with a line of infused chocolates in Oregon and want to expand distribution to California, you set up a vertically integrated grow-MIP-retail operation in California and start producing and selling your chocolates there. (This option is a costly proposition.)

>> Partner with a vertically integrated company in the targeted state and have them produce and sell your products. In essence, you authorize the other company to produce your product using your recipe and package and sell it in their own stores or sell it wholesale to other state dispensaries.

>> Start an MIP in the other state. You can then sign agreements with growers to source the flower you need and sign agreements with retailers who want to purchase your product for resale.

TIP

If you have a great recipe and a knack for marketing and business, creating your own processed product brand may be the best segment of the cannabis industry for you.

Even with federal legalization in Canada, processed product brands struggle to conduct business across provincial divides. With current regulations, retailers can sell only to customers in the same province. As Canada introduces a wider range of products, including edibles, to its menu of options in 2019, these rules may change making it easier for processed product brands to expand distribution across Canada.

Profiting from cannabis with an ancillary business

You don't have to be in the cannabis business to profit from it. Several ancillary businesses (those that "never touch the plant") stand to benefit from the growth of the cannabis industry, including the following:

>> Fertilizer manufacturers

>> Nurseries

>> Manufacturers and sellers of grow lights

>> Heating, ventilation, and air conditioning (HVAC) companies and professionals who specialize in ventilation and circulation for grow operations

>> Breweries that sell their CO_2 to grow facilities

>> Packaging and labeling services

>> Security services and manufactures and sellers of security equipment

>> Marketing, public relations, and advertising firms

>> Real estate companies and investors

>> Law firms and consulting agencies that specialize in helping clients achieve and maintain compliance with the ever-changing cannabis rules and regulations

Addressing Common Challenges

The cannabis industry is brutal. Businesses are pressured from all directions. They can't get loans from federally insured banks or accept credit or debit card payments; they're not allowed to claim standard business deductions; they can't conduct business across state lines; and they struggle daily to comply with a long, growing, and ever-changing list of rules and requirements. You really have to wonder how any cannabis businesses survive — most don't. The profit margins are slim, and the room for error even slimmer.

In this section, we open your eyes to the many challenges you're likely to face if you decide to start your own cannabis business, so you're well aware of what you're up against. Our intent isn't to discourage you from pursuing the dream of owning and operating your own cannabis business, but to inform you of the challenges so you're in a better position to overcome them.

TIP

One of the best ways to overcome any business challenge is to bring on professionals to supplement your own talents and experience. You may be a wonderful business person with little knowledge of cannabis, or you may be a cannabis savant with little to no business acumen. By being honest with yourself about your own strengths and weaknesses and plugging any gaps with the requisite expertise, you can improve your chances of success exponentially.

Dealing with money issues

If you buy into the media hype about the cannabis industry, you may believe that starting a cannabis business is about the easiest way to earn a fortune in the United States. You may have been led to believe that it's the second easiest road to riches, next to winning the lottery or investing in Bitcoin.

The truth is that making money in the cannabis industry is challenging, and one of the biggest challenges is due to the rules and regulations regarding the money itself. Specifically, banking restrictions and taxes place a huge collective burden on any cannabis business, presenting a high cost of entry into the industry. In this section, we describe these challenges in greater detail.

Operating in an all-cash business (being barred from banking)

In U.S. states where cannabis is legal you may be unable to open a bank account for your business. Any federally insured bank is prohibited from profiting from cannabis. You may find one or two state credit unions that cater to the cannabis industry, but they have to clear a high regulatory bar, and they typically charge high fees.

Not being able to have a bank account for your business may not sound like a huge issue until you consider the ramifications, such as the following:

» All sales are in cash. You need a way to record all cash sales, and you need cash on hand to make change.

» Customers must pay in cash, so if they show up without cash, you may lose a sale. You may be able to have an ATM installed at your location, so customers can withdraw cash from their accounts, but you'll need an armored car service to pick up the cash and deliver it to you for accounting if you're operating more than one location.

>> ATMs in dispensaries are managed by third-party services that typically charge customers a fee for the convenience of cash withdrawals from their banks, which aren't necessarily connected to the ATM. Having to pay those fees makes the purchase more expensive.

>> Without a bank account, you can't pay your staff and vendors with a check. You'll be counting out cash to each employee and vendor, and if you're the vendor, you'll have to accept cash payments.

>> You have to pay your taxes in cash, which can be a huge hassle. Some state departments of revenue have you call ahead so they can escort you to the door with bags of cash.

>> Knowing you're running a cash business, potential thieves are more likely to target your business. You need to install a safe at each location for cash and product and have other security devices and protocols in place to limit theft and ensure the safety of your staff and customers.

Cash-flow can also become a challenge. While in a system with credit card purchases the charges are batched at the end of the day and sent electronically to your account available immediately, cash will require an armored car pick up, a double check by accounting and then a secure delivery to the bank before it is available for you to pay bills.

Individuals in the industry have had their personal accounts cancelled by banks when it is discovered they are in the cannabis industry. While this is becoming less pervasive with greater numbers of US states legalizing, it can still spook some professionals and investors and keep them from entering the industry.

REMEMBER

If you have a credit union account, any time they're being audited, you're being audited, so be sure to keep detailed accounting records.

In Canada, federal legalization has provided much greater banking flexibility, although initial bank accounts can be difficult to secure for cannabis businesses that aren't traded publicly. Canadian banks are still wary of cannabis businesses and have required additional information and credit verification with local vendors. In addition, due to trade agreements with the U.S. that bar monetary transfers from illegal activity, Canadian cannabis income may not be able to be brought into the United States at all or may be extremely heavily taxed.

Getting up and running without access to capital

The old saying "It takes money to make money" is even truer in the cannabis industry. You need to be independently wealthy or have access to wealthy investors who aren't looking for a quick return on their investment. States have gotten wise to the numbers of people who are interested in applying for cannabis licenses. The non-refundable fees can run around $60,000 just for the privilege of applying and they may require millions of dollars in bonds plus in-depth detail of your committed capital on the applications.

Finding the right investors is a major challenge. Most investors want to see a fast return on their investment, and they may require that you agree to loan and repayment schedules that drive you out of business faster than you went in. Plus, in some locations, investors must live in the state or at least have a residence in the state. Some large private investors have purchased condos in states in which they want to invest solely to comply with this requirement.

REMEMBER

Choose investors whose goals align with yours. Be sure they understand the time needed before they see profits and the tax implications not only for the business but for themselves as well. How big do you want to grow your business? Will you be looking to acquire other businesses or to be acquired? Are you planning to expand out of state if the opportunity arises? What type of other investment may be needed or welcomed in the future? Answers to these questions clarify your vision for the future and enable you to communicate that vision more clearly to prospective investors to ensure that you're on the same page.

WARNING

If you're working with individual investors or larger institutional investment groups that are targeting the industry, be very careful of the contracts you sign. Hire a very good lawyer who's familiar with the industry and is dedicated to serving your best interests. Hiring a lawyer to review all agreements is an additional cost, but it'll steer you clear of the most costly pitfalls.

Tackling taxation

Taxes seem to be synonymous with cannabis right now. Not only are customers of adult recreational products being socked with huge sales taxes, but businesses are often straining under the burden of high and recurring licensing fees. Whenever a state or municipality is facing a budget shortfall, legislators often start looking to cannabis as the solution.

In this section, we explain a couple of the more taxing issues you're likely to encounter in the cannabis industry.

TIP

Hire an accountant who understands all the cannabis connected taxes and exactly how to handle getting your taxes paid in a cash business.

280 E LEGISLATION AND THE FEDERAL TAX RATE ON CANNABIS BUSINESSES

According to Section 280E of the Internal Revenue Code business expenses in connection with the illegal sale of drugs are not deductible. Expenses such as payroll, rent, maintenance, professional fees, and capital improvements, are just a few of the many expenses deemed not deductible. As a result, if your cannabis business has income of $100,000 and expenses of $75,000, you end up paying federal income tax on that $100,000, not on the $25,000 of net profit.

Trade associations are working to minimize the excessive tax burden imposed by Section 280E and bring relief to the industry without securing federal legalization. However, until that time, plan on paying an effective income tax rate between 75 and 95 percent.

REMEMBER

Within the cannabis industry, federal effective income tax rates run between 75 and 95 percent, making them one of the biggest barriers to profitability in the industry.

STATE AND MUNICIPAL TAXES

Legislators have conjured up all sorts of ways to tax cannabis. For example, in Alaska, growers pay $50 per ounce when selling products to dispensaries or retailers. In California, growers pay $9.25 per ounce on the sale of cannabis flower and $2.75 per ounce of leaves, while retailers collect a 15 percent excise tax from customers. In Colorado, growers collect a 15 percent excise tax from retailers, and retailers collect a 15 percent sales tax from customers. Municipalities can tack on their own taxes.

REMEMBER

You must have a point of sale (POS) system in place that records the amounts collected and a system in place for remitting the amount collected to the various state and municipal taxing authorities. This system should also be fully cannabis compliant and designed for the industry, not a standard retail POS that has been modified.

TIP

Choose your location wisely. Because municipalities can tack on their own taxes, products may cost more in one area of the state than another, which can impact sales. Do your research and become familiar with the area and its tax rates specifically for cannabis before choosing a location.

Adhering to state and local laws

The predominant challenge of working in the cannabis industry is compliance with state and local rules and regulations that often change and may conflict with one another. These rules and regulations govern everything from hours of operation, to the amount of cannabis a consumer can purchase in a given day, to how green waste is disposed of, and much more. For example, Colorado requires that a specific protocol be followed if a staff member at a retail location accidentally drops a jar of flower. After the glass and flower have been removed from the floor, a trained staff member must grind up all the product and mix it with bleach and dirt to render it unusable and unrecognizable before placing it in a locked receptacle for pickup by the municipality.

To further complicate compliance, cannabis rules are changing all the time. Small rule changes may occur monthly with larger state regulatory overhauls occurring a couple times a year. While state rules take precedence for the most part, municipalities may set their own rules that are inconsistent with state rules or with rules in other municipalities. As a result, if your business operates in different municipalities, each location may need to follow different rules.

One area that's highly variable is the location signage rules. In some locations, you may be able to have a sign with your logo and perhaps even the green + sign, while other locations bar you from that identification. Coupons and discounts are another area with variations. Some municipalities won't allow any discounts for some customers (such as those with a coupon).

WARNING

Hire an expert in compliance or outsource compliance to a company that specializes in cannabis compliance in any and all of your business locations. Any violations can put your company in jeopardy.

In the following sections, we dig deeper into the topic of compliance. We encourage you to become familiar with the regulatory bodies in the locations you do business and provide guidance on key compliance issues.

Getting to know the regulatory bodies

As states, provinces, and countries legalize the growth, sale, and use of cannabis for medical and/or recreational purposes, they create governing bodies or assign marijuana regulation to existing government departments. The governing bodies in charge of cannabis may be associated with revenue, alcohol, tobacco, or gambling, or they may be created as a new division.

Identify the regulatory bodies in your state and municipality and explore their online resources to become familiar with the rules and regulations in your state and the municipalities in which you operate your business. Table 14-1 lists the regulatory bodies in states in which cannabis is legal for adult recreational use.

TABLE 14-1 **State Regulatory Bodies**

State	Regulatory Body	Website
Colorado	Marijuana Enforcement Division	www.colorado.gov/pacific/enforcement/marijuanaenforcement
California	Bureau of Cannabis Control	www.bcc.ca.gov
Oregon	Oregon Liquor Control Commission	www.oregon.gov/olcc
Washington	Washington State Liquor and Cannabis Board	lcb.wa.gov
Michigan	Bureau of Marijuana Regulation	www.michigan.gov/lara

Marijuana tracking and retail

One of state and local governments' biggest fears about the industry is *diversion* — legal product getting to the black market. Many of the rules created by the regulatory agencies are designed to keep diversion from happening. One of the primary tools for preventing diversion is the tracking system.

Each state has its own electronic system for tracking plant material from "Seed to Sale." Tracking codes and radio-frequency identification (RFID) tags are placed on plants at a certain height, and those numbers must follow the product every step of the way to the final customer.

Whatever type of cannabis business you're in, you're responsible for inputting tracking numbers into your state's system and being accountable for every single portion of that plant that passes through your possession, even green waste (discussed next).

Managing green waste

Green waste is any portion of the plant not allowed to be sold or used in your state. This can be stems, stalks, leaves, roots or byproducts from manufacturing processes. Most locations require that the green waste is made unrecognizable and unusable before being passed to the state or to a private waste disposal organization. For example, you may need to grind up unused plant matter and mix it with other substances such as dirt and bleach. In some areas, grow facilities are required to reclaim water to catch and eliminate any contaminants.

WARNING

Keep your dumpsters locked. Even if you don't dispose of any potentially usable product, you're going to have people dumpster diving to see if they can score some free product, and you can be held liable if they're injured or they find usable product and inspectors find out about it — not to mention the mess they may make throwing your neatly collected trash about the neighborhood and making noise at all hours and disturbing your neighbors.

Complying with packaging requirements

Every state has detailed rules and regulations for packaging and labeling products. Childproofing is now mandatory across all locations and will remain so, probably even with full federal legalization. Technology has created childproof packages for all types of products, even candy bars, and more innovations are in the works. Rules typically stipulate that all packaging must be opaque, so you can't clearly see the contents and that packaging not be attractive to minors or similar to the packaging used for certain commercially available products.

Labeling rules typically require the common or usual name of the product, a warning statement about possible adverse effects, a universal THC symbol on any products that contain THC, an indication that the product was tested by a third-party lab, an ingredients list, nutritional facts, the facility's license number and the batch number or lot code, the total quantity of specific cannabinoids in the package and per serving, when applicable, and so on.

REMEMBER

Packaging and labeling requirements vary by state and perhaps even by municipality. Check the current regulations, which you can usually find posted on the governing agency's website. Even if you're operating in the processed product brand segment of the industry, you must provide packaging and labels to your partner MIP if you're not doing packaging and labeling of your products yourself.

Complying with location requirements

One of the big cost centers of running a cannabis facility, regardless of the type of business (grow, MIP, retail) is ensuring the facility is compliant. Security is of major concern, but other requirements may also apply and may be specific to a portion of the business such as the following:

» Cameras with recording capabilities and a prescribed number of days of footage for all internal and external locations

» External lights on motion sensors or timers

» Locks, safes, secured cabinets, and even lockable refrigerators for items that must be stored cold

» Security personnel in some cases and situations

» Internal and external door locking mechanisms with badged or passcode access

» Barriers to the view of products in retail locations such as opaque exterior windows

- » Odor filters to mitigate the smell for neighbors
- » Chemical spill clean-up materials and eye washes
- » Security alarms for break-ins and gas alarms for extraction toxin build up
- » Separate and secured storage areas
- » Controlled delivery areas

Getting your products tested

If your business is a grow operation or MIP, you need to line up a third-party lab to test your products for potency, pesticides, molds, and other potential contaminants. Third-party testing isn't required by retail operations; however, retailers need to check the products they purchase to ensure that all product labels certify that such testing was performed.

REMEMBER

Investigate reputable labs in your area that have experience with marijuana testing. Find out how much product they need and how much lead time they require to conduct the necessary tests.

TIP

Keep a sample of each batch of product, so that if anyone or any agency challenges the safety or quality of one of your products, you can have the sample retested to prove your case.

Applying for licenses in other states

As more states and countries legalize marijuana, you have more opportunities to expand any cannabis business you currently have. Unfortunately, you may encounter some resistance when you attempt to expand into another state or country. In many jurisdictions, you may need to find a partner in that jurisdiction or invest in another company already operating in that jurisdiction to qualify as an applicant. Likewise, you may be contacted by business owners in other states or countries who are interested in expanding their operations in your locations.

In some cases, you may be required to purchase suitable property and hire staff before applying.

WARNING

Carefully research any company that contacts you about entering into a partnership so that the company can do business in your state or municipality. Be very wary of any company that requires you to invest or pay part or all of the application fee as part of the partnership agreement; even if you sign a contract to become a partner, the company's application may be denied, and you may lose your entire investment. Application fees can range from thousands to tens of thousands of dollars and are usually non-refundable.

Prior to applying for a cannabis license in your own state or another state, consider the option of hiring an application consultant, explore all costs involved, and size up the competition, as explained in the following sections.

Hiring an application consultant

Application consulting has become a new cannabis industry. You can hire a consultant to help you draft the application and get the operation set up to run in another location. They usually charge a flat fee because they can't guarantee that they can secure you a license. These fees can run as high as $50,000, which may include putting all the pieces in place to run a business in one specific segment of the industry, such as grow or retail only. It may also include connections with local investors, firms, elected officials, or partners with other resources if you're required to be vertically integrated.

This may seem to be an unnecessary expense to apply but consultants have been through the process before, and they know the process and the players. They can help to streamline the application process, improve your odds of gaining approval, and help you build your supply chain.

TIP

Choose your application consultant carefully. Get recommendations from other cannabis companies in the industry. When interviewing consultants, ask in which states they've helped clients apply for licenses and their track record for winning approvals. A reputable consultant will not take more than one client in a state to avoid competing against themselves and their other client.

Getting your finances in order

Prior to applying for a license, you need to create a business plan complete with detailed budget showing that you have the capital in place to cover the costs of starting and running a cannabis business. The process of creating a business plan is beyond the scope of this book, so check out *Creating a Business Plan For Dummies*, by Veechi Curtis (Wiley), for detailed guidance.

REMEMBER

Include in your budget the cost of consultants, land and building purchases, staff hires, and secure bonds even before you apply. The fees are hefty and non-refundable so be aware that you could lose your investment before you even break ground.

Sizing up the competition

When you're looking to expand into another location examine how that government is handling the expansion. If the government is opening the doors wide to an unlimited number of licenses, your odds of obtaining a license are high. However, you can expect to encounter stiff competition moving forward, because the market will quickly become saturated. On the other hand, if the government plans to issue a very limited number of licenses, the playing field often favors well-funded organizations that have dotted all their I's and crossed all their T's. Winning one of those licenses would be a steep uphill battle.

In some locations, such as Saskatchewan and Ontario, Canada, getting licensed is a matter of winning the license lottery. Winning a license requires more luck than due diligence, which results in many licenses issued to winners who have no idea how to start or run a cannabis business and are lacking the capital to survive the long and rocky road to success. Shortly after the winners are announced, established companies rush in and try to cut deals with the winners to help them run their operations in exchange for a future buy-out of all or a portion of the business.

REMEMBER

The lottery system typically stipulates that a license winner can't sell out right away and actually hold the license, operating as a business for a certain amount of time, such as a year. During this time, bigger players often move in and try to sign agreements to serve as operating consultants with the ability to buy out or share ownership with the smaller company after the wait time expires.

Staffing for Success

The cannabis industry is evolving quickly and some may say "growing up." The days of cobbling together a crew of friends and acquaintances to build and run a successful cannabis business are over. Nowadays, you need a staff with experience and expertise that span everything from botany and chemistry to business management, marketing, sales, accounting, communications, and human resources (HR).

In this section, we provide guidance on how to staff your cannabis business for success. You find out about the key positions you need to fill, the training you must provide, and the basics of getting your personnel certified to work in the industry.

Canada has specific rules regarding employment that differ from those in the United States, along with residency and work visa requirements that dictate local hiring.

TIP

You can certainly follow traditional recruiting practices to find the people you need, but if you're looking for a shortcut, consider engaging the services of a firm that specializes in recruiting for the cannabis industry, such as Vangst (vangst.com).

Filling key positions

Although you can fill some roles in your business with less experienced workers, fill key roles with people who have the knowledge and expertise to hit the ground running. In this section, we present key positions you need to fill along with insight into why these positions are so important.

Compliance

Your company's very existence rests on the competence of your compliance team, so hire an expert who has plenty of experience with dealing with compliance issues in the cannabis industry and a solid track record of success. Give this person the resources she needs to build a strong team of lawyers and field compliance staff.

Your compliance team will be working with regulators directly and responding to issues or challenges. The team needs to develop an intimate knowledge of the rules and regulations and be plugged into the various governing bodies to monitor and quickly respond to any new rules or revisions. Companies have been known to be compliant one day and non-compliant the next due to an unforeseen rule revision or an administration change at the regulatory body.

Accounting

Although all business accountants need to be able to crunch numbers and produce a variety of financial reports, accountants in the cannabis industry face unique challenges, especially in the U.S., where cannabis is a cash-only business.

To lead your accounting department, hire an accountant who has experience in the cannabis industry. A qualified candidate can help with all financial aspects of the business, including setting up the point-of-sale (POS) system, keeping the books, figuring out how to secure loans and investment capital, creating a system for paying taxes, and so on.

TIP

Because of the preponderance of cash in the cannabis industry, hire an accountant who's trustworthy and pays close attention to details. Be sure to conduct a thorough background check and have your books audited regularly by a third-party accounting firm.

Security

Someone in your company needs to focus on security, because cannabis companies (including grow, MIP, and retail operations) are all at a heightened risk of being robbed. You can find plenty of stories in the news about thieves driving cars or trucks through doors or walls in attempts to steal cash and product from retail locations and grow operations. Some locations have been robbed during operating hours.

To protect your business, customers, and staff, you'll need locks, safes, security cameras, and alarms along with the expertise to install security equipment and train the staff on security protocols and all security requirements for the cannabis industry. For example, state and municipal cannabis rules and regulations may stipulate that video from cameras be retained for a certain number of days before being erased or written over, and that footage be made available to regulators upon request.

TIP

Because security cameras are usually required around the exterior of buildings, local law enforcement may request access to footage in the case of an unrelated issue nearby. Complying with their requests is a great way to demonstrate that you're a good neighbor.

If you decide to manage security in house, hire someone who's familiar with the unique security challenges and regulations in the cannabis industry. Another option is to outsource security to a firm that has experience securing various types of cannabis businesses.

Marketing, sales, and communications

Whether you're in the grow, MIP, brand, or retail segment of the industry or all of them at once, you need experts in place to market and sell your products and to communicate effectively with the press and the public:

» **Marketing:** Marketing in the cannabis industry is particularly tricky due to regulations on marketing to minors and the fact that cannabis consumers are so varied. Consumers differ in regard to whether they're buying for adult recreational or medicinal purposes, as well as their level of experience. Appealing to all prospective consumers without alienating a specific group can be very challenging. At the same time, the marketing team needs to avoid any semblance of marketing to minors; for example, state rules typically require that at least 70 percent of the viewers or readers of a publication or outlet be people 21 years or older and that no more than 30 percent are minors. The publication or outlet should be able to provide demographic information to ensure compliance but the cannabis company is responsible for viewing that information.

» **Sales:** Sales managers and staff must be aware of all rules and regulations governing the sale of cannabis products. In addition, like the marketing staff, sales people need to evaluate prospective buyers and adjust their messaging accordingly. For example, a salesperson who treats a medical marijuana user like an adult recreational user is likely to lose a customers.

» **Communications:** Cannabis is a hot issue and will continue to be so for some time. The media are interested and may have an actual bias depending on the outlet. Staff your communications team with professionals to help you navigate these waters. Being unclear or getting misquoted can stir up trouble with both regulators and the communities in which you do business.

Though communications professionals can help ensure accuracy in the press and position you in the best light with strong messages, the first amendment to the U.S. constitution guarantees freedom of the press. You may not like what they write, how they mention you, but it's their right to do so. Even if you choose not to be quoted or interviewed for a story, that doesn't mean they can't reference your company. If you want to have the material exactly as you want it, advertise. Of course, you may not be permitted to do that either.

Providing the necessary training

Although you certainly want to hire people who have all the knowledge and skills required to perform their jobs, not all personnel will have the requisite knowledge of cannabis and the rules and regulations governing the industry. You must train them or hire someone to provide that training. Training should cover the following three areas:

>> **Rules and regulations:** Different rules and regulations are relevant to different segments of the business (grow, MIP, and retail) and to different positions in the company. If an employee can break a rule or regulation by doing or failing to do something or by performing a certain task improperly, she should know about it.

Adding to the challenge of training all employees is the fact that rules and regulations may differ across locations — in different states or municipalities.

>> **Products:** Budtenders must have a general knowledge of cannabis and its effects (and variations for individuals), along with more thorough knowledge of specific products. They need to be able to explain the difference between different strains, between flower and concentrates, and between different consumption methods. They also need to be able to evaluate a customer's needs and their desired effects and recommend suitable products.

>> **Safety and security:** All staff should be made aware of the fact that the cannabis industry is attractive to criminals. They need to understand security risks and protocols and know what to do in the event of a robbery. Personnel who work in extraction must also fully understand and follow safety precautions in any areas where dangerous extraction processes are performed.

>> **International staff training:** With legalization in Canada, the U.S. has recognized that some staff hired in Canada may be travelling to the U.S. for training and other cannabis business activities. At this point, international trade agreements may bar travel for those purposes and create a challenge for U.S. based companies that intend to bring staff to the states for those purposes.

Getting your people certified: Badging

All staff must be badged or authorized to work in cannabis by your government regulatory body. Most regulatory agencies issue two levels of badge: one for key personnel or decision makers and another for regular staff members such as budtenders or trimmers. The badge may require an interview at the location, a fee, proof of residency, and a background check with fingerprints. All company principles need a higher-level badge, and investors may need some type of authorization as well.

Badges are usually good for two years, after which time the badge holder must renew it and pay the renewal fee.

For details on how to apply for a badge, check the website of the cannabis regulatory agency in your state. There you should find a list of minimum requirements to qualify for a badge, guidance to help choose the right type of badge for the jobs you're considering, and an application you can download and print.

Setting Up Shop

After laying the groundwork for your cannabis business and receiving your license, you're ready to begin setting up shop. You need to choose a facility, start to establish your supply chain, build a website, and purchase and implement a point of sale (POS) system.

In this section, we bring you up to speed on the basics of getting all the pieces in place, so you'll be ready for opening day!

Choosing a facility

Real estate is a key component of the cannabis business. Regardless of the segment of the industry in which your business operates, you're likely to need a facility. In some cases, you can rent but in others you may be required to buy. Research rules and available properties carefully, so you're sure that a particular location is suitable for your needs. Of course, the location must be zoned for business, additional rules specifically for cannabis businesses may prohibit certain locations from being used. For example, most jurisdictions have setback rules that specify the minimum distance a cannabis business must be from schools, residential properties, childcare facilities, correctional facilities, and other marijuana businesses.

Suitable facilities vary according to the business type:

>> **Indoor grow facility:** If you're planning an indoor grow facility, you may need a warehouse, preferably in an industrial park far from any residential properties. You may be required to install special air filters to reduce odors but even with those in place, smells escape, and residents who are sensitive to those smells will complain.

>> **MIP:** If you're establishing a MIP, consider your distance to your flower supplier as well as to your retail locations. You may need to do safety modifications for any extraction space to ensure safety and pass all fire and safety inspections.

>> **Dispensary/retail store:** If you're planning to open a retail store, you have several factors to consider including parking, street access, car and foot traffic, size, office space, storage space, ability to secure the property, and the local demographics.

Establishing your supply chain

Prior to starting any wholesale or retail operation, you need to establish your *supply chain* — a system of suppliers and services required to obtain or manufacture a product and deliver it to customers. While the different segments of the cannabis industry collectively form a supply chain consisting of grow, MIP, and retail operations, each segment has its own supply chain, as well.

Your supply chain may include buyers and sales people as well as couriers that transport product.

Tackling transportation issues

Transportation can be particularly challenging in the cannabis industry. You may create your own courier division or outsource the task. Whether you choose to keep transportation in-house or outsource it, be sure that your equipment protocols or those of any transportation companies you're evaluating cover the following:

>> All drivers must be properly trained not only to perform their job duties but to maintain safety, security, and compliance.

>> Vehicles and cargo areas and surrounding areas are equipped with security cameras with live feeds. Live feeds also help track vehicles and are invaluable in an emergency situation.

>> Drivers are informed that all speed limits and all traffic rules must be observed at all times. Technology is available to alert managers if a driver is driving erratically or exceeding the speed limit.

>> Efficient loading protocols are in place for pickups and deliveries with frequent route changes to deter thieves.

>> Vehicles should be replaced every few years due to wear and tear from high mileage driving. In the long run buying or leasing a new vehicle is less costly than maintenance costs on older vehicles, which increase exponentially over 70,000 miles.

>> A system is in place that ensures compliance with state rules for routes and delivery times along with regulations for filing manifests for the state and using the government's tracking system. In some locations, all deliveries must be completed within the day, and specific transportation hours may be indicated. In the event that a package is declined at a location, perhaps for manifest irregularities or ordering mistakes, that package may need to be returned to its original location within the same timeframe. Most states prohibit any product in vehicles overnight for security purposes.

>> Effective and efficient packaging techniques are in place to ensure efficiency. Delivering half empty boxes, for example, is inefficient.

>> Rules stipulate that cash be transported only by specially trained experts or personnel in armored cars. Couriers should never be used to transport large amounts of cash.

REMEMBER

Always prioritize people over cash or product. Drivers should know to walk away from any dangerous situation.

Acquiring the necessary equipment

Regardless of the type of cannabis business you plan on starting, you'll need specialized equipment. Table 14-2 provides a general idea of the types of equipment required for the different cannabis business types. (This list isn't exhaustive.)

Of course, all business types require security equipment, as well, including security cameras, safes, and burglar alarms.

Examine your equipment needs thoroughly and conduct in-depth research into manufacturers, specific products, and sellers. Machines and other equipment represent a huge expense, but they also provide the means for generating profit, so consider not only the cost but also the potential return on investment.

TABLE 14-2   **Equipment Needs for Different Cannabis Businesses**

Business Type	Equipment Needs
Grow (indoor)	Grow lights
	Tables
	Air circulation equipment
	Product transport dollies
	Compliant trash collection receptacles
	HVAC equipment
	Watering/fertilizing systems and timers
	Water reclamation systems
	CO_2 systems
	Thermometers
	Hygrometers
	pH meters
	Pest management systems with showers
	Staff working clothes
	Washing machines and dryers
	Tracking RFID or other system readers
	Tracking tags
	Shears, scissors, and snips
	Safety gear such as goggles and respirators
	Sifters, twisters, drying racks
	Green light systems
	Humidity systems and sensors
	Cure buckets
	Product scales
	Packaging supplies
	Security cameras
	Door locks with badging systems
	Emergency equipment

(continued)

TABLE 14-2 *(continued)*

Business Type	Equipment Needs
MIP	Extraction machines
	Stills
	Processing and work tables
	Refrigerators
	Industrial kitchen equipment
	Safety sensors and alarms
	Compliant trash collection receptacles
	Product scales
	Packaging supplies
	Security cameras
	Door locks with badging systems
	Emergency equipment
	Respirators
	Air filtration devices
	Safety gear such as goggles and respirators
Dispensary/ retail store	Display cases
	Safes, locking cabinets, and locking refrigerators
	Compliant trash collection receptacles
	Cash registers
	Automated teller machine (ATM)
	ID checker
	Product scanners
	Security cameras
	Door locks with badging or keypad systems
	Emergency equipment

Creating a website/blog

Every business should have an official website/blog that provides the business the means of establishing an online presence. After all, if you don't take control of your company's reputation online, others will by posting comments and ratings about the company on various social media venues. A basic website that contains location and contact information, an about us page, the company's mission statement, and perhaps product information is sufficient to help with marketing and to provide suppliers and prospective customers the means to contact the company.

When designing and developing the company's website, make it a full team project, so everyone has the opportunity to give their input. Marketing should take the lead with considerable input from those in charge of compliance, but by making the website a team project, you ensure that all areas of expertise are involved in content development and accuracy.

REMEMBER

Your website must have an *age gate* — a statement asking visitors whether they're over 21 and allowing or blocking access to the site based on the visitor's response.

Building your point of sale (POS) system

Point of sale (POS) technology for retail has been around for many years but the cannabis industry has specific requirements that include regulatory and compliance pieces not applicable to other businesses. When you're in the market for a POS system, look for cannabis-specific systems, which are growing in complexity and effectiveness. Several players in this market, including Cova and Flowhub, have been working with established cannabis businesses to recognize and code through the kinks.

Traditional POS systems built for traditional retail don't have the compliance components necessary. Choose a system built from scratch for the industry instead of one adapted from the traditional retail world.

TIP

Opt for a system from a company that offers top-notch customer service. You want a company that can help you get the system up and running and is available when you encounter technical difficulties.

Maintaining a Positive Public Image

Not everyone likes cannabis in general and many people don't want operations in their town or neighborhood. Even after legalization you may find many people rooting for you to fail. One of the best ways to combat this negative cheering section, in addition to being totally compliant, is to be a good neighbor and a strong corporate citizen. While that may be important with any business, it is even more so in the cannabis industry.

In the following sections, we offer some general guidance on how to put your best foot forward.

TIP

Make sure you and your teams are volunteering in your community and supporting local non-profit organizations. Although volunteering is a good practice for any business, it may be required of cannabis employees in some locations. In these locations, staff can't be compensated for their time — they must truly volunteer it.

Attending community hearings

Part of your application may be a public hearing in your chosen location on the public's desire for your business. Even in locations where a public hearing isn't required of other businesses, it may be required for yours. This is a great opportunity to make friends with your neighbors and demonstrate the value that you bring to the community. Be prepared and be respectful of everyone who shows up at the hearing, especially the more vocal attendees with whom you may most strongly disagree.

Handling public affairs

Part of the success of your community hearings and your welcome in the area may rest with your outreach to constituents, local groups, and elected officials. Be positive and proactive. Invite your neighbors to your space. Work with your local public officials and elected leadership by bringing them to your location and answering any questions they have. The old adage holds true: It's better to make friends *before* you need them.

Communicating with the press

Cannabis isn't yet its own beat with reporters dedicated to writing cannabis columns, as they do with City Hall or business or sports, but it's not that far off. Some reporters at local, national, and international outlets are trending in this direction — specializing in writing about the cannabis industry.

Due to the growing interest in cannabis, you can expect to get a cold call at any time from a member of the press corps, especially in response to proposed cannabis legislation, a recent robbery of a cannabis business, or an incident of non-compliance. You need to be prepared. Engage the services of an in-house staff person or agency that has experience with cannabis and the press. They can help you draft messages and train you for interviews. Also, designate one person on your team to be the spokesperson. If you get very nervous just thinking about being in front of the cameras, choose someone other than yourself to serve as your company's spokesperson — someone with a cool head who's dignified and well-spoken.

Catering to the customer

A word about the customer. Cannabis consumers are the financial drivers for the entire industry. They're an evolving demographic that has morphed with legalization and changes to the stigma of cannabis use. The initial proponents and activists presented a cannabis culture more closely aligned to the images of Cheech and Chong, while today's cannabis user may be far from that perception or be steadfast in their belief that the scene is just as important as the product.

As a cannabis business owner, especially in the retail environment, you'll need to address a varied array of customers. You'll need to adapt to this varied demographic or specialize to attract your desired shopper. Be prepared to accommodate and adapt to a varied cast of characters, including the following:

>> **The cost conscious or money-is-no-object consumer:** Price is key for some, either bargain basement and interested only in the deal of the week or the high-end consumer willing to pay a premium for quality and service.

>> **The younger consumer:** This person may be familiar with the lingo and looking for the scene shopping experience. She may be a regular consumer and know exactly what she wants or know how to evaluate products on her own that match her needs.

>> **The longtime older user:** Many individuals who may have consumed years ago have reentered the market with legalization. They may not be familiar with the strength, product selection, or lingo in today's market, but they're not novices and require a respectful yet educational approach.

>> **The new older user:** With the changes to stigma and the emergence of information about CBD and health benefits from cannabis, more consumers are investigating marijuana. They may be very nervous walking into a dispensary and may not want anyone to know they're using the product. This consumer needs a welcoming, educational, and patient approach.

>> **The patient:** Patients are seeking symptom relief and better quality of life. The product selection and staff are a key for them as they may already know what works or be in the process of figuring it out with your help.

Chapter **15**

Finding Work in the Cannabis Industry

obs abound in the cannabis industry, and openings extend far beyond the obvious job descriptions of growers, extraction experts, and budtenders. Cannabis companies are in need of a wide range of general business and cannabis-specific knowledge and skills. A quick search on Indeed.com or other job boards reveals job postings for master growers, greenhouse managers, retail managers, marketing professionals, business analysts, lighting system designers, farming associates, dispensary managers, laboratory chemists, operations managers, production managers, delivery drivers, brand ambassadors, law enforcement officers, software developers, cannabis attorneys, food production facility managers, kitchen crew members, social media managers, budtenders, trimmers, packagers, and even professional joint rollers.

In this chapter, we describe some of the unique and not-so-unique positions available in the cannabis industry, steer you toward sources of job listings, and provide a few suggestions for improving your odds of getting hired. Chances are good that if you want a job in the cannabis industry, you can find an opening that's a good fit for your knowledge, skills, and interests.

REMEMBER

Because of the federal tax situation for cannabis businesses, the industry isn't exactly rolling in money, so don't expect to earn any more in this industry than you would in any other. Compensation is fairly comparable for positions that require a similar level of education and skills. As the cannabis industry matures, you can expect the same benefits offered in more traditional industries, such as health insurance, retirement plans, paid time off, training, and advancement.

Scoping Out Job Opportunities

If you want to work in the cannabis industry but aren't really sure what you want to do, you've come to the right place. In this section, we describe some common positions in the hopes that you find one or more that match your knowledge, skills, and interests.

Grow master or grower

Obviously, the cannabis industry needs people who have the knowledge and skills to grow cannabis. A *grow master* (or master grower) may design the grow facility (or enter an established location) and oversees growing operations at the facility, which includes sourcing; cloning; transplanting; pruning and training plants; setting up and maintaining lighting, ventilation, and irrigation systems; controlling diseases and pests; developing new strains; and ensuring third-party testing. Larger organizations may have a post-harvest role that takes over from the point the plant is cut down, or the grow master may also oversee for harvesting, drying, and curing flower. Think of the grow master as the captain of the ship — the person who coordinates the efforts of everyone else at the grow facility.

Depending on the size of the grow facility, the master grower may have one or more growers who perform more of the daily tasks related to growing, harvesting, and curing the plants.

If you have a degree in agriculture, botany, agronomy, or horticulture and experience working on a farm or in a greenhouse, or you have a green thumb and a passion for growing healthy plants, consider applying for a position as a grower. The master grower position requires a similar education background but much more experience related specifically to growing cannabis.

Cultivation technician

Cultivation technicians work under the direction and supervision of a master grower or a grower. They clone, plant, transplant, trim, water, and fertilize plants and maintain the cleanliness of the work area and tools.

Because cultivation technicians do much of the grunt work in a grow operation, this is a very physical job that involves a lot of walking, stooping, bending, kneeling, and lifting.

Trimmer

The trimmer or bud trimmer position is an entry-level job that requires manual dexterity and attention to detail. Trimmers perform the tedious task of removing the stem and leaves from the bud without wasting any of the precious bud.

The good news is that these positions don't require a college degree or professional training, starting out as a bud trimmer is a great way to get started in the industry. The bad news is that the job is tedious, and the wages may be minimum or just above, though in larger operations benefits may be included.

Joint roller

Yes, who would've thought you could turn your knack for rolling the perfect joint into a satisfying career. Joint rollers can earn $20,000 to $40,000 depending on demand in the area and the speed and quality of their rolls. However, responsibilities also include weighing and packaging product and keeping the work area impeccably clean.

In many of the larger production facilities joints are called "cones" and rolling skills are not required. Papers are pre-purchased in cone shape and simply must be filled and have the tops twisted.

Cure associate

The cure associate ensures the proper drying and curing processes for the flower prior to packaging, determining the need and executing intervention efforts such as *fluffing* (to air out the buds), emptying dehumidifiers as needed, and verifying weights. A cure associate may also be responsible for monitoring and managing cure rooms with daily checks on humidity and temperature; testing product as needed; cleaning screens and buckets; and verifying decisions by team and leads about product disposition.

Nutrient chemist

Large grow operations may mix their own nutrients to fertilize plants. A nutrient chemist develops the recipes for the various nutrient blends and must have a strong knowledge of soil composition, chemistry, and horticulture specific to cannabis plants.

You'll need a degree in chemistry, botany, horticulture, agriculture, or a related field and specialized knowledge related to plant fertilizers to qualify for this position.

Extractor

An extractor uses various equipment and solvents to pull the active ingredients from cannabis plant material (flower or trimmings) to create hash and other concentrates. This is a skilled role that may require previous experience or education working with the machines and processes involved in extracting concentrates or oils from the plant matter.

This job is one of the highest paying skilled labor jobs in the industry, but it's also one of the most dangerous, because the solvents used in some extraction processes can be very volatile. The right candidate for this job knows not only techniques for maximizing extraction potency but also techniques for ensuring proper ventilation and preventing explosions.

Quality assurance manager

Quality assurance is crucial to providing customers with safe, effective cannabis products. Each segment of the industry (grow, MIP, and dispensary/retail store) may have its own quality assurance manager, but for vertically integrated companies, a single quality assurance manager may be in charge of all three divisions.

The right candidate for this position needs a clear understanding of the various grow, manufacturing, testing, and packaging processes to be aware of all the points along the supply chain that can impact product quality and safety. The manager must collaborate with experts in the grow, MIP, and dispensary operations to establish procedures that ensure the quality and safety of all products and compliance with applicable regulations. To qualify for this position, you must have an analytical mind and pay close attention to details.

Dispensary manager

A dispensary manager has a long list of job responsibilities related to facilitating all dispensary operations, including the following:

>> Establish and maintain relationships with suppliers — grow and MIP divisions or companies

>> Hire, train, and schedule budtenders and other dispensary staff

>> Ensure that the dispensary is safe and secure

- Coordinate deliveries from grow and MIP divisions or companies
- Decide which products to carry and set prices for those products
- Stay abreast of all state and local cannabis laws
- Keep impeccable records
- Cooperate with cannabis regulators, inspectors, and law enforcement if any issues arise
- Ensure compliance with all rules and regulations governing dispensary operations

REMEMBER

Like the manager of any business, a dispensary manager must be very well organized and have people skills. In addition, a dispensary manager must be well-versed on all cannabis laws related to the sale, possession, and use of cannabis products. Most organizations require previous retail experience in any industry with a preference for cannabis expertise.

Budtender/sales associate

A *budtender* is a sales associate who interacts directly with the end customer or patient. Budtenders must be knowledgeable about cannabis in general, the specific products on display at the dispensary, the sales systems, and compliance rules.

To qualify for the position, you need to be well groomed, courteous, and eager and able to learn about cannabis in general and a variety of products. Excellent communication skills are also essential. You must be a good listener and be able to quickly evaluate the needs or desires of prospective customers, whether they're adult recreational or medical marijuana users.

The budtender/sales associate role is an entry-level position for most cannabis companies but still requires state authorization and badging. In Canada, certification of knowledge is required and may be provided or paid for by the hiring company.

Dispensary receptionist or cashier

The first person a customer or patient meets when entering the dispensary is the receptionist, and the last person is the budtender or in some cases the cashier. The receptionist is responsible for greeting customers and checking IDs to ensure all customers are of legal age and have appropriate paperwork (for medical patients and caregivers).

Receptionists and cashiers are both entry-level positions that require candidates to be well-groomed and courteous. In addition, because cashiers will be handling mostly cash transactions, they need to be good with numbers and trustworthy.

Packager

A packager or packaging associate works in a grow or MIP facility, weighing, labeling, and packaging various cannabis products; counting products; and filling out forms. Trimming bud may also be one of the job responsibilities.

A successful candidate for a packer position generally must meet the following requirements:

>> Strong attention to detail

>> Proficiency in basic math

>> General computer software skills

>> Ability to use a scale to weigh products

Packaging can be physically demanding. You may be spending long hours on your feet and have to bend, stoop, and lift throughout the day.

Edibles chef

An edibles chef whips up new recipes for edible products and oversees the industrial kitchen in a MIP facility. They must discover innovative ways to use cannabis infused butters and oils, along with concentrates, to create edible products for both medical and recreational use.

First and foremost, this position requires the candidate to be a chef, but unlike a chef at a restaurant, the edibles chef must adhere to the rules and regulations imposed on the cannabis industry in addition to food safety protocols and regulations. The edibles chef must ensure that products are properly tested, packaged, and labeled with accurate nutritional and potency information.

Courier/delivery driver

Some cannabis companies have their own couriers or delivery drivers to transport product from the grow operation to MIP, from MIP to the dispensaries, or from the dispensaries to customers. Some delivery companies also provide this service to cannabis companies and/or deliver product directly to consumers. Qualified candidates for these jobs typically need to be over the age of 21 and have a driver's license and a clean driving record. A commercial driver's license (CDL) isn't usually required.

Drivers must also be reliable and courteous and pay close attention to detail. Delivery mistakes can result in non-compliance issues.

Buyer

A buyer typically works for a chain of dispensaries to find and order products from MIPs and processed product brands. Responsibilities include the following:

>> Establish relationships with sales representatives of a wide variety of cannabis products.

>> Evaluate products and select those that are likely to appeal to and serve the needs of the dispensary's clientele.

>> Compare prices among suppliers that offer the same or similar products.

>> Secure purchase approvals as necessary.

>> Create and submit purchase orders.

>> Receive, verify, and input invoices into operations software.

>> Process daily accounts payable and accounts receivable transactions.

The right candidate for this position has an intimate knowledge of the needs and tastes of cannabis consumers and can stay one step ahead of trends in the marketplace.

Sales representatives

Sales representatives may work for grow operations to sell plant material to MIPs and dispensaries or may work for MIPs or processed product brands to sell manufactured products to dispensaries. Responsibilities include the following:

>> Build and maintain strong customer relationships.

>> Evaluate customer needs and present products that address those needs.

>> Educate customers on the benefits of products.

>> Manage a sample inventory.

>> Plan, coordinate, and execute local education and sales events.

>> Input orders and invoice customers.

>> Identify, encourage, and facility market influencers to expand market share.

Compliance manager

The compliance manager plays a vitally important role in any cannabis company, ensuring the company abides by all state and local cannabis rules and regulations. Responsibilities include the following:

>> Complete and submit all applications for licensing and renewals.

>> Interpret and communicate all compliance rules and regulations to relevant management and staff throughout the company.

>> Continually research cannabis laws, regulations, and ordinances at the federal, state, and local levels and keep track of pending legislation and ordinances as they make their way through the lawmaking process.

>> Coordinate with internal teams, including grow, MIP, and dispensary operations to ensure compliance with any new or revised rules and regulations, including those that apply to grow, manufacturing, packaging, labeling, and sales.

>> Collaborate with external suppliers and partners to ensure they're in compliance with applicable rules and regulations.

>> Audit and review the company's systems to ensure compliance with existing and new rules and regulations.

>> Establish and maintain relationships with representatives of governing bodies and with regulators and inspectors, address any compliance issues that arise, and document all interactions.

Communications director

A communications director leads the development of the company's educational and promotional campaigns and fields any media inquiries. Responsibilities include the following:

>> If the company hires a public relations (PR) firm, serve as the daily contact to plan and facilitate press releases and address media inquiries.

>> Collaborate with marketing, compliance, management, production, retail and sales to develop internal and external messaging as well as vehicles for delivery.

- >> Manage internal and outsourced writers and audio and video content providers to roll out content and campaigns.
- >> Oversee the development of and compliance with brand messaging.
- >> Monitor social media to gauge consumer sentiment and identify any areas of concern.
- >> Serve as or work closely with the company spokesperson to ensure accurate and consistent communication with the public.

Human resources (HR) manager

The HR manager ensures that the company has the knowledge and skills in place to achieve its business goals. Specific responsibilities include the following:

- >> Partner with management across all business units to identify human resource needs.
- >> Recruit new talent to meet the needs of all business units.
- >> Develop and implement competitive compensation and benefits packages to optimize recruitment and employee retention.
- >> Plan, implement, and manage the company's HR platform for payroll and benefits.
- >> Collaborate with management across all business units to develop and execute a comprehensive onboarding and training system that's suitable for each location.
- >> Develop, communicate, and oversee employee evaluation and termination policies and procedures.
- >> Ensure compliance with all state and local HR rules, regulations, and national fair labor laws.

Trainers

Trainers are responsible for training and onboarding new staff for roles within the company. As a trainer, you may work for a cannabis company or for a company that specializes in providing training for people in the industry. Some businesses specialize in providing compliance training for all segments of the cannabis industry — grow, MIP, and dispensary/retail stores.

Public affairs administrator

A public affairs administrator acts as a spokesperson for the company and a liaison between the company and government entities, community leaders, and business organizations to protect and further the company's interests and reputation. As a public affairs administrator, you may do the following:

>> Lobby federal, state, and local legislators.

>> Create and execute public outreach campaigns.

>> Address and resolve concerns that arise with legislators and their constituents.

>> Identify issues that may increase political risk to the company.

Laboratory worker

Laboratory workers are needed both in house and at third-party testing facilities to ensure the safety and quality of cannabis products. If you like science, chemistry in particular, and think you'd enjoy working in a laboratory, this may be the perfect position for you. In this capacity, you'd essentially be running chemistry experiments to test for concentrations of cannabinoids, terpenes, and other active ingredients and for the presence of toxins and other contaminants such as pesticides, solvents, and mold.

Security manager or officer

Cannabis plus cash make the industry a prime target for criminals, which opens the need for security experts and personnel. Responsibilities vary depending on the job but may include the following:

>> Evaluating a company's security needs.

>> Developing security systems and protocols to mitigate risks.

>> Installing security systems.

>> Checking and verifying customer IDs and medical marijuana cards.

>> Standing guard at a facility or a dispensary to protect customers and staff along with the facility and its contents.

>> Riding along with managers or staff to make large cash deposits or to pick up or deliver large volumes of product.

Accountant

Cannabis companies need all levels of financial skills depending on the size of the company. Responsibilities may include anything from basic bookkeeping and preparing financial reports to developing and delivering financial forecasts and advising management regarding prospective capital expenditures.

Due to the fact that cannabis is a cash-only business and is subject to the governance of a variety of taxing authorities, accounting in the cannabis industry is more complex than with most businesses. As an accountant, you may be called on to evaluate a point of sale (POS) system that's effective in tracking cash payments, offer advice on reducing the company's tax burden, and find the means to pay taxes and staff in cash.

Marketing manager or team members

Generally, marketing in the cannabis industry isn't that much different from marketing in other industries except for the added complications of having to comply with cannabis rules and regulations for packaging, labeling, and advertising. Marketing responsibilities include the following:

>> Create or oversee website/blog design and development.

>> Review advertising materials for strategic alignment, accuracy, and compliance.

>> Keep projects on schedule within budget.

>> Serve as the liaison with stakeholders in other business units to gain input and approvals on marketing and advertising materials.

>> Monitor and respond to customer comments and complaints about advertising materials.

REMEMBER

Advertising in the cannabis industry is highly limited and restricted. As with cigarettes and alcohol, laws prohibit advertising to youth, and cannabis advertising outlets must verify that at least 70 percent of the audience where ads are placed are over the age of 21.

Facilities manager

A facilities manager ensures that the company's buildings and grounds are properly maintained and in good working order. This position is responsible for security, parking, cleaning, and maintenance of essential systems, including heating and cooling, plumbing, and networking. The facilities manager may handle some responsibilities in house and outsource others to specialized service providers.

Technology manager

The cannabis industry requires computer and technology support as in any other business. Responsibilities vary depending on the job but may include the following:

>> Computer and software purchase, setup, and support for all locations and leadership staff

>> Evaluation and implementation of point of sale (POS) systems for retail outlets

>> Oversight of state tracking technology use in all areas of the company

>> System support for company accounting

Exploring Jobs in Ancillary Industries and Professions

Cannabis companies provide plenty of opportunities for other businesses and professions outside of the industry, so you may be able to reap some of its benefits while avoiding some of its drawbacks, such as the extremely high tax burden and, in some cases, relatively low wages. Consider the following positions in ancillary industries and professions:

>> Accountant

>> Advertising agent

>> Application consultant (specializing in helping companies apply for cannabis licenses)

>> Architect/builder

>> Armored car service provider

>> Banking professional

>> Brand ambassador

>> Business analyst

>> Fertilizer/soil supplier

>> Glassware manufacturer

>> Grow/hydroponics supplier

>> Heating, ventilation, and air conditioning (HVAC) technician

- » Hydroponic system designer/supplier
- » Irrigation system designer/supplier
- » Lawyer
- » Lighting designer/supplier
- » Merchandiser
- » Operations consultant
- » Packaging and container designer and supplier
- » Public relations or public affairs specialist
- » Security officer
- » Security system designer and supplier
- » Courier/delivery driver
- » Social media manager
- » Software developer
- » State regulatory agent
- » Trainer
- » Web designer/developer

Finding Employers

Cannabis is a booming business, and employers are scrambling to find qualified candidates to fill their ranks. Given the explosive job growth, you may expect head hunters to be reaching out to you. Well, unless you've already built a strong reputation in the industry, that's probably not going to happen. However, you can find plenty of openings in the cannabis industry. Here are the leading sources to explore:

- » **Traditional online job boards:** Traditional websites, including Indeed (Indeed.com), Glassdoor (Glassdoor.com), and Monster (www.monster.com) all list open positions in the cannabis industry.

- » **Specialized cannabis job boards:** Several job boards list jobs in the cannabis industry exclusively, including Vangsters (www.Vangsters.com), Ganjapreneur Jobs (jobs.Ganjapreneur.com), and 420Careers (420careers.com).

- >> **Cannabis company websites:** Visit the websites of cannabis companies operating in areas where you currently live or would like to live and look for a Jobs or Careers link. Explore the website, to find out more about the company before submitting an application or scheduling an interview.

- >> **Cannabis recruiting agencies:** Several recruitment agencies specialize in the cannabis industry, including Vangst (Vangst.com), Ms. Mary Staffing (msmarystaffing.com), and Viridian Staffing (www.viridianstaffing.com).

- >> **Job fairs:** Attend local job fairs. While most job fairs have employers from a variety of industries, you may also be able to find cannabis career fairs sponsored by recruiters.

- >> **LinkedIn:** LinkedIn is great for networking with people in every industry imaginable, including cannabis. It provides a great way for prospective employers to get to know a little bit about you before any formal introductions. If you don't have a LinkedIn account, set one up today.

Improving Your Odds of Getting Hired

Landing a job in the cannabis industry involves many of the same techniques as those used for getting hired in other industries. You need to do your homework, so you're aware of the company's culture and its specific needs related to the position it's seeking to fill. You can then tailor your resume and your interview accordingly.

However, finding a job in the cannabis industry provides a few additional opportunities for improving your chances of beating out other candidates. In this section, we provide a few suggestions.

REMEMBER

Put your best foot forward. Provide a high-quality resume and show up for any interviews properly groomed, well-dressed, and on time with a positive attitude. Although some parts of cannabis culture are more informal than others, you're applying for a job with a business, so look and behave professionally.

Brush up on cannabis culture and law

Prior to interviewing for any job in the industry, brush up on cannabis culture and law. By developing an awareness of cannabis culture, you can present yourself as someone who's more likely to fit in at the company and be able to engage in a positive way with coworkers and customers. By demonstrating an understanding of cannabis rules and regulations, specifically those relevant to the position you're pursuing, you show that you respect the importance of compliance.

By "develop an awareness of cannabis culture," we're not suggesting that you binge watch Cheech & Chong movies, but that you explore the incredibly diverse demographic of marijuana growers, manufacturers, sellers, and consumers. Cannabis culture is not stoner culture. It includes white collar and blue collar workers, doctors, patients, mothers, fathers, grandparents, athletes, creatives, and others who consume for a wide variety of reasons.

Attend industry events

Attending industry events gives you an advantage in the following three ways:

>> **Networking:** You have the opportunity to meet people who are working in the industry face-to-face. You get to know a little about them and their companies, and they get to know a little about you. By networking effectively, you begin to build familiarity in the industry, and you're no longer an outsider.

>> **Knowledge acquisition:** As you visit booths, read the materials supplied, talk with people, and attend presentations and workshops, you begin to develop general and specialized knowledge that makes you more qualified for various positions and enables you to engage in intelligent discussions. You'll be much better prepared for interviews by attending even one industry event.

>> **Culturalization:** The single best way to develop an understanding of cannabis culture is to hang out with people who live it. Industry events expose you to the diverse people and the shared language, ideas, and values that are crucial for defining the culture.

Get your cannabis badge or state clearance

Getting your badge or authorization to work in the cannabis industry makes the decision to hire you much easier. The company doesn't have to take the chance that you may not pass the background check after they hired you, which instantly makes you a more desirable applicant.

Although the company you work for may pay the fee for obtaining a badge or authorization, we recommend getting your badge before you start your job hunt. Look on your state's website for information about requirements and the process for obtaining authorization. You may need to study up on the law yourself or obtain training. You then have to submit an application along with a fee, which can vary depending on your position in the industry (executives and managers generally pay more). The process typically includes a background check, finger-printing, proof of residence, and an interview with a state regulator.

Become a cannabis activist

A great way to become an active member of the cannabis community and prove your passion and dedication to the cause is to become a cannabis activist. Here are a few ways you can help the cause:

>> **Join and support an existing cannabis activist organization.** Search for groups online that are active in lobbying for legalization and are reputable. After joining, look for ways to volunteer. Volunteering is a great way to network while showing your commitment to the industry.

>> **Attend local government meetings.** Neighborhood organizations, city councils, county boards, and other local groups make many of the decisions that affect local rules and restrictions. Attend these meetings and express your opinions when appropriate to do so.

>> **Monitor the state legislature and contact your representatives.** Keep track of proposed cannabis legislation and let your legislators know whether you agree or disagree with certain bills. You're part of their constituency, which they're supposed to represent. Also be sure to vote for candidates who support cannabis legalization.

>> **Attend informal cannabis events.** Events include cannabis conventions, networking parties, support groups for medical marijuana consumers, and recreational classes. Attending events is a great way to express your support while networking with others who share your interest in cannabis.

Chapter **16**

Investing in Cannabis

The cannabis industry makes headlines around the world daily, and some of the most widely read articles are those about investing in companies that are part of the industry. Everyone's looking to cannabis to be the next big industry explosion. Investors at every level, from institutional to individual, want to get in on the ground floor. Nobody wants to miss out on the Green Rush, and everyone hopes to become a millionaire.

Headlines about the potential value of the industry in the U.S. feed this frenzy, citing estimates of between $90 and $100 billion, assuming all states have legalized cannabis for adult recreational use. These figures would put the industry in line with the market for alcohol. Investors rightfully see an enormous opportunity, but before you invest, do your homework.

In this chapter, we bring you up to speed on several important issues to consider before investing in enterprises that may profit from cannabis.

REMEMBER

No investment is a sure thing. The potential for scoring large profits in any industry is always accompanied by potential for equally large losses. Consult a well-trained and trusted financial advisor, preferably one who has intimate knowledge of the industry, before investing in any cannabis enterprise.

Sizing Up Current and Future Investment Opportunities

Regardless of the industry you choose to invest in — agriculture, energy, hospitality, manufacturing, technology, whatever — you want to know where the industry is (current conditions) and where it's headed (future prospects).

In this section, we provide insight into the current conditions in the U.S. cannabis industry, along with a host of important factors to consider before investing. We explain how the cannabis industry differs in Canada and how different factors are likely to come into play, as well. Finally, we look ahead to what the future holds for investors seeking to profit from cannabis.

Considering the current market

With any young industry, such as cannabis, investors can expect tremendous volatility; startups can rise and fall with little, if any, warning. It's like the early days of the tech boom, when smaller companies were scrambling to claim their piece of the pie.

What makes the cannabis industry even more challenging for investors to pick the winners from the losers are the legal restrictions and inordinate amount of regulation the industry must contend with daily. Established and growing companies can be shuttered in a day due to regulatory infractions without much legal recourse and an uphill climb in terms of public perception.

In this section, we look at the unique challenges that companies in the cannabis industry must overcome to be successful.

REMEMBER

For well capitalized organizations looking to expand, these challenges also offer tremendous opportunity. As single and small operators struggle to overcome these obstacles, well-run and well-capitalized organizations can purchase high revenue stores at much lower costs.

Fragmentation and licensing

The current market in the U.S. is highly fragmented with varying numbers of licenses in each legal state and a disparity among states that permit only medical or both medical and recreational use. Licenses are frequently divided between those different silos even in the dual markets, requiring businesses to hold both medical and recreational licenses for stores selling both even on the same premises. This licensing model may also apply to grow operations.

As an investor, you need to be aware of the licensing requirements, because they're an additional expense for businesses, chipping away at profits and return on investment (ROI). In most states, each license must be renewed and its corresponding fees paid annually. Adding to this expense are attorney fees and the costs in time and staff to ensure compliance with any rule changes.

These costs can be considerable given the fact that most license holders are small operators with only a few locations. For example, in Colorado, which is recognized as the most mature market in the U.S., only 500 companies are licensed, and the largest player, Native Roots, has only 20 stores. Likewise, the initial winners of the cannabis licensing lottery in Ontario, Canada, were almost entirely small players.

Changing regulatory environment

Rules continue to change in the cannabis industry within states as well as from state to state. Regulations determine everything from manufacturing and locations to advertising and product tracking. These regulations, in turn, greatly impact compliance, profits, and expansion opportunities. With such volatility in daily operations and risk, investment is a long-term play with plenty of uncertainty.

Capital

Because cannabis is a Schedule I drug, securing capital investment can be challenging. The industry is barred from banking with federal banks, making traditional business loans inaccessible, though some state credit unions have begun working specifically with cannabis companies.

As such, the majority of investment to date in cannabis companies has been with high-net-worth individuals — investors who can afford to wait and to weather any wild swings in a company's market value. If this isn't you, think twice about investing in cannabis start-ups.

Inexperienced operators

WARNING

Before investing in any cannabis enterprise, carefully research the business and the person or people in charge of running it. Check credentials and track records related to both knowledge of the industry and business acumen. Just because someone knows a lot about cannabis doesn't mean they can start and run a successful cannabis business.

Many of the early players in the cannabis industry were passionate about the plant and invested their own limited resources in the hopes of becoming hugely successful. Unfortunately, they had little to no business knowledge or experience, and their businesses suffered as a result.

Exorbitant tax rates

State and municipal taxes on adult recreational marijuana products are extremely high. While those costs are paid by the consumer, it raises the end price, which lessens demand. Further compounding the problem is the fact that high taxes coupled with lax law enforcement can drive consumers to the black market, where producers and dealers avoid taxes altogether and can offer certain products at significantly lower prices.

Federal taxes present an additional burden. Section 280E of the Internal Revenue Code dramatically impacts profit margins of cannabis companies, delivering a federal effective tax rate in the industry that ranges between 75 and 95 percent. Unheard of in any other legal industry, this code prohibits cannabis companies from claiming most of the traditional business deductions such as rent, payroll, utilities, investment, and maintenance. Instead of paying taxes on net profit, cannabis businesses essentially pay taxes on gross income.

REMEMBER

The cannabis industry isn't legal at the federal level and continues to operate in a precarious position, greatly influenced by the opinion and perspective of the U.S. Attorney General and the White House administration that's currently in power. The industry continues to advocate for legislative changes federally, as with the bi-partisan STATES act legislation, and within individual states that would improve profits, access for investors from outside particular states, and returns on investment, but success isn't guaranteed.

Exploring publicly traded stock on the Canadian market

While traditional investors may struggle to find investment opportunities on the U.S. stock exchange, they can find opportunities in Canada, where cannabis is federally legal. You can purchase stock in cannabis companies on the Canadian market the same way you would for companies in any legal industry in the U.S. However, to be a successful investor, you need to understand the environment in which Canadian cannabis companies operate and the unique challenges they face.

REMEMBER

Canadian cannabis companies had no experience selling a single bud in the adult recreational market prior to October 17, 2018, so they're likely to face the challenge of having inexperienced operators, even though cannabis is federally legal and the industry is well capitalized. To date, revenue, profits and share prices have not performed as well as many investors had hoped.

Also keep in mind that government involvement in the Canadian market varies from province to province. Some locations are completely coordinated by government agencies, while others have some form of public/private partnerships to facilitate and regulate production and sales. These variations create an uneven landscape that limits private retail access to the entire Canadian market.

In addition, although Canadian law allows online sales with delivery, intra-province delivery is currently prohibited. Retail operators must secure a license within the province in which they intend to sell. Regardless of how the media presents Canada's legalization of cannabis, the whole of Canada isn't open for private business and investment.

In Canada, Licensed Producers (LPs) are the product growers, and the industry is starting with very limited product offerings — mostly flower and non-combustible oil. Other products including edibles, which are scheduled to be allowed in 2019, likely will be added to the industry as it evolves, and these products are expected to be as popular in Canada as they are in the U.S. As a result, future branded companies that produce edibles, tinctures, and topicals can be a solid addition to your investment portfolio.

All LPs must sell through the government intermediaries, and wholesale costs are similar across the board. In the U.S., grow operations usually have the lowest profit margins of the three different cannabis company types — grow companies, brand manufacturers, and retail stores. Vertically integrated companies, which include grow operations and retail sales, are the exception, because they can sell their own products reducing costs and increasing profits. This may give vertically integrated companies an advantage, making them an investment to consider.

REMEMBER

Vertically integrated private companies are not directly authorized to operate in Canada, as they are in the U.S., though due to mergers and acquisitions, some companies are already moving in that direction, combining retail license holders with LPs. The grow segments of vertically integrated companies are prohibited from supplying their own retail locations directly and must go through the government exchanges. At this point, Canadian officials have allowed these mergers even without express rules authorizing vertical integration. Through supply chain agreements, these companies may have the same advantages in product selection and pricing to their "owned" retail locations as vertically integrated companies within the U.S. currently do.

Expectations are high in the Canadian market, and investors can find plenty of stocks in promising companies, but expect a great deal of volatility as the players ride the learning curve that U.S. companies have been navigating for nearly a decade.

And, although cannabis is federally legal, many Canadian entrepreneurs, like their southern neighbors, are inexperienced business people working alongside regulators who are in the initial stages of exploring the best means to secure the industry.

The other piece of the Canadian puzzle for your investment consideration is the ability to ship product from Canada to other countries that may soon legalize cannabis in one form or another. As these opportunities unfold, look for companies that have the foresight and capabilities to capitalize on them.

Looking ahead to the future market

The future of the cannabis market is going to remain volatile for quite a while, and the financial projections are not guaranteed. If you're planning to invest in the Canadian market, specific U.S. companies, or conglomerates, keep in mind that the industry is young and has yet to prove itself sustainable.

It may be best to watch and see what the market does for a while and where the industry heads before committing your hard-earned cash. Most important to watch will be how any given company's real earnings measure up to expectations. Are they beating revenue projections each quarter?

Performing Your Due Diligence

If you choose to buy stock in cannabis companies, perform your due diligence, as you would when buying stock in any companies, but tread even more carefully. The desire to score big has made some investors overnight millionaires but has dealt huge losses to many more. Here are a few guidelines to reduce your risks:

>> Avoid buying over-the-counter (OTC) unsupervised cannabis stocks.

>> Don't rely solely on articles, blog posts, or press releases for guidance.

>> Read and understand the company's financial filings usually provided on their websites; look for a section for investors. You can access the SEC via its Electronic Data Gathering, Analysis, and Retrieval (EDGAR) system at www.sec.gov/edgar.shtml.or the CSA, Canada's System for Electronic Document Analysis and Retrieval (SEDAR) at www.sedar.com. (For more guidance, check out *Stock Investing For Dummies*, by Paul Mladjenovic [Wiley].)

Seeking Private Investment Opportunities

Most of the private investment in the cannabis industry has been from early adopters who financed their own enterprises and from high net-worth investors willing and able to take big risks for the opportunity to score big returns. Traditional investors have steered clear primarily due to the risks and the long waits to see a return on their investment.

Also, the laws in some states limit investment in a company to those living in that state. To overcome these limitations, some investors have gone so far as to purchase residences in other states, while the industry pushes for legislation, such as the STATES Act, which would allow for investments across state lines without advocating full federal legalization.

WARNING

Some private investment firms offer individual investors opportunities to buy shares in private U.S. companies. However, perform your due diligence first. Investigate both the private investment firm and the companies it represents to avoid any scams or poor investment decisions. Keep in mind that projections and expectations aren't the same as real revenue numbers and proven track records. With new companies emerging in each state that legalizes, the risks are considerable.

TIP

If you're looking to invest in a private company, carefully examine market share among companies that operate in any give state. For example, Oklahoma recently legalized medical marijuana without setting strong limits on the number of licenses, which leaves the doors wide open for the development of new businesses. As a result, existing licensed operations, inside or outside the state, are likely to have the opportunity in the future to pick up existing licenses and expand as the market consolidates. If you can afford to wait for the return on your investment, investing in a well-run and well-capitalized cannabis company that recognizes and pursues these opportunities can be a smart move.

UNDERSTANDING THE STATES ACT

The Strengthening the Tenth Amendment Through Entrusting States (STATES) Act is a bill in the U.S. Congress that would honor the cannabis laws passed by the various states. The act would amend the Controlled Substances Act of 1970 to exempt individuals and corporations from federal enforcement when acting in compliance with U.S. state, territory (including Washington D.C.), and tribal cannabis law.

As of the writing of this book, the STATES Act has not been passed or signed into law. However, it represents a significant step toward legalizing cannabis at the federal level.

Considering Investments in Ancillary Businesses

Another way to invest in cannabis is to find opportunities in ancillary businesses — those that support the cannabis industry, including:

>> Dispensary directories

>> Informational websites

>> Design and public relations firms

>> Consulting companies

>> Courier and armored services

>> Banking with credit unions

>> Realtors

>> Packaging producers

The benefit to these companies is that they aren't restricted by the punitive federal tax regulations or the high sales taxes and fees from the states. Their returns on investments may be quite high while the industry sorts itself out.

Investing in Cannabis Real Estate

If you're willing to look for investment opportunities peripheral to the cannabis industry, consider real estate. Cannabis businesses need land and buildings to grow, sell, and distribute cannabis, so if you own any that's suitable and attractive to businesses, you can earn a handsome profit.

Buying, selling, and leasing properties for use by cannabis companies can be highly profitable if your facilities are the ones chosen by the cannabis operators. Several factors contribute to making cannabis real estate a potentially profitable investment:

>> **Regulatory set-back limit locations:** States and municipalities have set-backs for retail locations from schools, day care facilities, and from other retail or grow locations. As a result, suitable locations may be in demand, increasing their value.

>> **Specific property requirements:** Many regulations stipulate property requirements, such as set-back limits. By specializing in real estate that's suitable for companies in the cannabis industry, you can essentially corner the market and sell or lease to the highest bidder.

>> **Willing landlords are limited:** Other landlords may be reluctant to lease properties to cannabis companies due to the odors or the possibility of having to deal with disgruntled neighbors and intrusive inspections and regulators. Assuming you can deal effectively with these issues, you can charge a premium because your competition is limited.

>> **Future locations approved:** As more states and municipalities within legal states warm to the industry, the market for cannabis-friendly real estate is likely to grow, opening even more opportunities for landlords.

6

The Part of Tens

Discover ten tips for growing premier weed and boosting your harvest.

Explore ten ways to enhance your cannabis experience while avoiding any adverse side effects.

Get the most bang for your buck by discovering ten ways to buy top quality weed without losing your shirt.

Cook up your own infusions and extracts, edibles, and beverages with easy-to-follow recipes in the appendix.

Chapter **17**

Ten Tips for Growing More and Better Weed

Whether you're a commercial or home grower, you have two goals when you're growing cannabis — more and better. You want top-quality weed and lots of buds on your legal number of plants. To achieve these goals, you may have to overcome certain obstacles, such as funds to invest in resources and the limited amount of space you have.

In Chapters 11 and 12, we lead you through the process of growing and harvesting cannabis. In this chapter, we present ten tips for boosting your per-plant harvest.

Choose the Right Strain

Choosing the right strain is a key first step in achieving the desired results with your harvest. Your choice depends on several factors, including desired effects and aromas, available space, climate (if you're growing outdoors), and desired time to harvest.

Start by narrowing your choice down to one of the three primary strains presented in Table 17-1.

TABLE 17-1

Three Primary Cannabis Strains

Strain	Characteristics
Sativa	Tall
	Heat tolerant
	Cold intolerant
	Long buds; less dense
	Requires changes in amount of light to flower
	Heady, euphoric effect
Indica	Short
	Cold tolerant
	Heat intolerant
	Dense buds
	Requires changes in amount of light to flower
	Body-centered, relaxing effect
Auto-flowering (typically a hybrid of ruderalis along with indica and/or sativa)	Smaller plants
	Flowers automatically (without changes in amount of light)
	Shorter time to harvest
	Effects vary by hybrid

After choosing an overall strain, focus on the desired effects, aromas, and flavors. At this point, shopping for seeds or plants is like shopping for cannabis to consume (see Chapter 8). You want to compare CBD-to-THC ratios to find a strain that delivers the desired psychoactive and/or medical benefits and compare terpene profiles to evaluate other qualities, including aroma and flavor.

Although buying seeds online and having them shipped to you across state lines is illegal, you can find seed catalogues online that give you some idea of what's available. For each strain, the catalogue typically includes the hybrid mix, adult plant size, weeks to germination, weeks to harvest, THC and CBD content, typical effects, and the average grams per plant you can expect after harvest and drying.

TIP

If you're a novice grower, consider starting with an auto-flowering strain. The plants are more compact, you'll be able to harvest flower sooner, and you won't need to adjust the amount of light over the grow cycle to trigger budding.

Choose Top-Quality Seeds

Growing more and better weed requires that you start with top quality, *feminized seeds* — seeds specially treated to grow into female plants. If the seeds you plant aren't feminized, each seed has about a 50/50 chance of being male or female, meaning you'll have to dump about half your plants four to eight weeks after the seeds germinate (when you can tell the difference). Likewise, if the seeds are damaged or old, you're not going to achieve the best results. One male plant in a grow room can pollinate the entire room of females.

REMEMBER

To choose top quality seeds, find a breeder with a solid reputation and buy a strain with a long history rather than a new and relatively unproven strain.

Use High-Quality Soil

Soil plays a key role in both the quantity and quality of the harvest. It must be the right consistency to retain water, drain properly, and aerate the roots. It must also contain the nutrients the plant needs to thrive and have a pH of 6 to 7.

REMEMBER

Generally speaking, you want a basic potting soil for starting your plants, not a soil that's high in organic nutrients (which is too rich for seedlings). After starting your plants, use a rich, loamy soil that's suitable for growing garden vegetables, such as tomatoes. A loamy soil is a mix of sand, silt, and clay that's easy to work with, retains water and nutrients, drains easily, and smells alive (with microorganisms). Auto-flowering plants tend to prefer non-fertilized soil mixes, whereas indicas, sativas, and indica/sativa hybrids prefer soils higher in nutrients.

Whether you're growing plants in the ground or in containers, consult with the horticulturalist at your local nursery for soil recommendations. If you're planning to grow your plants in the ground, call first about soil testing. Your nursery may be able to examine soil samples from your site to determine which soil amendments, if any, would be needed to make it optimal for growing cannabis.

Upsize Your Containers

When you're limited in the number of plants you're allowed to grow, and you're growing plants in containers, one of the best ways to increase your per-plant yield is to increase the size of the containers. If your containers are too small for the strain you're trying to grow, the plant won't reach its maximum size. Table 17-2 provides some guidance for choosing the right-size container for the desired plant size.

TABLE 17-2   **Container Size Selection Guidelines**

Container size (gallons)	Plant size (inches)
2–3	12
3–5	24
6–8	36
8–10	48
12+	60

Maximize Bud Production with Topping, Training, and Scrogging

You can significantly boost bud production by encouraging your plants to grow more horizontally than vertically. Growing horizontally, the plant produces more buds, which are spread out to receive nearly equal amounts of light, so they all grow about the same size.

To encourage plants to grow horizontally, you can use one or more (or all) of the following three techniques, as explained in Chapter 11:

» **Topping:** By topping the plant, the *growth tips* (where the bases of the fan leaves attach to the stem) grow into separate stems that extend out from the main stem. You may top each secondary stem sometime later to encourage the growth of two new branches from each stem.

» **Low-stress training (LST):** As secondary stems grow (stretch), gently pull down on them and anchor them in place, so they grow horizontally. You can also tie branches to a trellis to encourage them to spread out.

» **Scrogging:** Place a grid (typically made of wire or string to produce three- to four-inch square openings) about four to eight inches above the plant, and train the branches to spread in different directions. When buds begin to form, gently tuck them up through the nearest square. This spreads out the buds, so they're all about the same distance from the light source.

WARNING

Although you can use these techniques with auto-flowering plants, their stems may not bend easily, making them susceptible to damage.

Use the Right Nutrients in the Right Amounts at the Right Times

Cannabis plants need a variety of nutrients: primarily nitrogen, phosphorous, potassium, calcium, magnesium, and sulfur (from the soil) and carbon, hydrogen oxygen (from air and water), along with tiny amounts of certain elements, including copper, iron, manganese, and zinc. (See Chapter 11 for general guidance on nutrients and fertilizers.)

TIP

By adjusting key nutrients (nitrogen, phosphorous, and potassium) over the course of the growth cycle, you can increase your yield:

>> **Vegetative phase:** High nitrogen, medium phosphorous, and high potassium to promote plant growth.

>> **Flowering phase:** Low nitrogen, medium to high phosphorous, and high potassium to promote bud development. Lower amounts of nitrogen starting about six weeks into the flowering stage also reduces the amount of nitrogen in the flowers; high nitrogen content can make the buds smell and taste harsh.

TIP

If you're growing in soil, as opposed to water (hydroponic), opt for organic fertilizers and nutrients until you're more experienced. Organic products, such as blood meal, bone meal, kelp meal, are broken down in the soil over time to provide the essential nutrients, so you're less likely to damage your plants by over-fertilizing them. Organic nutrients may also produce a flower that smells and tastes better than one grown with chemical fertilizers.

Get the Lighting Right

Proper lighting is a complex topic. Although cannabis is a sun-loving plant, it can get overheated, and it requires a certain amount of darkness that varies over its growth cycle. Here are a few lighting guidelines:

>> In the vegetative phase, plants do best with about 18 hours of light and six hours of darkness daily. Some growers suggest a light/dark cycle of six hours on and two hours off to maximize growth.

>> In the flowering phase, plants need 12 hours of continuous darkness daily, or they will not produce flowers.

>> If you're growing indoors with grow lights, position the grow lights the proper distance from the tops of your plants, typically as follows: high pressure sodium (HPS) 30–50 cm; compact fluorescent lamp (CFL), 10–50 cm; light emitting diode (LED), 15–50 cm.

>> To boost your yield, increase the light intensity, either by using stronger lights or moving the lights closer to the canopy (tops of your plants), but not so close that they burn the plants.

>> Provide adequate ventilation for any lighting you use to prevent overheating your plants and to provide plants with plenty of carbon dioxide (CO_2) to support their growth. Cannabis plants grow best at room temperature or slightly warmer (in the range of 70 to 85 degrees Fahrenheit).

Ensure Proper Ventilation and Circulation

Ventilation involves pushing stale, hot air out and pulling in cooler, fresher air. *Circulation* involves moving the same air around in a closed area. To keep your cannabis plants healthy, you need to provide sufficient ventilation *and* circulation. Ventilation helps to maintain the proper temperature and humidity, while circulation provides a gentle breeze that strengthens the stems. Together, ventilation and circulation prevent mold and pests while supporting essential processes in plant growth:

>> *Transpiration* — the movement of water through the plant and its evaporation. Ventilation and circulation accelerate evaporation, thus enhancing transpiration while preventing leaf mold.

>> *Photosynthesis* — the process by which plants use light energy to convert carbon dioxide (CO_2) and water into carbohydrates and oxygen. To perform this magic, plants need plenty of CO_2. Ventilation and circulation help deliver a steady stream of CO_2 while carting off the oxygen that's produced as a waste product.

>> *Respiration* — the process by which plants break down the carbohydrates produced through photosynthesis to fuel growth and repair. Respiration requires a small amount of oxygen, which combines with the carbohydrates, producing carbon dioxide as a waste product.

Be Patient Near Harvest Time

Generally, you want to harvest buds when THC content peaks. If you harvest any earlier, you reduce both the quality and quantity of your crop. If you harvest later, the THC begins to break down into CBN, which can negatively impact the quality of your harvest (unless you want lower THC and higher CBN content). To recognize when THC content is at its peak, take the following steps:

1. **Watch the stigmas (the hair-like strands that cover the bud). When they change from white to orange, shift your attention to the trichomes.**

2. **Carefully observe the trichomes using a handheld microscope. When most of the trichomes turn from clear to opaque and some turn amber, you're ready to harvest.**

    When trichomes turn amber, the THC is beginning to break down into CBN.

3. **Harvest your buds.**

    See Chapter 12 for details.

REMEMBER

Peak harvest time may vary according to strain and the desired effects. You may want to harvest when the trichomes are still clear or after more of them turn amber.

Dry and Cure Your Weed Properly

Properly drying and curing your cannabis flower enhances its quality while ensuring you don't lose part or all of your crop to mold or rot. See Chapter 12 for instruction on how to dry and cure your weed properly. Keep the following key points in mind:

» During the initial drying, maintain a temperature of 60 to 70 degrees Fahrenheit and humidity of 45 to 55 percent. Use a small fan to gently circulate the air.

» The initial drying period takes about 5 to 15 days. When the bud is crispy on the outside but bounces back when squeezed, it's ready to cure.

» Place dried buds in airtight containers to cure. During the first week, open the containers several times a day for a few minutes to allow the buds to breathe, then open them once every few days. Curing cannabis for two to three weeks is usually sufficient, but you may want to cure it for four to eight weeks for optimal results.

Chapter **18**

Ten Tips to Enhance Your Cannabis Experience

I f you're satisfied with your cannabis experience, skip this chapter. We don't want to mess with your success. However, if you've tried cannabis and aren't impressed or you've been consuming cannabis for some time and feel as though it's not having the same impact as it once did, consider following one or more of the ten suggestions we present in this chapter for enhancing your cannabis experience.

REMEMBER

Your cannabis experience involves more than the cannabis you consume and your consumption method. Other factors can impact your experience, as well, including the setting, the people you're with, and your mood and expectations.

Choose Top-Quality Products

Cannabis is like steak—your enjoyment of it depends a great deal on the quality of the product. Legalization and regulation help to ensure that you're getting what you pay for. Just be sure to purchase trusted brands from reputable dispensaries.

If you're buying flower, you can gauge its quality by carefully examining it. High quality weed is:

>> Densely packed if it's indica, or slightly looser if it's sativa. Avoid buds that have lots of leaves or an extremely loose structure that exposes the stem.

>> Colorful — mostly green with a wide variety of accent colors, such as orange, purple, pink, or blue. Avoid buds that are mostly brown, tan, yellow, or white.

>> Spongy — just enough moisture to make it soft and springy instead of dry and brittle. Because you won't be able to touch the product, you need to evaluate with your eyes and nose. If the flower looks brown, dry, and brittle, it's too dry. If it looks wilted or wet or smells moldy, it hasn't been dried and cured properly, so it's too wet.

>> Pleasantly pungent, indicating high terpene content. Avoid buds that smell like damp hay or have little to no aroma. If you like the smell, you'll probably like the product.

>> Frosty. Top-quality cannabis is covered in a thick coat of sugary resin.

See Chapter 5 for additional guidance on how to buy top-quality cannabis products.

Experiment with Different Strains

Like wines, which differ in color, alcohol content, aroma, and flavor, strains of cannabis differ in cannabinoid content and terpene profile. As a result, your experience varies with the strain you consume.

REMEMBER

Consult your budtender for guidance on strains that are likely to give you the desired experience. Discuss terpene profiles to more closely align with your goals. Try different strains and keep a record of those you've tried. You may discover that you enjoy a dozen or more strains, each for different reasons.

Try Different Consumption Methods

Your experience with cannabis differs depending on how you consume it; for example, you can expect a quicker onset and more intense high from smoking it than from consuming an edible product. You may also find that smoking is more conducive to social settings, in which you can pass around a joint, a vape, or a bong.

Sample different consumption methods for different purposes and in different situations or settings to get a feel for how the consumption method impacts your experience.

WARNING

When experimenting with different strains or consumption methods, start low, go slow, and consume in a safe place with people you trust. You can't predict how a different product or a different mode of delivery will affect you.

Try Hash and Other Concentrates

If you're looking for a more intense experience, consider trying concentrates (extracts), such as kief, hash, oil, resin, or tinctures. (See Chapter 2 for a description of the different concentrates.) These products contain higher concentrations of various cannabinoids and terpenes depending on the strain from which they're produced. Concentrates that have a low CBD-to-THC ratio produce an intense high, whereas those with higher concentrations of CBD and little to no THC have stronger medicinal properties with little or no psychoactive effect.

WARNING

Be careful when trying high THC concentrates for the first time. Products that produce stronger psychoactive effects have the potential of creating stronger adverse side effects, as well. Experimenting with concentrates under the guidance and supervision of a trustworthy, experienced, and sober friend is best.

Set the Mood

Just as a restaurant's ambience impacts the overall dining experience, mood can make or break your cannabis experience. To enhance your experience, set the proper mood by attending to the following factors:

>> **Mind-set:** Adopt a positive mind-set, especially if you're consuming any products that are high in THC. If you're already anxious, angry, or depressed, THC can make you feel worse.

>> **Physical setting:** Consume in a place you find appealing — your home, the home of a close friend, a campground that permits cannabis consumption, or another place where you feel safe and comfortable.

> » **The company you keep:** Consume alone, if you prefer, or with close friends, relatives, or colleagues you trust and whose company you enjoy.
>
> » **Sensory and intellectual stimulation:** Whether you enjoy reading, partying, watching movies, listening to music, or engaging in other activities that stimulate your senses, mind, and emotions, cannabis can enhance the experience.

Chill Your Bong

One of the big drawbacks of smoking cannabis is that the heat can burn your throat and lungs. By using a bong, you draw the smoke through water, which helps to filter and cool the smoke to a certain degree. To cool the smoke even more, add some ice to the water. The cooler the water, the cooler the smoke, and the deeper you can draw the smoke into your lungs. As a result, you intensify the high without feeling the burn!

Boost Your High with Certain Foods

Certain foods synergize with cannabis to enhance the overall experience. To boost the effects of cannabis, try the following foods:

> » **Mangoes:** Like cannabis, mangoes contain terpenes, including myrcene, which is believed to help the cannabinoids cross the blood-brain barrier. Consuming mango an hour or so before consuming cannabis may speed the onset of the cannabis and extend the duration of the high.
>
> » **Omega-3 fatty acids:** Consuming foods that are high in omega-3 fatty acids may also increase the speed of onset, intensity, and the duration of the high. Omega-3 fatty acids bind with the cannabinoids to help them cross the blood-brain barrier. Foods that are high in omega-3 fatty acids include eggs, olive oil, cold-water fish (such as sardines and salmon), nuts, and avocado.
>
> » **Dark chocolate:** People bake cannabis into their brownies for good reason — chocolate, particularly dark chocolate, slows the breakdown of *anandamide* (the brain's bliss chemical), thus increasing the duration of the high. Look for chocolate that's at least 70 percent cacao.
>
> » **Tea:** Black and green teas contain *catechin* — an antioxidant that binds with the brain's CB1 receptors to relieve stress and elevate mood. Tea and cannabis work synergistically to maximize bliss and relaxation.

Exercise Regularly

The fact that regular exercise enhances the cannabis experience is no surprise — cannabis must enter the bloodstream, and cardio exercise improves circulation. In one study, blood plasma levels of THC increased by 15 percent when study participants rode a stationary bicycle for 35 minutes.

Many athletes use cannabis for focus or muscle recovery. Some notable marathon runners have even signed up as representatives of specific cannabis brands. CBD taken after a workout can also speed the recovery of muscles that were broken down and help you feel better faster.

REMEMBER

While exercise may enhance cannabinoid absorption, the jury is out on whether cannabis improves athletic performance. Some people find that cannabis increases their pain threshold and lung capacity and eases their anxiety, which can help them get through their workouts. However, THC has a negative impact on hand-eye coordination and reaction times.

Break the Monotony

As with any activity, your cannabis experience can fade from ritual to routine. What was once an experience that heightened your senses and sensibilities becomes a habit added to your daily drudgery.

To make your cannabis experience special, break the monotony. Try different strains and consumption methods, consume in different settings with different people, and approach each cannabis session as a special occasion.

Take a Tolerance Break

In a way, cannabis consumption is subject to the law of diminishing returns — with regular cannabis consumption, you build a tolerance for it. Over time, the intensity and duration of your cannabis experience begins to wane, and you must consume increasing amounts to achieve the desired effects.

Fortunately, tolerance is reversible. All you need to do is take a *tolerance break* (*t-break*) — stop consuming or significantly limit your cannabis consumption over a period of a few days to a few weeks. You need to give your body sufficient time to eliminate the cannabinoids from your system and become acclimated to life without cannabis.

If you're a heavy daily user, cannabis can stay in your urine and fat-soluble tissue more than 30 days.

WARNING

After taking a tolerance break, start back with amounts that worked well for you early on and ramp up from there. If you start with the quantity you were consuming just prior to your t-break, you're likely to consume too much and have a negative experience.

Chapter **19**

Ten Tips for Buying Cannabis

One of the key benefits of cannabis legalization is that it's accompanied by regulation, which improves the quality, consistency, and safety of products sold to consumers. You can walk into any licensed and reputable dispensary with the assurance that you're getting what you pay for. The days of buying an overpriced bag of weed loaded with leaves, stems, and seeds are over — at least at legal business establishments.

To further ensure that you're getting what you pay for and receiving the product that's most likely to produce the desired effects, you need to be an educated and disciplined consumer. You must be able to choose a reputable dispensary, carry on an intelligent conversation with your budtender, read and understand the labels, and distinguish *dank* (top-shelf flower) from *schwag* (low-quality weed). In this chapter, we provide guidance on how to ensure you're getting high-quality products that deliver the desired experience for a fair price.

Choose the Right Dispensary for You

Although regulations ensure some degree of consistency across cannabis dispensaries, establishments vary in their level of product quality and selection and customer service. Do your homework to find the right dispensary for you within convenient access to where you live or work. Some dispensaries are known for low prices and some for high end products. You may need to travel a little bit based on your own needs and desires.

Here are some qualities to look for in a dispensary:

>> Professionally designed website with an *age gate* (the site prompts you to confirm that you're old enough to be on the site).

>> High customer ratings on Google My Business, Yelp, and other retail review forums.

>> Clean, comfortable, and secure reception area and budrooms.

>> Wide variety of high-quality product offerings.

>> Attractive, well-organized product displays.

>> Friendly, knowledgeable, and helpful staff.

See Chapter 6 for more about choosing and visiting a cannabis dispensary.

Find a Knowledgeable and Helpful Budtender

A budtender is like a matchmaker, but instead of helping you find the right mate, a good budtender helps you choose products that produce the effects and deliver the overall experience you desire. Shop for a budtender at least as carefully as you shop for a dispensary. Look for a budtender with the following qualities:

>> **Friendly:** A good budtender makes customers feel welcome.

>> **Patient:** Your budtender should be happy to answer any and all questions. You shouldn't feel rushed or foolish regardless of the number of questions you ask or the level of your knowledge.

>> **Passionate:** Every budtender should be passionate about cannabis and about guiding and educating consumers.

>> **Knowledgeable:** Every budtender should know the products and the rules and regulations governing cannabis sales, possession, and consumption. If your budtender struggles to answer your questions or provide the guidance you expect, try another budtender.

>> **Effective communicator:** A good budtender tailors his message to each customer's needs and level of knowledge and experience. Less experienced

customers shouldn't be made to feel dumb, and experienced customers shouldn't be treated like novice consumers.

>> **Professional:** Although "professional" may have different meanings for different clientele, your budtender should be neat and clean and treat both customers and products respectfully. For example, a budtender who respects the product will pick up bud with a pair of tongs, not his bare hands.

REMEMBER

Most budtenders rely on tips to supplement their wage. If you liked the service, drop a few dollars in the jar.

Describe the Specific Effect You Desire

Even the best budtender can't read your mind. Be open about how knowledgeable and experienced you are and about what you're looking for. If you're in the market for medical marijuana, describe the conditions you have or the symptoms you're experiencing. If you're in the market for adult recreational marijuana, provide as much detail as possible about your preferences; for example, whether you're looking for a more stimulating or relaxing high, whether you plan to consume alone or with others, your consumption preferences, and so on.

If you're new to cannabis and aren't sure what you're looking for, that's okay. A good budtender will ask questions and engage you in a discussion that reveals the information needed to guide you to the right products for you.

TIP

If you're returning to cannabis after a long absence, let your budtender know, so they can treat you with respect while bringing you up to speed on the latest terms and changes with products and delivery.

Buy Legal Cannabis

One of the huge benefits of legalizing cannabis is that it results in higher quality cannabis, so take advantage of this benefit by purchasing only legal cannabis (not buying on the black market). All legal products are tested by certified third-party labs. Lab testing serves the following two purposes:

>> **Determines the potency of the product.** The only way to determine cannabinoid content, such as THC and CBD ratios and amounts, and a product's terpene profile is via lab testing.

>> **Identifies any potentially harmful contaminants.** Lab testing ensures that a product doesn't contain harmful levels of pesticides, heavy metals, microbes, residual solvents, or other contaminants.

Visually Inspect the Product

Regardless of the product you're buying — bud, oil, edible, or even paraphernalia — visually inspect the product and its packaging as carefully as possible and reasonable. You won't be able to tell much about certain products, such as gummies, just by looking at them, especially because the product can't legally be opened prior to purchase or in the dispensary, but you can tell whether the packaging is intact and whether certain products are damaged.

Visual inspection is more important if you're buying flower/bud, because appearance can tell you a great deal about the quality of the product. High-quality bud looks alive and colorful — mostly green with a wide variety of accent colors, such as orange, purple, pink, or blue — not mostly (or entirely) brown. It's densely packed if it is indica (slightly less so if it's sativa), so you shouldn't see the stem that runs through the bud if you're buying indica. It should also look frosty, with a thick coat of sugary resin characteristic of the trichomes, which contain the cannabinoids and terpenes.

REMEMBER

Some states require that bud be pre-weighed and packaged, so the flower on display isn't the flower you get, although the flower you get should be from the same batch that's on display. The actual product you purchase will be sealed up in the store, and you won't have a chance to open it and inspect it until after you leave the premises.

TIP

The busier the dispensary, the greater the product turnover, so busy dispensaries are likely to have fresher products. If, after leaving the dispensary, you're dissatisfied with the product, bring it back to the dispensary *with the receipt* and your ID.

Smell It

Prior to purchasing flower/bud, give it a big whiff. It should smell sweet, fruity, or pleasantly pungent (skunky). The odor is a pretty good indication of how the bud will taste. If it smells bad, smells like damp hay, or has little or no aroma, don't buy it.

REMEMBER

Just because a certain strain "smells bad" to you doesn't mean it's poor quality cannabis. You may simply not like the aroma of certain strains. You shouldn't buy a product if you don't like the way it smells because you probably won't like the way it tastes, either. However, if it smells like mold or mildew, it probably wasn't dried, cured, or stored properly and has gone bad.

"Feel" It

High-quality flower is sticky and somewhat spongy. If you squeeze and release it, it should return to its original shape and not crumble in your hands. Of course, the law prohibits you from touching the flower prior to buying it, so you need to make your initial evaluation with your eyes and nose. The flower should be colorful and covered with frosty trichomes (an indication that it's probably sticky). If it's brown, it's probably too dry and won't be spongy.

You can't really tell if the flower is too wet just by looking at it, but if it smells like wet hay, it's definitely too wet. If you get it home, and it feels squishy instead of spongy, it's probably too wet. A good way to test whether flower is dry enough is to bend the stem; if the stem breaks instead of folding, it's probably dry enough. If the flower has any fuzzy white powder growing on it, it's definitely too wet; the excess moisture has created the perfect environment for mold. You shouldn't buy it, but if you already did, return it to the dispensary with receipt in hand.

REMEMBER

Another problem with cannabis that's too wet is that you end up paying too much for it. Wet cannabis is heavier than dry cannabis.

Taste It

Unfortunately, you're not allowed to sample most cannabis products prior to buying them. While some dispensaries have samples of gummies and other products that don't contain cannabinoids on display to taste, you can't sample flower or other products that contain THC.

Although you can't taste flower and certain other products before buying them, you can taste them afterward and keep track of what you like and don't like. Ultimately, the proof of high-quality cannabis is "in the pudding" — its aroma, flavor, and the effects it has on you.

Ask About the Cultivation Method

Prior to buying any cannabis products, ask about the cultivation method. Here are a few specific questions to ask:

>> Was it grown outdoors or indoors? Plants grown outside are exposed to rain, fresh air, and the full spectrum of light, making them the most natural option. However, flower grown indoor tends to be more aesthetically pleasing with higher THC levels and more pleasant aroma and flavor profiles.

>> Was it grown organically? Whether organic or chemical fertilizers were used may not significantly impact the quality of the cannabis, but controlling pests through organic methods rather than through the use of chemical pesticides ensures a healthier product, especially if it was grown outdoors.

>> Were plants grown in soil or hydroponically? Plants grown hydroponically tend to have frostier buds resulting in higher concentrations of cannabinoids and terpenes. Some consumers, however, prefer the flavor of plants grown outdoors in soil.

Compare Prices

As a cannabis consumer, you would be wise to pay more for quality product and customer service, but don't pay more than is necessary. Compare prices at nearby dispensaries before deciding where to shop. You may be able to get comparable quality for less. However, for the highest quality, hand trimmed product expect to open your wallet wide. It's all about your own budget.

Appendix

Cannabis Recipes

Combining cannabis with delectable foods is a concept that appeals to many consumers. Here, we deliver 17 recipes broken down into infusions, entrees, desserts, and beverages.

REMEMBER

Technically, all recipes we present are infusions, but here we use the term to refer to alcohol, sugar, butter, and syrup infusions that may be used as ingredients in recipes.

Infusions/Extracts

Rarely does a recipe include raw or dried cannabis bud, although it certainly may. In most cases, ingredients call for an extract such as cannabis-infused butter, oil, sugar, or syrup. You can purchase these ingredients at most dispensaries, but if you want to cook up your own infusions/extracts from scratch, you've come to the right place. Here we provide recipes for infused butter, sugar, and lavender syrup.

Buddha Budda

Sweet Mary Jane: 75 Delicious Cannabis-Infused High-End Desserts, a 2015 Random House title (978-1583335659)

Buddha Budda is cannabis-infused butter. You can spread it on toast or muffins, melt it on waffles or pancakes, or use it to substitute for butter in any of your favorite recipes.

REMEMBER

When you're creating your own extracts or concentrates, the potency of the finished product varies depending on the amount of flower you use and its potency. Some plant strains have higher concentrations of CBD, THC, and other cannabinoids than other plants do. This recipe includes three different versions, so you can gauge the potency to match your own needs and desires.

Yield: 1/2 cup (8 Tbsp or 1 stick) of Buddha Budda.

THC concentration: Varies based on strain, amount, and potency of flower

INGREDIENTS

1/2 cup (8 Tbsp or 1 stick) unsalted butter

1.5–6 grams cannabis buds, ground or finely crushed

Level 1

1.5 grams cannabis buds, ground or finely crushed

Yield: about 150 mg THC total

1 Tbsp = about 18.75 mg THC

12 edibles: about 12.5 mg THC each

18 edibles: about 8.3 mg THC each

Level 2

3 grams cannabis buds, ground or finely crushed

Yield: about 300 mg THC total

1 Tbsp = about 37.5 mg THC

12 edibles: about 25 mg THC each

18 edibles: about 16.6 mg THC each

Level 3

6 grams cannabis buds, ground or finely crushed

Yield: about 600 mg THC total

1 Tbsp = about 75 mg THC

12 edibles: about 50 mg THC total

18 edibles: about 33.3 mg THC total

Digital temperature gun
(It's the only way to test the temperature of the weed.)

Decent digital scale that weighs both grams and oz

Paint-straining bags or cheesecloth

Large bowl

Strainer

Rubber gloves

1 Decarboxylate the cannabis: Preheat the oven to 250°F. Place the cannabis in a small, heat proof baking dish and place in the oven. After 15–20 minutes, check the temperature of the cannabis with your digital temperature gun; once it has reached 250°F, let it bake for 30 minutes, checking the temperature frequently. (In addition to decarboxylating, you're removing any moisture left in the plant material.) If it goes over the correct temperature for too long, it will burn, the THC may convert into CBN, and you will lose potency. Remove from the oven and set aside to cool. If not using immediately, store the cannabis in an airtight container in a dark place for up to two months.

2 Melt the butter in a small saucepan over medium-low heat. Add the decarbed weed and bring the temperature of the butter up to 190°F. Cook for 30 minutes, using the digital temperature gun to check the temperature of the butter frequently and make sure it does not go over 200°F. DO NOT LEAVE UNATTENDED! (If by chance it does go over 200°F for a few minutes, don't worry, it isn't ruined. The THC is still in there. But excessive heating causes degradation of THC and may convert it to CBN, one of the cannabinoids responsible for the sedative effects of cannabis, or result in vaporization of the compounds. Inadequate heating isn't good either, as it causes the majority of the cannabinoids to remain in their acid form and thus unactivated. The density of the product, and the time and temperature of the oven, can also prevent some conversion, which results in unactivated cannabinoids. Adding the decarbed cannabis to the butter or coconut oil and heating it again ensures a better conversation.) Mostly, you want to keep everything at a simmer, not a boil. Just turn down the heat and watch it.

3 Take the saucepan off the heat and let it sit for 10 minutes.

4 It's now time to press. Place a strainer over a large bowl. Place a paint strainer or cheesecloth into the strainer, folding down the sides over the outside. Spoon the infused butter into it. Using a large spoon or potato masher, press as much as you can through the cloth. Then, using your hands (rubber gloves help here!), squeeze the bag. Press out as much of the precious liquid as you can. Measure the amount of liquid (infused butter) remaining. Expect a 25 percent loss; this is not a loss of THC, only of butter. Make up the difference with regular melted butter.

Buddha Budda can be stored in an airtight container for up to 8 weeks in the refrigerator. It also freezes well, so make more if you have the bud and freeze the extra batch in an airtight container for up to 6 months.

Hey Sugar!

Sweet Mary Jane: 75 Delicious Cannabis-Infused High-End Desserts, a 2015 Random House title (978-1583335659)

At Sweet Mary Jane, for the first few years we infused all our baked goods with *Buddha Budda* or *Coconut Bliss*. But, eventually, I wanted to try another technique. After some experimenting, I came up with the Idea of infusing sugar. It turned out to be a genuine innovation. The beauty of infused sugar is that there is much less cannabis flavor and color in the finished product. Many of the confections we sell use *Hey Sugar!*. We also sell packages of it for people to use to sweeten their coffee or tea, or to bake with at home.

Use the highest-proof alcohol you can find. If you have access to Everclear, use that. Otherwise, Bacardi 151 rum will do the trick (if not quite as well).

Hey Sugar! can be dropped into any hot drink. If you want to add it to a cold drink, heat a small portion of liquid, add the Hey Sugar!, stir to dissolve, and then add it to your drink. It can also be substituted for sugar in any of your favorite recipes.

As you will see in the following recipes, the amount of bud used determines the level of THC in the finished desserts, with three levels of dosing.

Yield for each of the following recipes is 1/4 cup of Hey Sugar!

INGREDIENTS

1.5–6 grams cannabis bud, ground or finely crushed (amount varies depending on potency desired, see below)

1/4 cup granulated sugar

high-proof alcohol (Everclear works best, but not every state sells it; if you can't purchase it, use Bacardi 151 rum)

Level 1

1.5 grams cannabis bud, ground or finely crushed

Yield: about 150 mg THC total

1 tsp = about 12.5 mg THC

Level 2

3 grams cannabis buds, ground or finely crushed

Yield: about 300 mg THC total

1 tsp = about 25 mg THC

Level 3

6 grams cannabis buds, ground or finely crushed

Yield: about 600 mg THC total

1 Tsp = about 50 mg THC

Digital temperature gun
(It's the only way to test the
temperature of the weed.)

Decent digital scale that weighs
both grams and oz

2 mason jars

Funnel

Coffee filter

Small heat-proof baking dish

Heat-proof glass pie dish

1 Decarboxylate the cannabis: Preheat the oven to 250°F. Put the cannabis in a small, heat-proof baking dish and place in the oven. After 15–20 minutes, check the temperature of the cannabis with your digital temperature gun; once it has reached 250°F, let it bake for 30 minutes, checking the temperature frequently. (In addition to decarboxylating, you're removing any moisture left in the plant material.) If it goes over the correct temperature for too long, it will burn, the THC may convert into CBN, and you will lose potency. If not using immediately, store the cannabis in an airtight container in a dark place for up to two months.

2 Remove the baking dish from the oven and reduce the oven temperature to 200°F.

3 Transfer the cannabis to a mason jar. Pour in just enough alcohol to cover it, and seal the jar. Shake the jar every 3–5 minutes for 20 minutes, then open the lid.

4 Line a strainer with a coffee filter and place it over a bowl. Pour the alcohol solution through the coffee filter to strain off the plant matter. Gently press with the back of a spoon or your fingertips, being careful not to break the filter.

5 Place the sugar in a heat-proof glass pie dish. Add the strained alcohol solution to the sugar and bake for 30 to 60 minutes, stirring well every 10 minutes, until all the liquid has evaporated and the sugar is evenly colored. (The color can range from light to dark amber.)

6 Store in an airtight container in a cool, dark place. There is no need to refrigerate. Hey Sugar! Is good for one year.

HOW TO CALCULATE DOSES

Creating infusions that contain a specific amount of THC, CBD, or other cannabinoids is challenging and may be nearly impossible to do if you've grown your own cannabis, because potency varies based on the plant strain, how it's grown, dried, and cured, and other variables. However, if you start with flower from a reputable dispensary, it should be labeled with the weight of the product (in grams) and the concentration of each cannabinoid (as a percentage). Using those two numbers, you can make your own cannabis-infused butter (such as Buddha Budda) and have a pretty clear idea of how much of each cannabinoid is in the entire batch. You just have to do the math:

1. **Multiply the number of grams of flower by 1,000 to determine the number of milligrams.**

   1 gram of flower is 1,000 milligrams; 2 grams of flower is 2,000 milligrams, and so on.

2. **Multiply the number of milligrams of flower by the percentage of a specific cannabinoid in the flower.**

   For example, if you have 2,000 milligrams of flower with 15 percent THC, you have 2,000 mg x 0.15 = 300 mg THC.

After doing the math, you know that if you use 2 grams of that flower and one stick of butter to make your Buddha Budda, you're going to have about 300 mg THC in the resulting stick of butter.

More basic math is required to determine the total amount of a cannabinoid in an entire batch of a recipe:

1. **Divide the quantity of infused product called for in the recipe by the total quantity of infused product you made to find the percentage of infused product you used.**

   For example, if a recipe calls for 4 tablespoons (Tbsp) of infused butter, and you made one stick of infused butter, 4 Tbsp ÷ 8 Tbsp (the number of tablespoons in an entire stick) = 1/2 or 50 percent.

2. **Multiply the result from Step 1 by the total amount of cannabinoid in the entire stick to find out the total amount of cannabinoid in the recipe.**

   For example, if the stick of cannabis-infused butter contains 300 mg THC, then half the stick contains 150 mg.

Now you're ready to determine the amount of cannabinoid per serving. Simply divide the amount of cannabinoid in the entire batch by the number of servings the recipe produces. So if a batch of cookies contains 150 mg THC and makes 12 cookies, 150 mg THC ÷ 12 cookies = 12.5 mg THC per cookie.

Tip: If you don't have specifics regarding the amount of THC in the flower you have, look up the strain online and see if you can find any information about it. Seed catalogues list the percentage of various cannabinoids in each strain, which can provide you with a ballpark figure. Not knowing other variables, the number may not be very helpful, though.

Infused Lavender Simple Syrup

Maxwell Bradford, Native Roots

Serving size should be based on desired THC content.

THC per serving (See "How to calculate doses" sidebar.)

INGREDIENTS

3 grams dried lavender

3 cups water

2 cups cannabis-infused sugar
(See the earlier recipe for
infused sugar.)

DIRECTIONS

1 In a small saucepan bring water to a boil.

2 Stir in dried lavender.

3 Simmer until fragrant and remove from heat.

4 Strain out all residual lavender using cheese cloth or a coffee filter.

5 Bring the now purple filtered lavender water back to a rolling boil.

6 Add infused sugar and continue to boil until all sugar granules have dissolved.

7 Remove from heat and let cool.

Entrees and Side Dishes

This appendix is packed with recipes for cannabis-infused desserts, but we don't want to leave you hanging when the dinner bell chimes. In this section, we provide a sampling of entrees and side dishes. Keep in mind, however, that all you need to do is follow your favorite recipes and substitute Buddha Budda wherever the recipe calls for butter or oil!

Caramelized Brussels Sprouts

Janielle Hultberg, Private Chef

4 to 5 servings of approximately 4 Brussels sprouts

THC per serving (See "How to calculate doses" sidebar.)

INGREDIENTS

2 slices uncured bacon (cut into pieces)

2 tbsp infused olive oil

1 lb fresh Brussels sprouts cleaned and cut in halves

1 small onion (halved and thinly sliced)

3 cloves garlic (minced)

1/4 cup balsamic vinegar (or apple cider vinegar)

2 Tbsp light agave or maple syrup

Salt and pepper to taste

NOTE: *You can substitute mushrooms, kale, green beans, or spinach for Brussels sprouts or use a combination of them!*

DIRECTIONS

1 In saute pan, on medium heat, cook bacon until starts to crisp, remove from pan & set aside drain off fat and add infused olive oil.

2 Add onions and cook until they start to caramelize.

3 Add garlic and Brussels sprouts and cook until both sides of sprouts start to brown.

4 Add vinegar, syrup, salt, and pepper, stirring occasionally until most of liquid is evaporated and sprouts are tender but not completely soft.

5 Serve hot.

Michelle's Medicated This Ain't Your Mama's Wack and Cheese

Michelle Karlebach, Nectar Cannabis

There are so many sweets on the edible market that it's nice to have a savory recipe as well. This is my all-time favorite comfort food recipe, with a kick, and a punch! P.S. Cheddar cheese is white.

Approximately 4 servings of one cup of pasta each

THC per serving (See "How to calculate doses" sidebar.)

INGREDIENTS

4 cups cooked macaroni (about 2 cups uncooked)

8 oz shredded cheddar (I use 4 oz Cabot extra sharp and 4 oz Cabot habanero cheddar, hence the kick)

1 cup sour cream

3/4 cup cottage cheese

1/2 cup skim milk

2 Tbsp grated onion

1 1/2 Tbsp melted medicated butter

1 egg slightly beaten

1/4 tsp pepper

3/4 cup corn, frozen or fresh

1/3 cup dry bread crumbs

1 Tbsp melted butter

DIRECTIONS

1 Preheat oven to 350°F.

2 In a large bowl mix together macaroni, cheddar cheese, cottage cheese, sour cream, skim milk, grated onion, medicated butter, corn, pepper, and egg.

3 Coat a 2 quart casserole dish with cooking spray and fill with mixture from bowl.

4 In a small bowl, mix together bread crumbs and 1 Tbsp melted butter and sprinkle over macaroni.

5 Cover and bake at 350°F for a half hour, then uncover and bake an additional 5 minutes or until it's set.

Spinach (or Baby Kale) and Chevre Goat Cheese Frittata

Janielle Hultberg, Private Chef

Number of servings depends on diameter of pan and number of slices cut

THC per serving (See "How to calculate doses" sidebar.)

INGREDIENTS

8 eggs

1/2 cup almond milk(regular or unsweetened not vanilla)

3 Tbsp extra virgin cannabis-infused olive oil or butter

6 sliced mushrooms (baby portabella, cremini, or button

1 large shallot, quartered and sliced

3 small clove garlic, minced

1/2 cup chopped spinach (or baby kale)

1/3 cup soft goat cheese

3 Tbsp chopped red onions

Sea salt and pepper

1 Preheat oven to 350°F.

2 Heat a skillet to medium-high. Add 1 Tbsp olive oil to the hot skillet, then add shallot. Sauté for a minute or so. Then add the garlic.

3 Add the sliced mushrooms and sauté for 5–10 minutes, until deep brown, to render out the moisture. Finally, add the spinach or kale to the skillet and sauté another 2–3 minutes.

4 Transfer the veggies to a plate and wipe the skillet with a paper towel.

5 Put the skillet back over high heat with 2 Tbsp olive oil. Mix eggs and milk with 1/2 tsp salt and fresh pepper to taste. Whisk until frothy.

6 Briskly swirl the skillet around as you pour in the egg mixture — this creates a crust on the outer edge. Then add the mushroom and spinach mixture back to the skillet and crumble the goat cheese over the top.

7 Remove from heat and place in the oven for 15–20 minutes until cooked through.

8 Slide out of pan onto a cutting board and cut into wedges.

Desserts

Based on the number of recipes we received for cannabis-infused desserts, most people seem to prefer to take their cannabis after or between meals. In this section, we present cannabis-infused dessert recipes that represent a diverse range of desserts from cookies and brownies to cakes and pies, along with sweet sauces to dribble on ice cream and other dessert favorites.

Almond Cutout Cookies

Janielle Hultberg, Private Chef

Serving size depends on the size of the cutout for the cookies

THC per serving (See "How to calculate doses" sidebar.)

INGREDIENTS

8 oz unsalted cannabis-infused butter, cold and cubed

5 oz powdered sugar

1/2 tsp salt

11 oz gluten-free flour blend

4 oz almond meal

2 egg yolks (save whites for icing)

DIRECTIONS

1 Cream butter and sugar and add egg yolks one at a time.

2 Add powdered sugar, salt, flour, and almond meal and continue mixing until dough forms a ball.

3 Wrap in plastic wrap or put in Ziploc bag and refrigerate for 30 minutes.

4 Preheat oven to 350°F.

5 On lightly dusted (with arrowroot powder or corn starch) board/counter/table, roll dough to desired thickness, cut out, and bake until lightly golden.

Chocolate Chip Oatmeal Cookies

Janielle Hultberg, Private Chef

Serving size depends on size of cookie

THC per serving (See "How to calculate doses" sidebar.)

INGREDIENTS

1/2 cup unsalted cannabis-infused butter (See "Buddha Budda" recipe.)

1/2 cup coconut oil

3/4 cup palm sugar

1/4 cup agave syrup

2 eggs plus 1 egg white

1 tsp vanilla

2 1/4 cups gluten free flour blend

1/4 tsp baking soda

1/2 tsp salt

2 1/4 cup gluten free oats

1 cup dark chocolate chips

1/2 cup chopped nuts of your choice

Optional: You may replace chocolate chips with 1 cup craisins or any other dried fruit. You may also add 1/2 tsp cinnamon.

DIRECTIONS

1 Preheat oven to 350°F.

2 Grease baking pan or line it with parchment paper.

3 Mix all ingredients until thoroughly blended.

4 Using a spoon, scoop batter onto greased pan or parchment paper, spacing about 2 inches apart.

5 Bake for 10–15 minutes to the desired crispness.

6 Remove from oven and transfer to cooling rack.

7 Eat warm or store in airtight container in refrigerator or freezer.

French Toast Cupcakes

Sweet Mary Jane: 75 Delicious Cannabis-Infused High-End Desserts, a 2015 Random House title (978-1583335659)

Makes 12 servings

THC per serving: Please see "How to calculate doses" sidebar.

INGREDIENTS

Cupcakes

1 1/2 cups all-purpose flour

1 cup sugar

1 1/2 tsp baking powder

1 tsp ground cinnamon

1/2 tsp ground allspice

1/4 tsp freshly grated nutmeg

1/2 tsp salt

1/2 cup Buddha Budda, slightly softened (See the "Buddha Budda" recipe.)

1/2 cup sour cream

2 large eggs

1/2 tsp maple extract

4 slices bacon

Topping

1/4 cup all-purpose flour

1/4 cup sugar

2 1/2 Tbsp unsalted butter, cut into 1/2-inch pieces and chilled

1/2 tsp ground cinnamon

1/4 cup chopped pecans

DIRECTIONS

1 Prepare the topping: In a medium bowl, combine the flour, sugar, butter, cinnamon, and pecans. Using your fingers, mix in the butter until no pieces are larger than a small pea. Cover and refrigerate until ready to use.

2 Preheat the oven to 350°F.

3 Line a 12-cup muffin tin with paper liners.

4 In a large bowl, whisk together the flour, sugar, baking powder, cinnamon, allspice, nutmeg, and salt. Set aside.

5 In a large bowl using an electric mixer on medium speed, beat together the Buddha Budda, sour cream, eggs, and maple extract until completely smooth. Reduce the mixer speed to low and add the flour mixture. Beat until just combined.

6 Fill each well of the muffin tin three-quarters of the way with batter.

7 Divide the topping evenly and sprinkle it over the top of each cupcake, gently pressing it into the batter with your fingertips.

8 Bake for 20–25 minutes or until a toothpick inserted into the center of a cupcake comes out clean.

9 Let the muffins cool in the tin for about 15 minutes, then transfer to a wire rack to cool completely.

10 Cut the bacon into 12 pieces total and press a piece onto the top of each muffin. If you are going to freeze these, omit the bacon.

Store the bacon-topped cupcakes in an airtight container in the refrigerator for up to one week or in the freezer for up to three months. Reheat in the toaster oven for extra deliciousness.

Key Lime Kickers

Sweet Mary Jane: 75 Delicious Cannabis-Infused High-End Desserts, a 2015 Random House title (978-1583335659)

Makes 24 truffles

THC per serving: Please see "How to calculate doses" sidebar.

INGREDIENTS

6 Tbsp heavy cream

2 Tbsp unsalted butter

1/4 cup Hey Sugar! (See the "Hey Sugar!" recipe.)

10 oz good-quality white chocolate, coarsely chopped

8 drips pure key lime oil

Graham cracker crumbs, for coating

Key lime oil can be found in craft shops and natural food grocers, or ordered online.

DIRECTIONS

1 Weigh the bowl that will hold the finished ganache and write down this number.

2 Set up a double boiler with 2–3 inches of water in the bottom pot and bring the water to a simmer. Pour the cream in the top section and heat until it begins to simmer gently.

3 Stir in the butter, corn syrup, and Hey Sugar!. When well combined, add the white chocolate; stir well. When the ganache is smooth, remove the top section of the double boiler from the heat and add the key lime oil, stirring to combine.

4 Wipe the water off the bottom and sides of the pan (you don't want any water dripping into the ganache) and pour the ganache into the bowl you weighed previously. Place in the freezer for 45–60 minutes, or until the ganache is firm but pliable.

5 Place the graham cracker crumbs in a shallow bowl. Line two baking sheets with parchment paper. Weigh the ganache, subtract the weight of the bowl, and divide by 24: This is your per-truffle weight. Using a spoon, scoop out the ganache, weigh to make sure it's the correct portion, and set on one of the prepared baking sheets.

6 Using your hands, quickly roll the ganache into balls and then roll in the graham cracker crumbs to coat completely.

7 Set the truffles on the second prepared baking sheet. Cover and store in the refrigerator for up to 5 weeks.

Truffles are best served at room temperature.

Merciful

Sweet Mary Jane: 75 Delicious Cannabis-Infused High-End Desserts, a 2015 Random House title (978-1583335659)

Makes 18 brownies

THC per serving: Please see "How to calculate doses" sidebar.

INGREDIENTS

Vegetable shortening, for greasing the pan

3/4 cup Buddha Budda (See "Buddha Budda" recipe.)

1/4 cup (4 Tbsp or 1/2 stick) unsalted butter

10 oz semisweet chocolate

4 oz unsweetened chocolate

6 Tbsp unsweetened cocoa powder

6 large eggs

2 1/2 cups sugar

1 tsp salt

1 Tbsp pure vanilla extract

2 cups all-purpose flour

Drizzle

1/2 cup white chocolate chips

1/4 tsp vegetable shortening

1 Preheat the oven to 350°F and grease a 10-by-15-inch baking pan.

2 In a small saucepan, melt the Buddha Budda and butter together over low heat. Add the semisweet and unsweetened chocolates and stir until the chocolates have melted. Whisk in the cocoa powder and remove from the heat.

3 In a medium bowl, whisk together the eggs, sugar, salt, and vanilla until well combined. Add the chocolate mixture and whisk well. Fold in the flour.

4 Pour the batter into the prepared pan. Bake for 18–20 minutes, or until a toothpick inserted into the center comes out with a few moist crumbs clinging to it. Let cool completely before cutting into 18 equal-sized bars.

5 Prepare the drizzle: In the top section of a double boiler, melt the white chocolate and the shortening over simmering water. Stir continuously until the chocolate has melted, being careful not to get any water into the chocolate or it will seize.

REMEMBER

Chocolate should melt into a smooth, satiny pool, but it's temperamental and won't tolerate moisture. If even the tiniest bit of condensation drips down the inside of a pan, or if steam escapes from the bottom of the double boiler, the chocolate will react badly, becoming a grainy mess; this is known as "seizing."

6 Dip a fork into the melted chocolate and drizzle it over the tops of the brownies.

7 Let the chocolate set. Wrap tightly in aluminum foil and store in the refrigerator for up to 1 week or in the freezer for up to 3 months.

Michelle's Bombass Balls (or Just the Chocolate Sauce

Michelle Karlebach, Nectar Cannabis

15 servings based on quarter-sized patties

THC per serving (See "How to calculate doses" sidebar.)

INGREDIENTS

For patties:

1 cup (about 10 to 12) pitted medjool dates

1 cup cashews

3 Tbsp creamy almond butter

1 Tbsp maple syrup

1 cup shredded coconut (or 1/2 with 1/2 cup of hemp hearts)

Pinch of sea salt (optional)

For chocolate sauce:

1/4 cup maple syrup

1/2 cup raw cacao or cocoa powder

1/2 cup melted coconut oil (the desired amount of medicated coconut oil should be included in this quantity. If you use only medicated coconut oil, you will have very strong patties!)

1/2 tsp cinnamon

1/4 tsp chili powder

Himalayan salt

DIRECTIONS

1 In a food processor, mix cashews until crumbly.

2 Add dates, almond butter, and maple syrup and continue mixing. Transfer to a bowl.

3 Place shredded coconut into a shallow bowl or a plate.

4 Roll mixture from food processor into balls about the size of a quarter and flatten gently between hands to form a patty.

5 Press the patties into coconut mixture to coat.

6 Place patties on a tray or sheet lined with parchment paper and pace in the freezer for about 20 minutes.

7 Whisk together ingredients for chocolate sauce in a bowl.

8 Dip most of each frozen patty into chocolate sauce and place on parchment paper. Place tray back in freezer.

9 Double dip! Re-dip the patties into the remaining chocolate, sprinkle Himalayan salt on top, and then return to freezer until hard.

Makes about 15 servings depending on how big your balls are!

Store in an airtight container in either fridge or freezer.

Enjoy and please do so responsibly.

Michelle's Medicated Blueberry Pie

Michelle Karlebach, Nectar Cannabis

This pie is what started my love of edibles! Cannabis and blueberries really complement each other beautifully. It also takes about 10 minutes to get it in the oven if you opt for store-bought crust, so it's fast and easy! If you're vegan, you can use medicated coconut oil instead of the butter with a vegan pie crust recipe.

Approximately 6 to 8 slices in a 9-inch diameter pie

THC per serving (See "How to calculate doses" sidebar.)

INGREDIENTS

6 cups fresh or frozen blueberries (You may substitute some pitted cherries, too!)

1 Tbsp lemon juice

1/4 cup all-purpose flour

1/2 cup white sugar

1/4 tsp cinnamon

2 Tbsp medicated butter, cut into small pieces (You may substitute medicated coconut oil)

Double recipe for pie crust, or buy roll-out kind from the store

DIRECTIONS

1 Preheat oven to 425°F.

2 Mix blueberries, lemon juice, flour, sugar, and cinnamon in a bowl.

3 Roll out the bottom pie crust in a pie dish.

4 Transfer blueberry mixture into the bottom pie crust and dot pieces of medicated butter along the top.

5 Place top crust over blueberry mixture, tuck the top dough over and under the edge of the bottom crust, and pinch together.

6 Cut slits into top of pie. (Consider cutting slits into the pattern of a smiley face!)

7 Place the pie on the middle rack for 20 minutes at 425°F, reduce heat to 350°F, and bake for 30–40 minutes longer.

Allow to cool completely before serving.

No-Guilt Nosh

Janielle Hultberg, Private Chef

Number of servings depends on serving size of ball

THC per serving (See "How to calculate doses" sidebar.)

INGREDIENTS

1 cup dates

1 cup raw almonds

1 cup raw walnuts

2 Tbsp cannabis-infused coconut oil (or infused butter)

1 Tbsp flax meal

1 Tbsp water

Shredded coconut

DIRECTIONS

1 In food processor blend all ingredients except for the shredded coconut until you can form balls out of dough.

2 Roll a small portion of dough between the palms of your hands to form a ball about the diameter of a quarter.

3 Roll the ball over the shredded coconut and place it on parchment paper.

4 Store in airtight container at room temperature for up to a week or in the freezer for up to 3 months.

Sesame Seed Cookies

Janielle Hultberg, Private Chef

Approximately 24 cookies

THC per serving (See "How to calculate doses" sidebar.)

INGREDIENTS

2 1/2 cups sesame seeds

1 cup palm sugar

2 Tbsp dark agave syrup

8 oz unsalted cannabis-infused butter, room temp

2 eggs

Pinch of salt

1/8 tsp baking powder

1 1/3 cup gluten-free flour blend

DIRECTIONS

1 Grease baking pan or line it with parchment paper.

2 Preheat oven to 350°F.

3 Toast sesame seeds until lightly golden and let cool.

4 Cream together butter, sugar, and syrup, scraping the bowl often.

5 Add eggs, one at a time, scraping the bowl a couple of times.

6 Add salt, baking powder, flour, and seeds, and mix well.

7 Using a teaspoon, scoop the cookie dough out on the baking pan or parchment paper spacing at least 2 inches apart.

8 Bake 6–8 minutes until golden. They'll be crispy when cooled.

Beverages

After all this coverage of entrees and desserts, you must be getting thirsty. Unfortunately, we have only a couple recipes of beverages to quench your thirst. The good news is that one of them is for brewing your own tea. Everyone should have a good recipe for cannabis-infused tea stuck to their refrigerator door!

Energizing Masala Chai Cannabis Tea

Verté Essentials

4 servings

5–10mg cannabinoid per serving

INGREDIENTS

8 oz water

4 oz hemp, coconut, or other nut milk

1–4 Tbsp natural sugar

1 Tbsp coconut oil

5–7 cardamom pods, smashed

1 stick cinnamon

4 black peppercorns

1 slice (dime size) fresh ginger

2 Tbsp black tea leaves (or equivalent tea bags)

20–40 mg cannabis sativa oil or extract

DIRECTIONS

1 Bring water and milk to a simmer with spices in a medium saucepan.

2 Reduce heat to lowest setting and add tea.

3 Steep about 3–5 minutes, stirring occasionally, until tea takes on a deep, tan color.

4 Strain into a cup and stir in sugar to taste.

Infused Lavender Lemonade

Maxwell Bradford, Native Roots

Makes 2 cups

THC per serving (See "How to calculate doses" sidebar.)

INGREDIENTS

1 dozen or so lemons (enough for two cups juice)

1/2 cup sugar

1 cup infused lavender syrup (See the "Infused Lavender Simple Syrup" recipe.)

DIRECTIONS

1 Juice the lemons until you have two cups juice without seeds.

2 Add sugar.

3 Add infused lavender syrup.

4 Stir until sugar is dissolved.

Index

Rubin, Alan L. (author)
Diabetes For Dummies, 157
ruderalis, 13
rules and regulations, 281, 209. *See also* laws
"runners high," 172

S

safety, 19–20
safety and responsibility
  about, 121
  dosing decisions, 124–132
  health and safety risks, 122–124
  maintaining, 132–133
  overconsumption, 134–136
  training staff on, 281
  underage development, 136–137
sales department, 280
sales representatives, 297–298
salves, 117
sativa
  about, 13, 14
  characteristics of, 320
  compared with indica, 125–126
  structure of, 28
Sativex, 119, 169
scams, 83–84
Schedule I drug, 9, 45, 68, 74, 87, 262–263
Schedule II drug, 68
Schedule III drug, 68
Schedule IV drug, 68
Schedule V drug, 68
schizophrenia, 170
Screen of Green (ScroG) kits, 208, 220–221
scrogging, 220–221, 322
sebostatic, 146
sebum, 146
Section 280E legislation, 271–272, 310
security manager/officer, 300
security team, 279–280
sedatives, cannabinol (CBD) as, 37

seedling stage, in growth cycle, 190, 195
seedlings, planting, 212
seeds
  about, 29–30
  choosing, 321
  germinating, 211–212
  inspecting, 82
  obtaining, 209–211
  planting, 209–214
segmenting, as indoor cultivation consideration, 192
seizures, 158, 180
sell-by date, on product labels, 15
selling limits, state laws and, 50–51
sensory stimulation, 330
serving size, for edibles, 116
Sesame Seed Cookies recipe, 358
Sessions, Jeff (Attorney General), 47
sexual dysfunction, 170–171
shake, 105
shatter, 41
shisha, 108–109
shucking, weighing after, 230–231
side dish recipes, 346–349
side effects, 122–124, 182
size, inspecting, 82
skin conditions, 171–172
sleep, cannabis for improving, 157
slightly acidic soil, 206
smell, 82, 336–337
smoking
  about, 16–17, 101–103
  homemade devices, 109–110
  hookahs, 108–109
  long-term complications from, 123
  one-hitters, 108
  with a pipe, 103–105
  pre-rolls, 105–108
  pros and cons of, 130
  rolling joints, 105–108

About the Author

Kim Ronkin Casey is a professional in the public relations and communications arena. For more than 20 years, she has been creating internal and external communications campaigns for industries as diverse as the U.S. White House to multiple United Nations Ministerials and Fortune 500 companies, nonprofits and most recently in the cannabis industry.

Ms. Casey has led in-house corporate communications and PR divisions. She also has extensive agency and independent consulting experience. Currently she consults in the cannabis industry and is excited to see where the ride will go. She has the unwavering support of her family and lives in Colorado with her husband, Scott, and their two daughters, Sarah and Rachel, at around 7,400 feet in altitude — high enough that no cannabis needed.

Dedication

I would like to dedicate this book first to my family without whom I couldn't have seen the finish line. To my husband, Scott, who reminds me not to try to eat the elephant in one bite and sings off-key when needed. To my children for their patience — they may not want to tell their friends their mom is in pot, but maybe I'll be cool as an author. And to my mother, who always believed I could do anything.

In addition, to all of the relentless cannabis advocates around the world. There would be no industry — and hence, no book — without you!

Author's Acknowledgments

Sometimes it takes a village to build a book, which certainly was the case with this book. Special thanks to Senior Acquisitions Editor, Tracy Boggier, for kick-starting the project, choosing us to write this book, and serving as the diligent and patient shepherd in keeping everything moving in the right direction. Special thanks also to everyone who contributed their effort and expertise in suppling specialized content, including

Jason MacDonald

David Forester

Nelson Oldham

Kristen Bartsch

Adam Cole

Chris Colon

Ryan Gonsalves

Thanks also to those who shared their recipes and figures to include in the book:

Karin Lazarus, Sweet Mary Jane

Janielle Hultberg, Private Chef

Michelle Karlebach, Cannabis Nectar

Maxwell Bradford

Native Roots

Mary's Medicinals

Leafly

On the editorial end of this project, we give a special shout out to Chrissy Guthrie who carefully and patiently edited the manuscript and guided all the pieces through production to ensure that everything came together at the end and, miraculously, on time! And we also give thanks to our production editor, G. Vasanth Koilraj, for shepherding this book through the layout process.

Publisher's Acknowledgments

Senior Acquisitions Editor: Tracy Boggier

Editorial Project Manager and Development Editor: Christina Guthrie

Copy Editor: Christina Guthrie

Production Editor: G. Vasanth Koilraj

Cover Image: © Norman Posselt/Getty Images

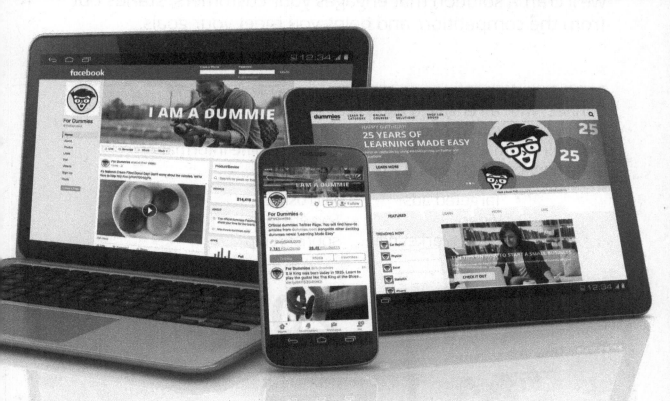
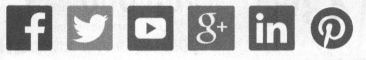

Leverage the power

Dummies is the global leader in the reference category and one of the most trusted and highly regarded brands in the world. No longer just focused on books, customers now have access to the dummies content they need in the format they want. Together we'll craft a solution that engages your customers, stands out from the competition, and helps you meet your goals.

Advertising & Sponsorships

Connect with an engaged audience on a powerful multimedia site, and position your message alongside expert how-to content. Dummies.com is a one-stop shop for free, online information and know-how curated by a team of experts.

- Targeted ads
- Video
- Email Marketing
- Microsites
- Sweepstakes sponsorship

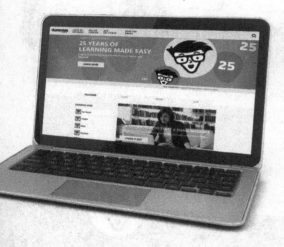

20 MILLION PAGE VIEWS EVERY SINGLE MONTH

15 MILLION UNIQUE VISITORS PER MONTH

43% OF ALL VISITORS ACCESS THE SITE VIA THEIR MOBILE DEVICES

700,000 NEWSLETTER SUBSCRIPTIONS TO THE INBOXES OF

300,000 UNIQUE INDIVIDUALS EVERY WEEK

# of dummies

Custom Publishing

Reach a global audience in any language by creating a solution that will differentiate you from competitors, amplify your message, and encourage customers to make a buying decision.

- Apps
- Books
- eBooks
- Video
- Audio
- Webinars

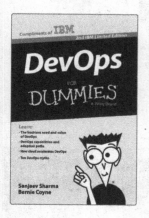

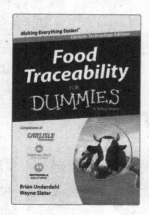

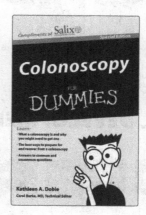

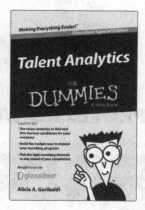

Brand Licensing & Content

Leverage the strength of the world's most popular reference brand to reach new audiences and channels of distribution.

For more information, visit **dummies.com/biz**

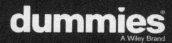

PERSONAL ENRICHMENT

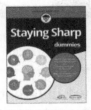
Staying Sharp
9781119187790
USA $26.00
CAN $31.99
UK £19.99

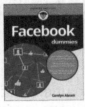
Facebook
Carolyn Abram
9781119179030
USA $21.99
CAN $25.99
UK £16.99

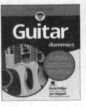
Guitar
Mark Phillips
Jon Chappell
9781119293354
USA $24.99
CAN $29.99
UK £17.99

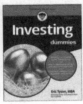
Investing
Eric Tyson, MBA
9781119293347
USA $22.99
CAN $27.99
UK £16.99

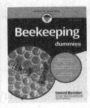
Beekeeping
Howland Blackiston
9781119310068
USA $22.99
CAN $27.99
UK £16.99

Digital Photography
Julie Adair King
9781119235606
USA $24.99
CAN $29.99
UK £17.99

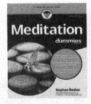
Meditation
Stephan Bodian
9781119251163
USA $24.99
CAN $29.99
UK £17.99

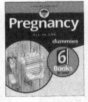
Pregnancy
9781119235491
USA $26.99
CAN $31.99
UK £19.99

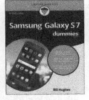
Samsung Galaxy S7
Bill Hughes
9781119279952
USA $24.99
CAN $29.99
UK £17.99

iPhone
Edward C. Baig
Bob "Dr. Mac" LeVitus
9781119283133
USA $24.99
CAN $29.99
UK £17.99

Crocheting
Karen Manthey
Susan Brittain
9781119287117
USA $24.99
CAN $29.99
UK £16.99

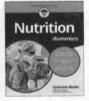
Nutrition
Carol Ann Rinzler
9781119130246
USA $22.99
CAN $27.99
UK £16.99

PROFESSIONAL DEVELOPMENT

Windows 10
Andy Rathbone
9781119311041
USA $24.99
CAN $29.99
UK £17.99

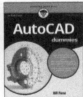
AutoCAD
Bill Fane
9781119255796
USA $39.99
CAN $47.99
UK £27.99

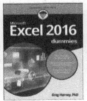
Excel 2016
Greg Harvey, PhD
9781119293439
USA $26.99
CAN $31.99
UK £19.99

QuickBooks 2017
Stephen L. Nelson, MBA, CPA, MS in Taxation
9781119281467
USA $26.99
CAN $31.99
UK £19.99

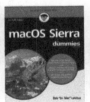
macOS Sierra
Bob "Dr. Mac" LeVitus
9781119280651
USA $29.99
CAN $35.99
UK £21.99

LinkedIn
Joel Elad, MBA
9781119251132
USA $24.99
CAN $29.99
UK £17.99

Windows 10
Woody Leonhard
9781119310563
USA $34.00
CAN $41.99
UK £24.99

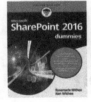
SharePoint 2016
Rosemarie Withee
Ken Withee
9781119181705
USA $29.99
CAN $35.99
UK £21.99

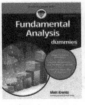
Fundamental Analysis
Matt Krantz
9781119263593
USA $26.99
CAN $31.99
UK £19.99

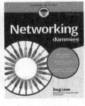
Networking
Doug Lowe
9781119257769
USA $29.99
CAN $35.99
UK £21.99

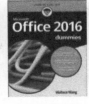
Office 2016
Wallace Wang
9781119293477
USA $26.99
CAN $31.99
UK £19.99

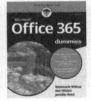
Office 365
Rosemarie Withee
Ken Withee
Jennifer Reed
9781119265313
USA $24.99
CAN $29.99
UK £17.99

Salesforce.com
Liz Kao
Jon Paz
9781119239314
USA $29.99
CAN $35.99
UK £21.99

Coding
Nikhil Abraham
9781119293323
USA $29.99
CAN $35.99
UK £21.99

dummies.com

dummies
A Wiley Brand

Learning Made Easy

ACADEMIC

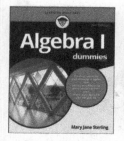

9781119293576
USA $19.99
CAN $23.99
UK £15.99

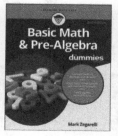

9781119293637
USA $19.99
CAN $23.99
UK £15.99

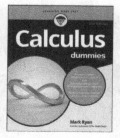

9781119293491
USA $19.99
CAN $23.99
UK £15.99

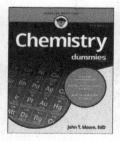

9781119293460
USA $19.99
CAN $23.99
UK £15.99

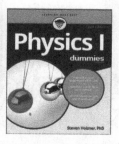

9781119293590
USA $19.99
CAN $23.99
UK £15.99

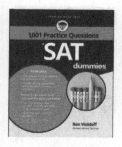

9781119215844
USA $26.99
CAN $31.99
UK £19.99

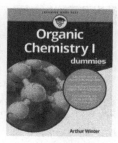

9781119293378
USA $22.99
CAN $27.99
UK £16.99

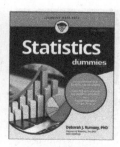

9781119293521
USA $19.99
CAN $23.99
UK £15.99

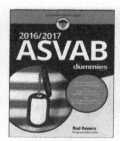

9781119239178
USA $18.99
CAN $22.99
UK £14.99

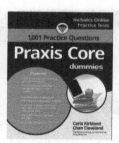

9781119263883
USA $26.99
CAN $31.99
UK £19.99

Available Everywhere Books Are Sold

dummies.com

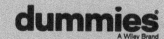

Small books for big imaginations

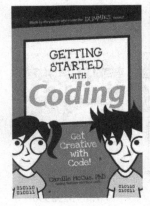

GETTING STARTED WITH Coding
Get Creative with Code!
Camille McCue, PhD

9781119177173
USA $9.99
CAN $9.99
UK £8.99

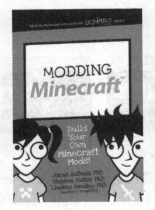

MODDING Minecraft™
Build Your Own Minecraft Mods!
Sarah Guthals, PhD
Stephen Foster, PhD
Lindsey Handley, PhD

9781119177272
USA $9.99
CAN $9.99
UK £8.99

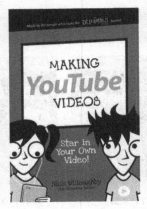

MAKING YouTube® VIDEOS
Star in Your Own Video!
Nick Willoughby

9781119177241
USA $9.99
CAN $9.99
UK £8.99

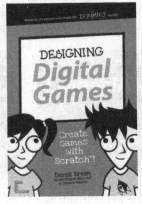

DESIGNING Digital Games
Create Games with Scratch™!
Derek Breen

9781119177210
USA $9.99
CAN $9.99
UK £8.99

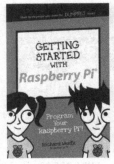

GETTING STARTED WITH Raspberry Pi®
Program Your Raspberry Pi®!
Richard Wentk

9781119262657
USA $9.99
CAN $9.99
UK £6.99

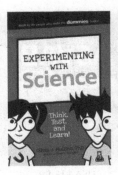

EXPERIMENTING WITH Science
Think, Test, and Learn!

9781119291336
USA $9.99
CAN $9.99
UK £6.99

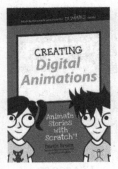

CREATING Digital Animations
Animate Stories with Scratch™!
Derek Breen

9781119233527
USA $9.99
CAN $9.99
UK £6.99

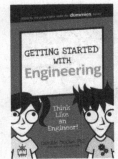

GETTING STARTED WITH Engineering
Think Like an Engineer!
Camille McCue, PhD

9781119291220
USA $9.99
CAN $9.99
UK £6.99

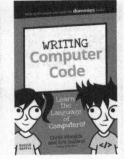

WRITING Computer Code
Learn the Language of Computers!
Chris Minnick and Eva Holland

9781119177302
USA $9.99
CAN $9.99
UK £8.99

Unleash Their Creativity

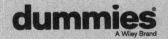